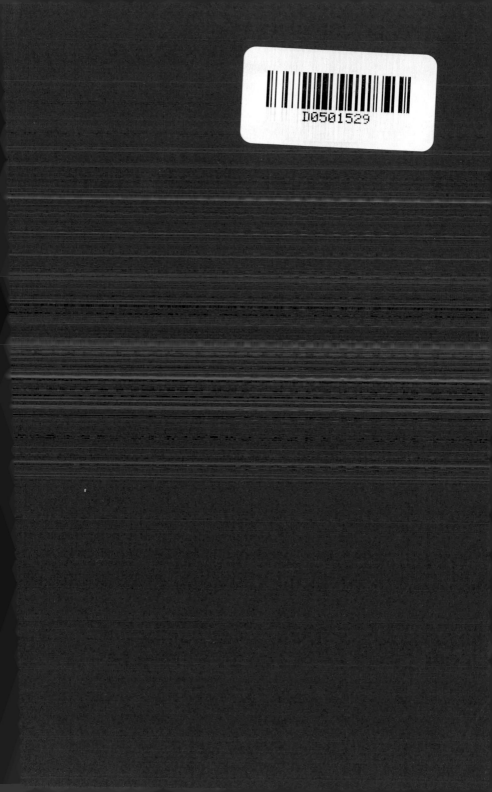

D0501529

BELLEVUE

HARPER & ROW, PUBLISHERS

New York, Evanston, San Francisco, London

1817

DON GOLD

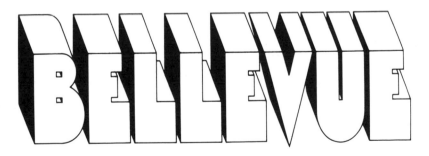

A Documentary of a
Large Metropolitan Hospital

The quotation from Emily Dickinson (on page 387) is reprinted by the kind permission of Little, Brown and Company and The Harvard University Press.

Portions of this work originally appeared in *Today's Health*.

FIRST EDITION

Designed by C. Linda Dingler

Library of Congress Cataloging in Publication Data

Gold, Don.
  Bellevue.
  Includes index.
  1. Bellevue Hospital, New York. 2. Hospital care.
I. Title.
RA982.N5B516   362.1'1'097471   74–15825
ISBN 0–06–011588–2

75 76 77 78 79 10 9 8 7 6 5 4 3 2 1

To my son Paul, with love

CONTENTS

PREFACE

The first time I ever entered Bellevue, I sat in the main waiting room for several hours, watching. I saw old black men with canes; pregnant women; teen-age boys in bright clothes and shredded sneakers. Volunteers reporting for work. Unshaven men and tattered old women from the streets. Well-dressed persons in search of care without high cost. Bald heads. Wisps of gray hair. Afros. Old suits and old Levi's. Crutches. Eye patches. Bandages. Shopping bags stuffed with belongings.

I watched a Housekeeping aide in a blue uniform sponge each bench very slowly, as if determined to destroy every germ on it, or pass his entire day on that assignment. He assessed his work, stepped back, walked away, came back, resumed sponging. He took his time.

I watched doctors meet and listened to them talk. At Bellevue, I realized immediately and confirmed later, small talk is almost nonexistent. So are other things. The verb "to die" is not spoken often.

I noticed that most water fountains didn't work, that most clocks firmly bonded to walls seem to have stopped years ago, that the public bathrooms were disaster areas.

As I spent more time at Bellevue, I realized that its main buildings, interconnected, had spread across the landscape like architectural afterthoughts, without a hint of ingenuity or planning. After a while, the place takes on a grim, drab tone. It is vulnerable.

It has been attacked in the press, from the *New York Times* to the *Village Voice*, with regularity. A state audit charged its staff with inefficiency, failing to account for missing narcotics, inadequate food-storage facilities. "We observed rodent holes in biscuit mix and spaghetti containers," the state audit reported.

I tried to find out for myself. I spent months at Bellevue, in almost every service. I talked to hundreds of people who know it well. I watched and listened and took notes. If a name is used in this book, for a doctor or a nurse, it is a real name. Patients' names and identities have been deliberately altered, but patients, too, talked to me freely. My own role was never disguised.

Everything in this book happened as it is described regardless of existing rules and regulations; the words that people say in it were said that way. There is no fiction here, no adornment. There is drama at Bellevue, and drudgery.

The process of selection is an expression of the writer's opinion. I have tried to be fair to Bellevue, showing it at its best, saving a life, and at its worst, losing one. For me, Bellevue was neither the abyss of inferior medicine nor the best hospital in the world, although it might have been simpler to begin with either supposition. And if Bellevue seems to be the central character in this book, it is the people in it who matter most.

This is, more than anything else, a book about people: doctors, nurses, students, administrators, technicians, patients. It is about their skills and their emotions and how they get along with each other under the stresses a hospital imposes. My method, I suppose, is that of the old journalism. My hope is that by looking at the people of Bellevue we may discover something about ourselves.

D.G.

BELLEVUE: HISTORY

Bellevue historians make a case for the hospital's being the first public hospital in the United States. They may be correct. There is evidence that its history goes back to 1658, when five company workshops of the Dutch West Indies Company were donated for use as a hospital. That hospital was moved, in 1700, to Warren and Broadway. In 1736, the Publick Workhouse and House of Correction was built on the site of New York's old city hall; on the top floor was a six-bed infirmary, usually thought of as the beginning of Bellevue.

In 1811, Mayor DeWitt Clinton supported the purchase of part of the old Kip's Bay Farm and, in addition to it, an area at what is now Twenty-eighth Street and the East River known as Belle Vue Place. On the land, a group of structures, including a hospital, were erected; they became known as the Bellevue Establishment.

It assumed the name Bellevue Hospital in 1825, after it had been enlarged to cope with the victims of a yellow-fever epidemic in 1819. By 1870, Bellevue had twelve hundred beds, an outpatient department and twenty-four-hour ambulance (horse-drawn) service. In 1898, a training school for nurses was established. By the turn of the century, future construction was inevitable. A new Bellevue was erected in 1904 and the buildings that still stand today were begun. The seven-story A&B building went up in 1908, Pathology in 1911, three others in 1916 and 1917. The Psychiatry building went up in 1935, the Administration building five years later, until the First Avenue acreage could not contain any more.

In 1966, the new Bellevue construction was begun; it was dedicated in 1973. In 1970, the hospital's management was taken over by the New York City Health and Hospitals Corporation; that same year, the AES (Adult Emergency Service) building was added to the complex.

Among the "firsts" that Bellevue claims are:

The first recorded instruction in anatomy by actual dissection, in 1750

The first use of the hypodermic syringe, in 1856

The first outpatient department in the United States, in 1867

The first hospital-based ambulance service in the world, in 1869

The first emergency pavilion, in 1876

The first American school of nursing patterned on the Florence Nightingale method, in 1873

The first hospital Caesarean section performed in the United States, in 1887

The first cardiopulmonary laboratory in the world, in 1940. It led to the Nobel Prize for Dr. Dickenson Richards and Dr. André Cournand, for establishing the process of cardiac catheterization, in 1956.

In the past, both Cornell and Columbia provided medical services to Bellevue; since 1968, the New York University Medical School has been the exclusive source of doctors and medical services.

BELLEVUE: VITAL STATISTICS

Bellevue is the fourth largest hospital in America and the largest in Manhattan. It has more than 1,500 beds in the old hospital. Approximately 30,000 patients are admitted annually, another 100,000 are treated by its Emergency Service. Almost 400,000 visits comprise the clinic schedule each year; there are 79 separate clinics. By law, it must accept all who seek medical aid.

The hospital has an attending staff of 1,000 physicians. Approximately 450 interns and residents serve Bellevue through its affiliation with N.Y.U. There are 700 nurses at Bellevue. The nonmedical staff numbers more than 6,000.

More than two million laboratory tests on inpatients are processed each year. More than 7,000 operations are performed annually. The pharmacy processes 250,000 prescriptions for inpatients a year, more than 365,000 for outpatients.

Seventy-five percent of Bellevue's patients reside in Manhattan, the vast majority of those in lower Manhattan. The majority of Bellevue patients are Puerto Rican and black.

The new Bellevue, on the eastern edge of the twenty-acre campus, cost taxpayers $160 million. On its twenty-five floors, there will be more than 1,000 beds, plus space, eventually, for psychiatric patients. The new Bellevue has: high-speed elevators, piped-in oxygen and suction at bedside, 4-bed, 2-bed and 1-bed rooms replacing the old 26-bed open wards, bathrooms adjoining each patient room, vast clinic facilities (600 rooms), chute disposal of trash and soiled linen, streamlined food service and more. The Bellevue complex covers 10 square blocks, contains 14 buildings and has 75 separate entrances.

Its presence expands Bellevue's capacity and capabilities and enhances the link of medical facilities along First Avenue, from

Twenty-third Street to Thirty-fourth Street. From south to north, they are: the federal hospital run by the Veterans Administration; the public hospital, Bellevue; and a private voluntary hospital, University Hospital. N.Y.U. provides the attending and house staff for all three.

THE PROFESSIONALS

Bernard Weinstein	Executive Director, Bellevue
Dr. Dirk Berger	Psychiatry (Ward NO-6)
Dr. Kenneth Kirshbaum	Psychiatry (clinic)
Dr. Lanie Eagleton	Chest Service
Dr. Diane Rahman	Obstetrics
Dr. Robert Nachtigall	Gynecology
Dr. Bruce Mack	Neurology
Dr. Kalmon Post	Neurosurgery
Dr. Eugene Fazzini	Pathology
Loretta Chiarelli, R.N.	Emergency Ward
Dr. George Feldman	Medicine
Dr. Sol Zimmerman	Pediatrics
Dr. Mary Williamson	Surgery
Tom Spencer, R.N.	Adult Emergency Service

BELLEVUE

MONDAY

Nursing Service Report

C&D laundry chute out for three days.

The telephones are out of order on C–2, D–2, B–4 and A–4. I&K and Psychiatry could not make telephone calls out but were able to receive calls.

On B–2 last night there was an altercation between two patients: William Wharton and Robert Black. Wharton received a one-inch laceration under the left eye which required six stitches. Mr. Black was transferred to C–3. They were quiet after that.

Recovery Room—Barry Zelko, 20 years old—traumatic amputation of right arm. He apparently fell from a subway platform—his condition is satisfactory.

Observation Unit—Carly Warren, nurse's aide from Psychiatry, questionable occipital fracture. She was injured on duty yesterday when a patient shoved her against the wall. She is having a neuro work-up and her condition is satisfactory.

Bernard M. Weinstein leaves his house, his wife and his two children in Fairlawn, New Jersey, at 8 A.M., to join the traffic procession into Manhattan. As his six-month-old Chevrolet Monte Carlo weaves through the inevitable congestion, he divides his attention between the news blaring from the radio and the woes that may await him on the job.

Weinstein is a meticulous dresser and keeps his blond hair precisely groomed. At five feet, nine and a half inches, 150 pounds, he is not a large man, but he appears to be larger than he is. He is a jogger, an occasional tennis player. He is in good shape for his 42 years.

He has to be. Weinstein is the Executive Director of Bellevue Hospital and has been for six years, the first nonmedical administrator in its history. It is a complicated, demanding job. Weinstein must keep track of Bellevue's 6,000 employees, the more than 1,000 members of its medical staff (interns, residents, nurses), a total of 240 job classifications and an annual budget of $81 million.

Weinstein was born in Boston (in an ambulance, actually) and raised in Winthrop, Massachusetts. He has a bachelor's degree in public health from the University of Massachusetts and a master's from the University of Pittsburgh. He has been an administrator at several New York hospitals; he came to Bellevue after serving as Assistant Director at Mt. Sinai Hospital.

Credentials aren't enough, however, to master a place like Bellevue. It takes sheer endurance. Each morning, as Weinstein's Chevy glides toward Bellevue, he must know what he will confront that day. He can't wait to find out. A firm and honest man, Weinstein has solved some of his problems by being direct, by avoiding pomposity and by turning what would be raw anger in another man into action rather than brooding.

This morning, Weinstein knows he can look forward to several matters awaiting his attention. Over the weekend, phone calls from aides have alerted him. He pulls into the hospital garage, drives to the roof and finds one of the last spaces. There is no elevator, so he walks down, into the adjoining Administration building, to his office.

He enters the building without looking to his left or right. He does not see Bellevue as others, as strangers, might see it. Stretching along First Avenue, its haphazardly designed buildings bear some resemblance to a prison. Only bars are absent. Several inner courtyards, grassy islands, provide some relief, but for the most part Bellevue sprawls from one antiquated building to another, like a grim, decaying maze. There are new apartment buildings and relatively new hospitals in the neighborhood, but Bellevue personifies the past, both in its sense of permanence and tradition and in the depressing presence of its architecture. Weinstein does not pause to consider any of this. He is beyond that stage in his appreciation of Bellevue.

It is 9 A.M. and his secretary, Rose LaMarca, loyal and properly protective, has typed his agenda for the day: calls to make, letters to write, meetings to attend. Weinstein has a cup of coffee, follows it with a stick of Dentyne. Then he's off to check out a heating problem in the new hospital with his chief engineer.

When Weinstein arrives in the lobby of the new hospital, he notices that the chief engineer has kept his coat on, an omen. He pats Weinstein on the back and says, "We're runnin' this place on a bag of tricks, every time the sun goes in or out. But don't worry, today we're *over*heated."

Together, they survey the heating in the Pediatrics clinic. The engineer dips a thermometer toward a heating vent.

"It's not right," he says. "If this were a cold day, we'd be in trouble. We'll find out what's wrong and fix it immediately."

They walk through other rooms in the clinic. From a lukewarm room, they enter one that is torrid.

"How do you like our sauna?" a nurse asks them.

Two steamfitters are pounding away at some pipes.

"We brought in twelve of these guys on Saturday," the engineer tells Weinstein.

"You can feel variations in temperature as you walk along," Weinstein says.

The pair goes up to the thirteenth floor, where the newly installed heating and cooling equipment is located. It is a maze of pipes, ducts, computers for detecting fires and monitoring hot and cold gusts. A computer operator punches a few buttons and tells Weinstein that in the clinic area the temperature is 76, 77 and 85. The engineer looks more and more like Charlie Brown in agony.

In the lobby again, a few minutes later, Weinstein tells him, "Put down on one piece of paper your eight biggest problems with the physical operation of the building."

Weinstein returns to his office through a door marked "Private." He has a large desk. Behind it is a conference table for eight surrounded by bookcases. There are three large windows, not one of which offers a distracting view, nothing more appealing than the back of the garage.

It is almost 10 A.M. and Weinstein begins a series of phone calls.

He discusses the Methadone Maintenance program with the Director of Psychiatry.

"I'm not going to change the regulations of the hospital based on confusion," Weinstein tells him.

They change the subject. "Good, good. Same bullshit again," Weinstein says. "I don't have to read the *Times*. Other people do and they always tell me what is important. Okay. Let's see what happens. Right. 'Bye."

A doctor arrives for an appointment. He is late. He is flustered. Driving down from a distant suburb, he's been in his car since 6:30 A.M., humbled by traffic. He wants to talk to Weinstein about a paramedical training program he's been running at Bellevue, giving staff employees the chance to learn new skills.

There are almost one hundred people in the training program, including clerks, nurse's aides, a few with college degrees, a few college dropouts, a few blacks.

Weinstein dispenses with small talk.

"I had a visit from some people in our central office," he says, "and they said you had made disparaging remarks about the quality of our people in training here, expressed negative feelings about minorities."

The doctor seems unmoved. "We're not training them to push machines," he says, firmly but without rancor. "It's more sophisticated than that. Present-day training has little to do with the old techniques. It is hopeless to try to bring those old-timers up to date."

"Those in labor here have a passionate commitment to upgrading," Weinstein says. "And they have that right. You decide who goes into your program. However, I can see some bad rumbles starting. We should seek out qualified students in our system. So you have to be very astute in your efforts, very orderly and diplomatic in what you say."

"I think we should make the opportunity available, but the ones we have in the program now can't be upgraded," the doctor insists. "When we tried to train them, it was a farce. You can't teach them anything new."

Weinstein doesn't want to waste more time in rhetoric. "Okay, thanks for coming down," he says. "I want to give it more thought. I'd like to see notices posted around here to inform people about the opportunity. Then you can screen them without being criticized, as long as you view them objectively."

When the doctor leaves, he's replaced by the head of Bellevue's ambulance service (run by the HHC), in uniform, wearing an Emergency Medical Service badge. During the weekend the disaster bus, a mammoth emergency vehicle, was unable to respond to a fire call because its battery was dead. Regular ambulances went instead. Weinstein asks him what happened.

"It was one of those mornings when everything went wrong," the officer says. "Now, we start it every morning and each shift has to check it to see that it works right."

"We've got to avoid getting a legitimate call and being unable to respond because of mechanical failure," Weinstein tells him. "We need a backup plan, a couple of ambulances ready to go."

"Actually, the bus should be in our garage, but it doesn't fit. It's too big," the officer says.

"Do you store spare batteries in the garage?"

"Yeah, we've got 'em," the officer smiles. A front tooth is missing.

"Okay, I'll ask the night administrator to check it out. Thanks a lot," Weinstein says. The officer leaves and is replaced by Kevin Porter, a young, round-faced, long-haired administrative specialist who supervises two of Bellevue's old buildings, F&G and I&K. Along with a male nursing supervisor, Weinstein and Porter take off to tour Porter's buildings.

As they walk briskly toward the first ward, screams emerge from it. The nursing supervisor recognizes the sound. "That's our twenty-four-hour screamer," he says. The screamer is a 26-year-old severely retarded quadriplegic in a wheelchair. He has been at Bellevue for two years, a disposition problem.

Weinstein asks a nurse on the ward, "Is it a matter of constant treatment or a matter of rehabilitation?"

"Both. As you see him now, that's how he is. It's difficult for us. And he doesn't understand us," the nurse answers.

"We sent him to a nursing home," Porter says, "and he was sent back minutes later. Now his mother wants to care for him at home."

Throughout the dialogue, the patient has continued to scream. Weinstein winces. The nurse does not.

"Let's try it, with some Home Care assistance," Weinstein says to Porter. "Any hang-up in such an arrangement?"

"Well, the mother isn't so stable, but it is worth a try to send him home, with support," Porter says.

"Custodial care, that's what he needs," the nursing supervisor adds, not distracted by the patient's shrieks.

Weinstein asks the ward nurse if she has any problems he can handle for her.

"Well, not much you can't see for yourself," she says. "The lighting on the ward is inadequate. We have trouble seeing to change dressings. And another patient has been on the ward for more than two years and he smokes in bed and turns on the television late at night."

"Just like he's at home, eh?" Weinstein says. He sees a wall that is crumbling. "Ah, that wall has a way of decorating itself. Any special problems?"

"The heat," the nurse says.

"Too hot?"

"Too cold. The patients complain."

"Anything else?"

"The floor. It comes out in patches."

Weinstein makes notes. This is the old Bellevue. He is used to it but not bored by it.

The three men walk to another ward. Most of the patients, all women, are resting silently, but one old black woman sees the group enter.

"Polyps, that's what I got," she says. "My granddaughter, she know all about it. I got it and I don't know but she know all about it. I'll get me another operation soon. I am feeling better."

"Good luck," Weinstein says to her, smiling.

"I'll need it," she says.

"We *all* need it," he says.

Weinstein turns to the nurse on the ward. "You getting all you need to take care of your patients?" he asks.

"Well, I need paper towels and plastic bags and pajamas," she says.

Weinstein makes more notes on a small pad.

"You get all that, you'll be a happy woman?" he asks, laughing.

"And the patients will be happy, too," she replies, stiffly.

The men walk down to the prison ward, which is being repainted. Weinstein strolls through it, past beds filled with male prisoners both sick and surly. One inmate, with "PERDON MADRE MIA" tattooed across his back, is watching Abbott and Costello on TV, oblivious to Weinstein and the others. A rock radio station at full volume competes with Abbott and Costello. Porter turns to Weinstein and says, "I think there's a need in our prison system to take care of paraplegics in a long-term way."

"You're dreaming," Weinstein says.

Weinstein walks back to his office. It is 11:55 A.M. He talks to Porter, who walks along with him, about what they saw, what must be done. Later, Weinstein will send out a memo assigning the chores, as he does after all tours and meetings requiring follow-up action.

"None of these things was new to you?" he asks Porter.

"No," Porter answers.

Porter leaves. Weinstein decides he'd better block out a few minutes for lunch. He orders a tuna-salad sandwich and coffee, from the Bellevue snack bar.

The snack bar, the only place outside of the hospital cafeterias, which aren't open to the public, where food can be bought, is run by the Auxiliary to Bellevue Hospital Center, Inc. The Auxiliary, active since 1906, takes donations of time and money —some as large as $50,000. It mounts an annual appeal, in the form of a simple, direct letter; it scorns parties, dinners, dances and conventional fund-raising benefits. It canvasses the neighborhood for contributions. It is not an organization run by an elite. "We believe in work, not social activity," one member puts it. "If you can't give money, we'll be just as happy to have some of your time."

The Auxiliary, working out of a tiny office on Bellevue's main floor, participates in the daily life of the hospital. Besides the snack bar, which makes a profit of $50,000-$60,000 a year (it would be $30,000 more if the city hadn't prohibited the sale of cigarettes on hospital premises), the Auxiliary assists in running an Upper East Side thrift shop. The funds raised are used to set up a cancer-testing program, a blood-replacement program, a day care center, and patient libraries and book carts. The Auxiliary supplements staff salaries, provides funds for nonmedical departments, like Occupational Therapy, gets money to needy patients, and gives Christmas presents to all the patients at Bellevue. It also supplies newspapers and supports workshops, arts and crafts programs and entertainment for patients.

At 2 P.M. Weinstein assembles his immediate staff in his office: Joe Moreinis, the business manager; Madeline Bohman, the Deputy Director; Doris Lesser, Director of Staff Services; Betty Kauffman, the Director of Nursing; Susan Wick, an administrative assistant; and Gerald Niedziolka, an administrative resident, a young man working on his master's degree, getting practical experience at Bellevue.

Lesser is in her early forties. She is short, with closely cropped salt-and-pepper hair, dark-complexioned, glasses, serious and smart. Kauffman does not wear a nurse's uniform; her face is familiar enough around Bellevue. She is an authoritative middle-aged veteran of many hospital wars, but she has the voice of a teen-age girl. Her hair is short, curly gray-brown and she wears glasses, too. Bohman, formerly a nurse, has risen to the number two spot in the Bellevue administration through the ranks, picking up her master's degree along the way. She has gray hair, is in her forties, wears glasses and is a heavy smoker. She is earthy and knowledgeable. Wick is the youngest, in her thirties, attractive and efficient; her job is to spare Weinstein the trouble of dealing with many details he can easily delegate to her. Moreinis, dignified, dapper, husky, with gray hair and glasses, is an expert at profit-and-loss matters, without being pedantic about it. He has been an associate of Weinstein's for years and was called to Bellevue after Weinstein settled into his job. Niedziolka is there simply to observe, to learn.

The meeting is the epitome of expeditiousness, although it is clear that these people like and respect each other. The conversation moves crisply from point to point.

There's been a bequest to Bellevue from the will of a grateful patient. Such bequests have brought more than $200,000 to the hospital during the past few years.

A resident in Psychiatry has forwarded a request to reduce the clinic fee for one of his patients, from $30 to $10 per visit. Weinstein's staff has investigated and discovered that the patient can afford to pay the $30 fee.

"When they're in private practice, they say it's therapeutic to pay. Here it's not so important," Weinstein says.

Bellevue must accept all patients. But it does charge them.

Most inpatients at Bellevue are covered by insurance: Medicaid, Medicare, Blue Cross and others. Such insurance covers all of, or most of, the $130-a-day charge. Bellevue will settle for less if the patient is uninsured and has limited income; it will accept whatever the patient can pay over an agreed-upon period of time.

Clinic patients pay from $2 to $36 per visit, based on family income and size; Bellevue trusts the patient to complete an accurate statement about both. If the patient is covered by Medicaid or Medicare, it pays the entire cost of clinic visits.

Patients who can afford to pay, do so. The average clinic fee, however, is $4–$5.

There's a suggestion to replace wall sockets in the ICUs (Intensive Care Units) with safety receptacles. It would cost more than $2,000.

"Are we going to get it done just in time to move out and into the new building?" Weinstein asks.

No, it can be done quickly, Lesser tells him. He approves it.

A proposal by the Director of Radiology, which the medical board will review, calls for the miniaturization of X-ray films, for greater storage and easier retrieval. It could cost approximately $140,000.

"Will it save money in staff and space?" Weinstein asks.

No one knows yet. Weinstein asks for more research before he's satisfied.

Various budget matters are covered. Moving equipment and twelve thousand linear feet of patient records to the new hospital will incur a $35,000 moving-company bill, Lesser reports.

A plan to move inpatients from old to new Bellevue is being typed for Weinstein's perusal.

A director of a service wants another clerk in his department.

"He says there's no one to answer his phones," a staff member says.

"If it becomes acute, let me know," Weinstein says, smiling.

Metropolitan Hospital on the Upper East Side has been asked to define what sort of adult and adolescent treatment it is capable of providing. It is an effort to cut down the flow of referrals to Bellevue. Metropolitan has not yet responded.

Weinstein shows a floor plan for the medical prison ward in the new Bellevue, occupying much of the eighteenth floor. It pleases those present, although the subject is a controversial one and, Weinstein knows, will come up again this week.

It is 4 P.M. when the meeting ends. Weinstein signs letters his secretary has been working on, requisitions requiring his approval. There is a request to purchase several cardiac pacemakers.

"Do you know those pacemakers they put into people's hearts?" he asks his secretary. "Well, they're $1,150 each." He approves the requisition, runs off to shave in a room he keeps for himself in the residents' quarters.

It is almost 5 P.M. by the time he gets into his car for a drive to Metropolitan Hospital. He is to attend a meeting of city hospital administrators, complete with dinner from the Metropolitan kitchen. He is looking forward to the meeting but not to the meal.

Dirk Berger gets up in his Queens apartment at 6:30, troubled. His wife is asleep. So are his two children. He sips a Tab and tries to clear his head. Last night he got a phone call telling him that a former patient on his ward in Bellevue Psychiatry had committed suicide. The tragedy preyed on his mind all night and he could not help feeling guilty about it.

Berger is the chief resident in Psychiatry. A 30-year-old New Yorker, he went to college at Yeshiva University, to medical school at Catholic University of Louvain in Belgium. After interning at St. Mary's Hospital in Montreal, he came to Bellevue. He is now in his fourth year there, his second as chief resident. The psychiatric residency is three years; Berger elected to stay on for the additional year.

Five feet ten and weighing a trim 160 pounds, he is handsome, blond, with blue eyes. His hair is curly and fashionably long, his clothes fashionably bright, but his personality remains tranquil. He does not shout.

This morning, as he drives his 1971 Plymouth Cricket through Queens toward the East River, he knows that the suicide will be only one of dozens of crises he will have to deal with. It is bad enough. The others could be worse. On Ward NO–6, which Berger runs, there is little time to be self-indulgent, to contemplate the fate of the New York Rangers or the music of the Beach Boys, two of Berger's private obsessions. On NO–6, every day is a taunt.

NO–6 is the psychiatric ward that treats patients from the Murray Hill Mental Health District, patients who live in the area bounded by Fourteenth Street, Forty-second Street, the Hudson River and the East River. NO–6 sees them as constituents, not as strangers passing through. Berger's staff includes five first-year residents, two full-time attending physicians, three social workers, two activity therapists, a head nurse and four staff nurses, a mental health assistant to work closely with the community, a psychiatric technician (an aide with special training in dealing with psychiatric patients) and a group of nurse's aides and practical nurses.

For most psychiatric patients at Bellevue, the average stay is two to three weeks. Seventy percent of the patients are discharged. The rest are sent on to state hospitals. On NO–6, Berger and his staff work hard to treat the patients and, just as important, to keep in touch with them once they leave the ward, to continue treating them as outpatients.

When Berger arrives on the ward at 8 A.M., many of the thirty-two patients there are shuffling through the corridors. The ward itself is in the shape of a block "C." Berger enters through a locked door at the center of the longest corridor. To the right is the women's wing, to the left an identical men's wing. In the center is a large community room, where patients sit during the day, have their meals, listen to the radio, play cards, look out the windows, which face a small courtyard and First Avenue.

Each wing contains dormitories and small rooms for sleeping, seclusion rooms for violent patients (bare except for a thin mattress on the floor, and locked whether occupied or not), bathrooms with showers. To the right of the entrance is Berger's office, an office for his secretary and a conference room for staff meetings, patient consultations and group therapy sessions. Beyond those rooms is the nurse's station, filled with records and equipment, and a small cubicle for the ward clerk, who cuts her way through hospital protocol to process patients in and out. At the tip of each arm of the "C" is a recreation area, with games to play, couches, chairs.

For Berger, the ward is the focal point of his life as a doctor. For patients and visitors, it can be an unsteadying and cheerless setting. Patients keep in motion, like competitors in a slow-motion walking race. They line up in front of the medication room, opposite Berger's office, to receive their drugs. They linger outside the kitchen or the linen room. They sit, endlessly. They rave.

Berger feels tested by them, not intimidated. He knows that NO–6, one of seven adult wards at Bellevue (there are wards for children and adolescents and a prison ward, run by the Department of Correction, as well), is the best Bellevue has to offer. It is a training ward and that means that Berger has five residents to treat patients. He has the best and largest staff, and the fewest patients, among the wards at Bellevue. Other wards can offer medication and can "contain" the patients. NO–6 does more. It shelters those in its community who cannot endure the psychic threats of the city. It helps them to cope and it offers them a refuge if they cannot. The patients know that when they leave NO–6, they can return to the doctors and staff who cared for them. Berger *knows* his patients, their delusions, their frailties, their frustrations, their hopes. He has inspired his staff to share his concern.

It is that concern which makes any failure, like the suicide reported to Berger, an invisible wound on the doctors' nervous systems. Today, at 8:30 rounds, it is evident.

Rounds, in Psychiatry, take the form of a staff meeting to evaluate each case. Today there are twenty staff members present, including residents, nurses, social workers, activity therapist. The head nurse reads through patient charts, sums up what took place on the ward over the weekend. The others listen.

"Not too bad a weekend," the head nurse says. She is young, dressed, as is everyone else, in her own clothes rather than medical uniform.

She recites specifics.

One male patient took a shower, played cards, took his medication. He was "kind and cooperative." His blood pressure was stable.

Berger nods.

Another patient had left a rehabilitation center in another state and was uncomfortable in Bellevue's custody. He was upset that his family had not contacted him. Berger tells a social worker to notify his family.

A third patient, an old man, looked pasty and seemed to be sleepy, but paced relentlessly through the halls of the ward.

A patient asked to take a shower, then stayed in the shower for forty-five minutes. She was dragged out.

"That one," the head nurse says in anger, "she antagonized everyone. She cursed and kicked other patients and refused her medication. She really carried on. She was terrible."

Berger says nothing.

One of the drug addicts is making progress. Berger knows the man; he spoke with him last week.

"He verbalized perfectly," Berger tells the group. "He told me, 'The pressures come from inside me.' He is sick and the methadone isn't working. He is better off on tranquilizers than on the drug he abuses." Berger suggests that the patient be discharged, observed, kept on tranquilizers.

The head nurse continues. One patient's wife visited him and put her arms around him. He fled. "The wife can't believe he's so aggressive at home and so calm in the hospital," the head nurse says.

She mentions that one of the female patients lurks around the nursing station. "I have the feeling she is going to try to choke me," she says.

Some patients stay in bed all day. Some don't eat. Some are hostile. One old woman protrudes her tongue and drools. The head nurse reports that the woman tried to tell her fortune.

"She predicted that your hands would get wet," Berger says, smiling.

The others in the room report, too, on patients they're treating:

"She was quite concerned that no one in her family knew that she was at Bellevue. Her sister found out and visited her. It upset her."

"One patient told me that there wasn't anything wrong with him, that he'd come here to rest."

"His IQ is 64. The psychologist says he's not psychotic, but that he has difficulty in reality situations. I don't think Thorazine is indicated. He's received it twice and it simply made him awfully sleepy."

Berger listens, cautions, gives advice. He participates without dominating. It is clear that all those present respect and like him.

The suicide comes up. The resident who had treated that patient is glum. Berger is, too. There was no indication in the patient's history to justify the suicide, Berger says.

"She was anxious when she was discharged, afraid she couldn't make it on the outside," a social worker says.

"She was a chronic state-hospital patient. And she did ask one of us, 'Did you ever feel like killing yourself?' But when she left, she sounded cheerful and said she hoped to make it out there," a resident adds.

"She just didn't look like one to do it," Berger says. "She may have given us some hints, but we didn't pick them up." He reminds the staff that she had three children.

After the meeting, Berger attends another meeting, one held twice a week with staff and patients in the large open area at the center of the ward. Most of the patients are present. A few shuffle aimlessly, wearing the bulky white hospital slippers that scrape softly against the worn corridor floor. Others sit, numbed by drugs or reflecting in their faces an unquenchable inner anger. They all sit in a large circle. Berger encourages them to talk about anything that relates to the ward and their life on it.

Charges fly from all parts of the room.

"I'm talking to a friend of mine when this guy comes up and hits me," says one black woman. She is thin. Her ill-fitting, brightly colored dress sags around her ankles, above her stained sneakers.

"Lies. Bullshit. Lies and bullshit," says a black man near her, but not to her. To the air, a generalized indictment.

Others are encouraged to speak, to win equal time.

A fat black woman, her face frozen in anger, bounces in her chair to get attention. "We should have Kool-Aid instead of ice water," she shouts defiantly.

The thin black woman, forgetting the man who defamed her, joins the cause. "And put the damned Kool-Aid in a big jug, like one of those things they put coffee in, not a damned little pitcher." She is clutching her purse in one hand, a deck of cards in the other.

A young black man joins the dietary rebellion. He is sick of peanut butter and jelly. He finds an ally in the thin black woman.

"Let's get us some cheese spread instead of peanut butter and jelly," she shouts. "Or Spam—you know, that stuff that comes in a can."

Berger interrupts: "We'll find out what's available from Dietary."

The young black man resumes. He urges that leftover pie and cake be kept on the ward, for snacks at night. He inspires the fat black woman to have a reverie.

"When I was here before, they had the most delicious chocolate cake I ever ate," she says, remembering the taste, the texture.

"Ice cream and cake. Now that's a party," shouts a voice from a far corner.

"Keep your voice down," screams a man. "Why, the language

you use." He is talking to the thin, agitated black woman. Unexpectedly, while Berger leans forward anticipating escalation, she does not go into a frenzy. She is contemplative.

"I agree with you," she tells her critic. "It's not nice of me. I do have a temper. And these nurses and doctors disturb me."

The man is not satisfied. "You annoy everybody here. You play the radio too loud. I'm talking about how you deal with the people you live with."

The chubby Kool-Aid advocate changes the subject: continuity is not a characteristic of these meetings.

"When I'm sleepin', patients take flowers from all over the place and shake them under my nose. Now, I'm a pollen sufferer and I just can't have flowers around me."

"The flowers ought to be put in a special place, where they can be seen without bothering anyone," Berger tells her and the others.

The thin black woman is no longer reticent. "I don't give a damn about the radio," she screams. "I don't try to take it over. I just sit any Goddamned place I want to sit."

"And the TV set," another patient says. "Why you got to watch cartoons if that is what is on?"

Berger proposes that the patients form a TV viewing committee, to list programs and vote on who gets to watch what.

An old woman sits in her chair and, rhythmically every few seconds, tries to rise slowly out of it. A nurse behind her whispers, "Mrs. Morgan, please," and gently pushes her back into the chair. They do not exchange glances.

Berger summarizes what has been said. He tells the patients how important it is to discuss their problems, to express their anger. His manner is calm, his language simple; they understand him.

After the meeting, Berger holds a brief meeting with a few members of the staff. The thin black woman, he tells them, is retarded; when she is picked on, she reacts. It was good that she sat through the entire meeting. She didn't run. The pollen sufferer is getting better. She used to complain about being raped and robbed, not about ice water. But what about the ice water? Kool-Aid needs ice and the building's electrical system won't support an ice machine. Berger remembers that one staff member has "an ice connection." He suggests "we get some buckets and rip off some ice."

Berger goes to his office. It is drab, furnished with old furniture collected from even older offices and classrooms. He is joined by the first-year resident who worked over the weekend. Berger wants a report. He pops open a can of Diet Pepsi and listens.

The resident talks about one woman who troubles him. "She is really bad. Look at her today. I raised her Thorazine when her behavior got so bizarre."

"Raise it again," Berger says. "She isn't groggy."

One patient is disturbed by the drug he's taking. "Change it," Berger says. "His head has taken enough."

The resident describes another case. "I remember that one," Berger says. "He seemed grossly psychotic, delusional, hearing voices. Escaping from five men with knives. Schizophrenic. But now he's calm, better. Stop the drugs."

The resident is exhausted after a weekend on duty. He gets up and tells Berger to call him at home if anything comes up. At 11 A.M., it is time for another meeting.

One of three staff teams assigned to a specific group of patients assembles in Berger's office. One of the team's tasks is to evaluate patient progress by classification: (1) patients without privileges; (2) transitional patients; and (3) patients who are allowed periodic passes into the outside world or are ready for discharge. The team includes a resident, a nurse, a social worker and several aides. The resident, a woman, outlines the cases for Berger.

A young man, who has given three different names and ages, has been admitted to the ward three times in a year, asking for medication for insomnia. He is asking to see a lawyer, demanding to be discharged. He is psychotic, the resident says, and is on Thorazine. He complains about being on "dope." He wants to be transferred to a ward with "pretty young girls." The nurse says he's "completely obnoxious." The social worker adds that his mother is coming to visit him.

"She could help us, if she's not crazy, too," Berger says.

Next case: a 65-year-old woman who, according to the resident, is not psychotic, just depressed. "She is completely logical, has a good sense of humor and is a pleasant old lady." Nevertheless, Berger points out, she made a serious attempt at suicide, an overdose of Valium and Seconal. The social worker notes that the woman is not on welfare and does not have money or clothes.

"How can we let her out in the street, just like that, with no family?" the social worker, a young woman not long out of college, asks.

"She has good reason to be depressed," Berger says. "She'll get better here. No antidepressants. Vitamin B–12. Librium."

"She says she's buried a series of husbands and she's finished with marriage," the resident adds.

"Is she Jewish?" Berger asks, jokingly.

The group decides to keep the woman occupied, with activities and work projects, and to find shelter for her, so she can leave the hospital.

A teen-age black girl, an orphan since the age of five, has lived with a foster family that preferred its own children to her. She moves in and out of reality.

"Today she seems very well," the resident reports. "She came to talk to me. But her hands and legs are rigid, which she says is from the drugs we're giving her. I get five calls a day from the family, to release her or move her to a private hospital. I've tried to explain that she'll get more attention here. And she wants to go to college. I've told her that if all goes well I'll say she had depression, period. She worries about her family, which she feels she owes much to yet hates."

"We must deal with that guilt. About turning down the foster family. We can say it is more therapeutic for her," Berger says. "Whatever, we better take a good, long look."

A black man, an alcoholic in his forties, was picked up by railroad police at Penn Station. "He will be a headache," the resident predicts. "He says he's a cook on weekends and he says he earns $18,000 a year. He says he was in the Army for twenty-two years and made ninety-two parachute jumps, but he won't discuss his Army discharge."

"He got here because the Long Island Railroad police didn't want to bring charges, didn't want to waste time having to appear in court," Berger tells the resident.

"He loves vodka and he loves to gamble."

"Watch for the DTs."

"His memory is often exact, but he *is* psychotic. It is hard to follow him."

"He's drunk. The question is what is beneath that?"

"He wants out."

"Good. Let him see a lawyer. Don't give him medication unless the DTs appear. Watch him. He may be a quick discharge. I'll see him myself this afternoon."

"Okay. I'll give him some Librium. Ten mg. three times a day."

The meeting ends at noon. Five minutes later, Berger is at another one, in an office on a floor below NO–6.

As a part of his work, and the work of NO–6, with the community, Berger spends time at the Aberdeen Hotel on West Thirty-second Street. Many of the occupants of that hotel were sent there from NO–6, to have a place to live while continuing to get treatment. Berger visits the hotel every week, to see those patients. This rambling meeting is with a social worker, an activity therapist and a psychiatrist who work at the Aberdeen. They talk until 1:15. Berger, for the first time during the day, looks weary. He has slumped in his chair for most of the meeting, letting the others tell him what's going on at the Aberdeen. Now he goes back to the ward, to his own office. The patients have had their lunch. Berger has his: a large container of diet soda.

Afterward, he strolls to the men's wing of NO–6, to see Charlie Johnson, the man picked up in Penn Station. He chats with the man for a few minutes, then discusses him with the resident on the case.

"He smells of booze and has red eyes," Berger tells her. "I'll give him twenty-four hours. Right now, he's in a rage about being here. And I tend to believe him. He hasn't lost control. The nurses will want to medicate him. I'm disinclined. If he sleeps it off, it'll be certain he didn't belong in Bellevue in the first place."

At 2 P.M., there is another team meeting: resident, nurse, social worker and aides. Again, a rundown of patients and their status.

A 21-year-old man, one of thirteen children, has a history of getting into fights. He's been shot at least once. He has a seizure disorder. He's been arrested for petty larceny and for molesting an 8-year-old girl. No convictions. The Bureau of Child Welfare got involved when he was reported for having sexual intercourse with his sister. His IQ tested out at 64. That defines him, in Berger's scale, as "moderately retarded." According to the resident, he has "a limited ability to interpret reality and is a problem on the ward." No one feels he is psychotic, however, which means that his case must be disposed of.

"When I called his mother, she told me she didn't want him at home. She told me to keep him," the resident says.

Berger says, "He needs a structured environment, permanently. Not a Willowbrook or a state hospital, where they don't want him or where he can just walk out. There is no place for him now, so he could easily wind up on the streets again."

"Perhaps he can be settled down by activity therapy?" the social worker asks.

"Let's watch him on the ward," Berger says.

"If that fails, we'll have to refer it to Family Court," the resident says.

"I suppose he could act out sexually on the ward. Thorazine will zonk him. He won't be able to get a hard-on," Berger says.

"I'd like to get him off the ward."

"It'll take time."

The resident pauses, seems uncomfortable. He tells Berger that he's heard that patients are having intercourse on the ward at night. He is serious, almost unnerved by the revelation.

"Sure there's screwing on the ward. Homosexual and heterosexual. The very sick ones tell us about it later. The others don't. There's nothing to do about it, if it is done in private."

It is after 3 P.M. when the meeting adjourns. Berger wants to talk to two patients. They are contrasts in psychotic styles.

Berger finds the first, a ward patient, sitting alone in the recreational area at the end of the men's wing. He is a black man, middle-aged, and is sitting on a bench staring at his feet. He is wearing a blue-and-white seersucker robe, soiled pajamas and shower sandals. He does not seem to be receptive. Berger tells him who he is, softly, gently, without any psychiatric jargon. The man tells Berger his story.

He had been assaulted by a group of men in the Port Authority bus terminal and had thrown a trash basket at them. Berger listens. The man was arrested by police for throwing the basket and because he seemed to be drunk and angry was taken to Bellevue Psychiatry.

Berger tries to find out what is real and what is not. The man deals, successfully, with a series of questions about his own life. Can he remember simple facts? Berger invents a name and address and asks the man to remember and repeat them. The man cannot. Berger tries a simple subtraction problem. The man cannot do it. Berger tells him a brief tale about a kidnaped sailor, a story designed to test memory. The man cannot repeat it. He can describe the night he entered Bellevue and his description straddles the line between reality and unreality. A group of men were following him, were attacking him, were in turn attacked by police armed with bricks. He had been drinking. He can drink a bottle of wine in two hours, eight or more in a weekend. Berger's manner, quiet and solemn, encourages the man to continue speaking. Finally, Berger thanks him and leaves.

"He's sick, but I don't know how sick," Berger tells the staff nurse. "It'll take more observation."

Back in his office, Berger greets the second patient, from the Aberdeen, a patient he's known, in and out of Bellevue, for several years.

Nathan Rothberg is 29, thin, sloppy, shrewdly intelligent behind a façade of glib cynicism. He dropped out of Yale a semester before graduation. He has not been able to hold a job. His parents were divorced. He sees his mother, whom he adores. His father is dead. He has come to see Berger for drugs, because his mother must go away on business and Nathan needs support. He lives on welfare at the Aberdeen and spends his time being harmlessly lecherous and engaging in petty thievery. Well informed about the law, he doesn't want to violate it flagrantly. An able amateur composer, he doesn't compose.

When he enters Berger's office, he taunts Berger. He tells him he's glad to see that he no longer bites his nails (Berger never has). He asks Berger how his wife is treating him in bed. Berger remains calm.

Nathan, who has taken the chair beside Berger, gets up and falls to his knees in front of Berger. "Oh, wondrous psychiatrist, bring me to salvation," he says. Berger assists him back into the chair. Berger tells him, sternly, to take himself more seriously, to lead with his strengths instead of his weaknesses. While Berger talks, Nathan maintains a frozen smile. Berger gives him a prescription, then escorts him to the door. After Nathan leaves, Berger turns to one of the residents standing nearby and says, "Terminal mental illness. But brilliant."

The resident has his own problems to talk about. The black 19-year-old orphan. Her foster father, a middle-class postman, the resident has learned, is moving to Arizona and wants to take his "daughter" with him. She has told the resident that she wants to stay in New York, go to college and marry her Puerto Rican boy friend. "It's tricky to interfere," Berger says, "but it's up to you to represent her best interest."

Another patient feels like killing the cop who brought him to Bellevue, the resident tells Berger. In fact, he feels like killing all cops. Berger shrugs. He looks tired and this is one case he expects the resident to deal with. They make their way into his office, where Berger falls into his decaying chair and delivers an instructive monologue to the resident.

"You know, the more raving and crazy they are when they arrive here, the easier they are to treat, in any psychosis, especially schizophrenics. And the younger, the better for us. A terrible stress, a sudden retreat from reality in a young person is easier to treat. Older, chronic cases don't respond as well or as quickly.

"Fortunately, this ward is special. We take back our patients when they need us. The other wards here take them back only within thirty days of discharge. We're after continuity."

It is late in the afternoon now. The resident is looking forward to going home; he eases out of Berger's office. A woman is waiting to see Berger. He invites her into his office.

She is a middle-aged Latin American whom Berger has been seeing for several years. With the help of her parish priest, he's managed to sustain her as an outpatient, although she carries a collection of delusions with her. She is tormented by the oddities and crudities of life in New York. So, at times, is Berger, so he is able to comfort her and send her out smiling. When she leaves, Berger checks with the nurses coming on duty for the four-to-twelve shift, strolls through the corridors talking to patients. Then, after 6 P.M., he heads for his car and the drive home to Queens. Through dinner and into his sleep, the events of the day circulate. The suicide. The black alcoholic. The orphan and her foster father. The dialogue at the ward meeting. The Aberdeen.

Kenneth Kirshbaum is 25, a second-year resident in Psychiatry. Born in Paterson, New Jersey, Kirshbaum was a chemistry major at the University of Pennsylvania, then went to N.Y.U. Medical School. He came to Bellevue from N.Y.U.

Kirshbaum is married to a schoolteacher; they live in Queens. He seems to be taller than he actually is (six feet one), because he is thin (148 pounds). His carefully combed dark hair and his glasses make him seem older than 25. He is a precise, neat, conservative man and an understated, straightforward, unpretentious doctor. With patients, he is never obscure, never given to psychiatric games or heavy-handed pedantry. He is a moralist who wants his patients to have happier lives. At Bellevue, that idealistic goal can be sustained only at the expense of the doctor's own well-being.

Kirshbaum's second year of residency is spent in the Bellevue psychiatric clinics. The walk-in clinic is set up to deal with short-term therapy for adults who simply appear at the clinic in need of help. Former inpatients, who knew Kirshbaum when he served on one of the wards, come in, too. Those who need regular care are sent on to the Mental Hygiene clinic, where patients have their own doctors on a continuing basis. During his second year, Kirshbaum will see both walk-in and MHC patients; there are satellite clinics for drug addicts, alcoholics, and patients who are in family or group therapy, as well as for children and adolescents.

Kirshbaum will consult to the general hospital as well and will teach clinical psychology to medical students from N.Y.U.

The clinics are in the basement of the psychiatric fortress, compounding the depression that some patients bring with them. Despite renovation, doubling the number of examining rooms to forty, and repainting the walls, the atmosphere is dark, placing an added burden on the spirit of the doctors. In the walk-in clinic, the doctors play psychiatric roulette; patients come in, enraged or catatonic or simply nervous, and are sent to the first available resident. The doctor has looked at the patient's chart, a catalogue of trouble, but he cannot be fully prepared for what the patient will do or say.

Last week the range of Kirshbaum's experience included a bulbous black woman who came charging in, leading an alcoholic son and a 26-year-old daughter, who was sucking her thumb and clutching a teddy bear. The mother wanted all three admitted. In the course of an interview with a drunk, the man threatened to kill Kirshbaum. Kirshbaum called for two guards, who found a large knife in the man's pocket. A woman came in to talk, but grew more menacing as the dialogue went on; a guard found two loaded revolvers in her shopping bag.

All of Kirshbaum's work is not so dramatic or threatening. Much of it is solid psychiatry, dealing with neurotics and watching out for psychotics, as the patients file into and out of his cramped office at a pace that might foment unrest in private practice.

Occasionally, Kirshbaum draws duty in the Psychiatric Admitting Office at night. The PAO is psychiatry's chamber of horrors, a procession of deranged, tormented, alienated and eccentric souls who have stumbled in for safety or been brought in by police, relatives, friends. For a doctor, it is a demanding, exhausting tour, relieved only by random absurdities.

The last time he worked the PAO at night, Kirshbaum was interviewing a patient when an ambulance pulled up. Kirshbaum went to meet it, anticipating an emergency. A man dressed only in a sheet emerged. He had been forwarded to Bellevue from another hospital and he carried a form marked "suicidal hysterical."

"I'm not crazy," he told Kirshbaum. "I got mad and I belted my wife. She expects it, for God's sake." He told Kirshbaum that when he got to the first hospital, escorted by the police, his wife seized his clothes. "How the hell do I get home in a sheet?" he asked. Kirshbaum phoned for a taxi. The man, in his judgment, was neither suicidal nor hysterical.

This week Kirshbaum is due for another shift in the PAO. He looks forward to it, because it can never be mundane and rarely is uneventful. Meanwhile, he will spend most of his time seeing patients less frenzied. The only departure from that schedule is an opportunity to learn at a 9 A.M. teaching conference for second-year residents. A senior staff member, an experienced teacher-psychiatrist, presides. Although attendance is voluntary, Kirshbaum feels that, for him, it is mandatory. It is a contemplative way to start his day, before the procession of neurotics begins.

Today the subject is "Borderline Cases" and the speaker-moderator is a senior N.Y.U. faculty member, psychiatrist and clinic supervisor. He has gray hair, glasses and cradles a pipe in his hand; he is dressed in tweeds, with a bow tie. He speaks softly.

The fuzzy state between neurosis and psychosis, he says, is often agonizing to define. There are plenty of terms in use:

"pseudo-neurotic," "ambulatory schizophrenic," "psychotic character," Helene Deutsch's "As-If Personality" and others.

"It's a difficult diagnosis to make," the psychiatrist tells the residents, "and the search for it can be a way of avoiding the study of the case itself."

"You've got to look at the patient," Kirshbaum says.

"Yes. There's a difference of opinion in the literature and there is debate about whether a neurotic can become a psychotic. Some doctors see the borderline case as a defined cluster of symptoms, but there's very little about it in the standard textbooks."

There are fifteen residents in the room. As the psychiatrist goes on, one doctor nods off, another files her nails and a third compulsively draws her thumbnail along the stripes on her pants.

"Where do you draw the line?" Kirshbaum asks.

"Well, one line of research indicates that you can define the borderline syndrome by the infantile, dependent attitude, the failure to progress, sensitivity to acceptance or rejection, obsessional or hysterical behavior and the presence of anger. I think you have to define it on the basis of the patient's whole history, style of life." The psychiatrist puffs his pipe. The room is silent.

"I had one who was in analysis for years," he says. "The patient got involved with her previous doctor. He asked me to see her, to break or dilute the transference taking place. A disaster. And I got the brunt of it. She had me up every night for an hour or two, threatening suicide. After two or three weeks, I told the other doctor that I couldn't go on.

"She had a twenty-year history of treatment and would select the best psychiatrists around. From one famous one to another. She could function, but she suffered from deep depressions. All the analysts took a crack and failed. After I gave up, too, she was hospitalized. Shock therapy. She saw her recovery as some sort of rebirth, a fantasy of being a new person with all her problems resolved. Still no delusions. Just periodic intense depression. She probably belongs in this borderline syndrome; because she wasn't isolated, she functioned."

Diagnoses today, he adds, are more subtle. "In fact, most of Freud's patients would be declared neurotic today. We have to think more consciously, more sharply. Definition is fundamental to diagnosis. Yet definitions differ. A schizoid here would be called a 'depressive' in England. And Karl Menninger has said that all diagnoses should be thrown out the window."

With that to think about, the residents move out of the conference room. Kirshbaum heads for the basement, to attend a unit meeting in the walk-in clinic. The unit to which he is assigned includes four social workers, three residents, a part-time director and two full-time attending psychiatrists. That group meets daily at 11:30, to discuss patients, their problems, possible courses of action. When it is over, Kirshbaum runs for a fast lunch in the cafeteria in Psychiatry, a steamingly hot room with overhanging pipes and commonplace food.

After lunch, Kirshbaum is scheduled to see clinic patients. His first today is a 49-year-old woman, Elizabeth Mack, who seems to be fighting against age by dressing out of *Seventeen* magazine, in jeans and a sequined T-shirt. Her chart reveals to Kirshbaum that she has been in Bellevue before, with a drinking problem, but she has been a loyal member of Alcoholics Anonymous since then. She works, but is "afraid and depressed."

"What brings you here now?" Kirshbaum asks.

She tells him that a few weeks ago she was at home alone when an intruder came crashing through her window. A stocky black man in his thirties, he had an Afro hairdo and a conspicuous gold tooth. He assaulted her, slashed her, urinated on her and fled, she tells Kirshbaum.

"It was terrifying and I was tempted to have a drink, but I resisted it. I do need your help, though, because I still think about it."

"It sounds to me like your depression came on after the mugging, which isn't surprising. That's a rattling experience for anyone." Kirshbaum is openly sympathetic.

"Well, it happened and that was it. I mean, where is there any safety? I told myself to forget it. But it just didn't go away."

"Your anxiety got more intense. And you had trouble sleeping. Are you still attending the AA meetings?"

"Yes, I enjoy them."

"Do you ever think of hurting yourself?" Kirshbaum asks. It is his euphemism for suicide. He tries to avoid being blunt.

"No. I'm just fearful. You know? I've put up a gate on my window now. But I find it hard to live behind it. Once I had shutters, a board and an iron brace. I made them myself. Now I have to live behind that new gate, even though I don't think that man will ever come back." She speaks softly, almost in a whisper, and she wrings her hands very slowly.

"It all sounds reasonable to me," Kirshbaum tells her. "Your fear will change in time. For your acute anxiety, so you can work, I'd like to give you some medication for a week. Then I'll see you again next week, during your lunch hour. Think about what we've said today and we can talk about it next week." He writes a prescription for Valium and hands it to her. As she leaves, another resident stops in front of Kirshbaum's door.

"Who was that?" he asks.

"Oh, she was mugged in her apartment. Bad stuff. What happened probably revived some old sexual anxiety. She needs reassurance, medication and a chance to talk. She should clear after not more than four visits."

The resident crosses his fingers and waves them at Kirshbaum, who smiles.

His next patient has been pacing outside the door, peering in. When the resident moves on to his own patients, Kirshbaum's patient rushes in.

His name is Bobby Warren and Kirshbaum knows him very well. He is 15, black, and, in the course of his life, has received more than twenty shock treatments. An inpatient at several mental hospitals, including Bellevue where Kirshbaum first met him on a ward, he seems to be managing in the outside world. When he was a child, he lived with two uncles; his mother and father lived apart. Now he lives with his father, who sent him to Bellevue when he became unmanageable at home. A bright student, his social behavior is infantile.

He is quite tall and wears a T-shirt that is emblazoned with "Property of the New York Knicks," and tattered jeans. He wears sunglasses. He sits, glumly, in the chair next to Kirshbaum's desk. Kirshbaum reminds him that he's happiest when there are rules to follow: Warren will cook if his father washes the dishes, or vice versa. He reminds Warren, too, that he doesn't always listen to Kirshbaum's advice.

"I listen when I want to, and when I don't want to, I don't listen," Warren says. "There are things I don't want to tell you."

"How would you behave, what would you do, if you had a son?" Kirshbaum asks.

"I'd never hit him. Never. I'd take him out. I wouldn't drink either. I hate liquor. I'd take him to ball games."

"I mean, if he had emotional problems?" Kirshbaum asks. He

sees Warren as primitively smart, with the emotional level of a 5-year-old.

Warren has made a long chain of paperclips on Kirshbaum's desk and slips the chain through his fingers like rosary beads. He thinks about Kirshbaum's question.

"Well, if I couldn't handle it, I'd take him to a doctor, not to a hospital. My father took me to a hospital *first*. I'd want a doctor to tell me how to handle it. I'd take him to *you* because I trust you."

He tells Kirshbaum that if he has a problem he will call Kirshbaum at home. "I'm calling you. I found your number in the book," he says, defiance in his voice.

"If you call it, you'll find it's been changed to an unlisted number," Kirshbaum tells him. "But you can always reach me through the clinic, day and night. They know where to find me." Like most doctors, Kirshbaum tries to preserve his private life without making himself unavailable in emergencies.

"Okay," Warren says. He has a wide smile on his face. That and his gawky movements make him look 15, whatever may be going on in his head to make him younger. As he leaves Kirshbaum's office he makes a slight waving motion with his hand and bounces an imaginary basketball out into the hall.

The boy is not delusional, Kirshbaum is convinced, but he does have acute paranoid episodes. He attacks other kids and can be violent. He needs every minute accounted for or he fills his time with trouble. Kirshbaum has gotten him into the public school in Bellevue Psychiatry (one of two at the hospital), where Kirshbaum can consult with his teacher. His father has been cooperative. Warren comes in regularly. Still in high school, he talks about college, which Kirshbaum finds heartening. His father talks about moving away from New York and that frustrates Kirshbaum. Kirshbaum doesn't have children, but this one consumes almost as much of his time as his own child might.

But there are more patients in the small waiting room. They stride into Kirshbaum's office every fifteen or thirty minutes. It is a busy day. After Warren leaves, Kirshbaum sees two regular patients who simply need reassurance, support. It is now almost 4 P.M. There are two more patients waiting to see him.

The first is a 24-year-old Italian who looks like a young Marlon Brando, short, solid, faintly aggressive. He wears a white T-shirt and chinos, soiled white socks and well-traveled moccasins. His name is Michael Gallo, but he is not, he has told Kirshbaum, related to the winemakers or the Mafioso. He is a former drug addict. Under heroin, his psychosis was masked. When he was detoxified, he had paranoid hallucinations. He seems to be making progress; he is calmer than he has been in previous sessions with Kirshbaum. The medication Kirshbaum has prescribed, Thorazine and Valium, may be working. Or he could be supplementing them with goods from the street. Kirshbaum can't tell.

"Are my medicines better than heroin?" he asks.

"Sure."

"And entirely legal."

"I'd still like to try Seconal," Gallo says.

"And become addicted again. You'll need more and more of it. Twenty, thirty a day, to get the same old high."

"Well, the Valium is good, it calms me down, but that Thorazine makes me dizzy."

"Continue on it for a while. It is helping you."

"Yeah," Gallo says, getting up in slow motion. In fact, the entire conversation has been a sluggish, slow one, with chunks of silence between comments. "Yeah," he says again, standing near Kirshbaum's chair. He glides out. Kirshbaum wonders if he is back on drugs, not the drugs he has given him.

The next patient's chart is on Kirshbaum's desk. She is Eleanor Golden, a 28-year-old woman from an upper-middle-class suburban family. She has a Ph.D. in English from U.C.L.A., but has not in any way used the degree or the experience. She's been a patient at both an expensive private hospital and Bellevue; she got to the latter when she couldn't pay her bills at the former. She arrived at Bellevue screaming and was in seclusion for two days before she could describe her problems to a doctor. Her father dominated her, encouraged her dependence. She married a man who proved to be vicious; rape within marriage became a fact in her life and the torment that edged her toward madness. As Kirshbaum reads the chart, a man armed with a large tank-type mechanism appears at his door.

"Any roaches in here?" the man asks.

Kirshbaum pauses, makes certain the man is not a patient on the loose, then says, "No, but when there are, they're gigantic." The man carts his tank to the next office.

Eleanor Golden enters. She is tall, conspicuously underweight, red-haired. Her face is strewn with freckles. She does not wear make-up. Her dress is a once-fashionable Scandinavian import, now on the verge of being shabby.

"You know I've been going through this awful divorce," she says.

"Yes, I know."

"And because of my history, there's a chance I might lose custody of our child. You know that?"

"Yes, I know that, too. What can I do for you?"

"Well, we've talked about all this for weeks. You've been of great help to me. Really, you have. In the past, when I got depressed, it was dangerous for me. Now it's begun to lift a bit. I don't feel *crazy.*"

"Good. I'm glad."

"I've got a job now. You know *that.* You know *everything.* I've got my own place and I'm furnishing it with stuff I like. Stuff *I* like. And I'm less of a slob than I used to be. This dress won't win any prizes, but it's an improvement over the rags I used to wear. Right?"

"Right."

"You might say I'm repairing my self-esteem. *You* might. I looked up a few old friends last week. I haven't done that in years. We had a very pleasant time together. I guess they didn't know I'd been crazy and I didn't tell them and they didn't know at all. I'm more alert these days, if that's the right word."

She rambles on, for twenty minutes, reconstructing her pride, asserting her health. Kirshbaum supports her, steadily, sincerely.

"Here's the best news," she says, leaning forward in her chair so that her face is over his desk, inches from his face. "I've tried some writing again. I did an article on flowers. I don't know if you know anything about flowers. Petunias, to be precise. Know what? A magazine bought the piece. I'm going to be published."

"That's marvelous," Kirshbaum says. "Wonderful. Keep it up. Keep it up."

She is smiling. Her voice quivers as she says, "Yes." She gets up, still smiling at her triumph, and leaves. When she's gone, Kirshbaum remains seated at his desk. He is still smiling, too.

The Chest Service at Bellevue is not a glamorous, fashionable or exotic enclave. A medical student projecting a need for veneration might prefer to go into surgery, where the mysteries of the cutting edge inspire respect, or psychiatry, where the intricacies of the doctor's thought processes comfort the tortured patients. It takes a special sort of zeal to lead a doctor into the Chest Service at Bellevue.

Lanie Eagleton, the Chest Service's chief resident, is such a doctor. Eagleton, 33, is a slim man, of average height, with thinning brown hair, who avoids the flashy clothes seen on some doctors around Bellevue. His white jacket is his favorite piece of apparel. Bespectacled, Eagleton has the manner of a seminarian, studious and precise. Although he is married, with two children, and has a home in Garden City, he spends most of his days, and most of his evenings, at the hospital. He has his own room there.

There is a small-town-doctor quality about Eagleton. Born in Olney, Illinois, he went to Hamilton College in Clinton, New York, and to Harvard Medical School. He was an intern and resident, for two years, at the University of Virginia Hospitals. He spent two years at the National Center for Health Statistics in Maryland before coming to Bellevue. After a year at Bellevue, he became the Chest Service's chief resident. Older than most of the other residents at Bellevue, Eagleton is more interested in academic medicine than in private practice.

The Chest Service was created in 1903, primarily to deal with TB. It still does, but TB, thanks to the development of medication, is under control; patients can be cured. The Chest Service wards that Eagleton knows so well are filled with patients suffering from other chronic pulmonary diseases: bronchitis, emphysema, bronchial asthma, lung cancer.

For the most part, they are old. Many of them have spent their lives on the streets, in flophouses, in decades of drink. They have compounded their ill health by neglect. They come to Bellevue coughing, spitting blood, in pain. For Eagleton, New York City is a witches' brew of irritants and allergens.

In the three wards of the Chest Service there are one hundred beds, not always filled. There is an outpatient clinic which sees 2,500 patients a year. On the wards and in the clinics, the tools are evident: machines to induce air into lungs, to measure lung capacity and condition, antibiotics and other drugs, oxygen tanks. Eagleton's knowledge of the field is encyclopedic. He has the dedication of a scholar, the fervor of a missionary, the patience of a veteran stamp collector.

Eagleton's day begins at 9 A.M., at a staff conference in the Chest Service library. Fifteen others on the staff, including interns, residents and attending physicians, are present. The library is an old room, filled with dusty books and journals, old tattered chairs, a sofa regurgitating its innards, a large conference table. A blackboard and X-ray viewing equipment are available.

Eagleton distributes the duty schedule for the month, assignments for all the doctors on the service. At the bottom of the schedule is the note: "Chief resident may be called at any time." It is the best indication of Eagleton's role.

The meeting begins with a first-year resident presenting two cases he has just seen. He illustrates his talk with X-rays. Behind the rib cage, the patches of dark and light tell the doctors what they want to know; they read them the way a careful cross-country driver studies his road map. Eagleton says little. He rarely interrupts, because he believes that the residents must have some autonomy. He will teach, gladly, if that seems appropriate, without ever being overbearing.

The first case is that of a 98-year-old man last seen two months ago, when he weighed 126 pounds. He has reappeared at Bellevue, complaining of pains in his lower back. Now he weighs seventy-three pounds. "He was disoriented, with a low-grade fever and an inability to produce any sputum for lab analysis," the resident points out.

The X-rays are not conclusive; the resident resists making a diagnosis. "We'll probably find a tumor and TB," Eagleton says.

"The man is awake and alert," the resident says, "he doesn't seem to be desperately ill."

"What do ninety-eight-year-old lungs usually look like?" one of the attending physicians asks.

"We don't see very many," the resident answers, seriously.

The second case is a Guatemalan stonemason who was visiting New York when he felt chest pains and began spitting blood. He came to Bellevue for help. "He seems healthy," the resident says, "but there seems to be disease in the right upper lobe." He points to the X-ray. The staff agrees that he's a candidate for two drugs he's never had before, but the man doesn't want to hang around New York. He wants to go back to Guatemala soon.

"Find out the largest hospital to which he has access down there and we can arrange to have the drugs shipped to it," one of the attending physicians suggests.

"Good idea," Eagleton says. The resident will follow up.

Normally, after the meeting Eagleton would go to the wards to do bronchoscopies, inspecting the interior of the tracheo-bronchial tree through a long, illuminated tube. Today his bronchoscope is being repaired by a medical equipment firm, which frustrates him. Such repairs sometimes take days. But Eagleton is not the sort to waste time. With his bronchoscope unavailable, he moves on to other responsibilities.

He joins a resident examining a patient, an alcoholic suffering from malnutrition. They study X-rays for a few minutes. Eagleton is not happy with the quality of the films. "Poor film. I'd take more, because I don't believe that one," he tells the resident.

The patient has TB and one lung has collapsed and is draining both air and pus. Surgery might be necessary, but Eagleton prefers trying medication first. He knows that the presence of TB hampers healing after surgery. The man has developed subcutaneous emphysema as well. The hole in his lung is leaking air into the pleural space and into body tissue, beneath the skin. Although the man is hooked up to drains, his body has become puffy. Eagleton feels his hand and arm. He feels bubbles under the skin, a spongy quality. If it gets worse, Eagleton can cut the skin to release the air.

Eagleton tours the Chest Service wards, checking with residents, visiting patients he knows. A man who has had liver surgery also has TB. An aged Oriental man was transferred to the Chest Service after drastic bowel surgery because he, too, was found to have TB. An old man who went on a drinking spree fell down and was brought to Bellevue. A routine examination revealed lung cancer. Surgery may not be appropriate. The man, a chain smoker, might not survive on one tobacco-stained and weakened lung. Radiation therapy or chemotherapy may be the best move.

Ward C-4, which Eagleton visits next, is the Chest Service's model ward. On C-4, there's an effort made to educate patients and develop a doctor-patient relationship which can endure, at the clinic, once the patient is discharged from the hospital.

More than half of the patients on C-4 spend an average of five months on it and two years in outpatient therapy. Chest Service patients are not cured rapidly; it takes time and attention. On C-4, there's a pool room, library, a room where movies are shown. Patients are taught to take care of themselves. The purpose is to get them well, so they can go into training or find a job. Eagleton knows that such idealism can be delusional. Too many of the patients wind up back on the Bowery. He'd like more help from Psychiatry in dealing with such personality problems, but Psychiatry is overworked and he can't always get help from there when he needs it.

Eagleton has been walking relentlessly through the wards. It is now 12:15, time for lunch. He joins three Chest Service residents in the doctors' cafeteria. Canned ravioli, wilted broccoli, a tired shredded salad, a slice of watermelon and milk. There is considerable conversation among the group about pulmonary disease. Eagleton does not waste time; he can teach over lunch, too.

After lunch, he hunts for new patients by surveying the population of the Emergency Ward. The EW is the ward where the worst emergency cases arrive. Cardiac arrests, trauma victims, strokes, shotgun wounds, knifings. It is a busy room, filled with nurses, and residents from many services. Eagleton winds his way through the white jackets and green surgical outfits, checking patient charts. Perhaps one of them will have symptoms that the Chest Service can treat.

Eagleton waves at a surgeon he knows. "Are you going to do that operation on Mr. Flint?" he asks. The surgeon shakes his head.

"That's okay," Eagleton says to one of his own residents who has tagged along. "If they won't open a chest for us, I don't fight them over it. I simply refer the patient to an outside surgeon. If he can't afford one, I'll do what I can right here."

There is one such case now, a psychiatric patient named Sarah Morgan, that bothers Eagleton. He has seen her X-rays and feels that exploratory surgery is essential. Surgery has resisted his appeal. They aren't convinced that her symptoms warrant surgery. He has gone to the chief of his service and to the chief of Radiology and both have supported him. Eagleton has called the Psychiatry resident on the case to tell him that he's making progress. The resident and the chief resident in

Psychiatry, Dirk Berger, have been adamantly demanding surgery for the woman.

Eagleton visits patients he's seen in other services, patients
who are in the wards of other services but who have needed a
Chest Service consultation done by him.

In the Surgical Intensive Care Unit he sees an elderly man he
had bronchoscoped. The man has survived abdominal surgery
and is now in postoperative care. When Eagleton enters the
ICU, the man is almost invisible, surrounded by a clutter of
machines and tubes. He is 65, but looks much older. He is
cadaverous, bald, tremulous.

"How are you doing?" Eagleton asks him.

The man has a nasal-gastric tube in his nose, a tracheostomy
with a tube in his neck draining secretion from his lungs, an
oxygen supply system, an IV (intravenous) tube in his arm and
a cardiac monitor. He does not reply to Eagleton's question.

"Well, he looks good," Eagleton says and continues his stroll.

As he's walking down a corridor, a large young black man
dressed in patient's blue pajamas stops him.

"Man, this bandage on my throat hasn't been changed in four
days, and let me tell you, baby, it is itching bad."

Eagleton thinks that the best treatment is often immediate
treatment. He doesn't want to make the man wait, so he stops
a passing nurse, gets what he needs and does the job himself.
"It would have taken a half-hour to find an intern to do that,"
he tells the nurse.

He moves on, to the Medical ICU, where he sees a man who
had entered Bellevue with several ailments at once: congestive
heart failure, respiratory arrest, pneumonia. Fluid had collected in his lungs and a tracheostomy had been performed to
remove it and make it easier for the man to breathe. The patient is now in the ICU bed. A plastic pipe emerges from his
neck, his face the mask of tragedy, his mouth wide open in a
kind of frozen cry. He flaps his arms and legs, points to his chest,
but cannot speak. He must tap a spoon against the side of the
bed to get attention. A resident comes up and asks Eagleton,
"Should we calm him down with Thorazine?"

"No. Everything that will sedate him is a respiratory depressant. Don't," Eagleton says firmly.

As he walks out of the Medical ICU, Eagleton asks the head
nurse about a patient he'd seen a week ago, a man who was
coughing up blood.

"Oh, he expired," the nurse says, routinely. Eagleton shrugs and walks over to another patient.

"How's your breathing?" he asks the man.

"Not so good. Not so good," the man answers.

Eagleton listens to his chest, checks his chart.

"He's much better, actually," he tells the nurse.

When he visits patients, Eagleton's commentary contains ritualized language.

"Still coughing up stuff? . . . How's your breathing? . . . Deep breath. Again. Again."

Several hours have passed since Eagleton began his rounds. He has spent most of that time in other services; he prefers to wait until the end of the day to see Chest Service patients. During the day, he's available to his interns and residents if they need him. They can find him easily enough. Like most doctors at Bellevue, he carries a beeper which alerts him to the phone when he's wanted.

At night, Eagleton can see Chest Service patients without the pressure of other matters. He can spend time with each one, study each case carefully. Since he sleeps at Bellevue most weekday evenings, he won't be distracted by the need to commute. He can concentrate during those quiet hours.

At 3:30, Eagleton joins a group of other Chest Service doctors for a conference with pathologist Eugene Fazzini, to cover a number of cases, some dead, some alive. Slides are shown, organs passed around, presentations made, findings debated.

Finally the organs, having been passed from doctor to doctor, are packed away. Fazzini washes his hands and the conference ends.

It is now after 5 P.M. and for Eagleton it is time to wander through the Chest Service wards. He'll have a quick meal, then go from bed to bed, conferring with nurses, talking with patients, studying charts, until late at night. Then he'll go to his own bed, in his tiny room at Bellevue, to get enough sleep to be alert at the 9 A.M. staff meeting tomorrow.

The first year out of medical school is the one in which the M.D. becomes a doctor. After four years spent mostly in classrooms, the first year of residency (or internship, if the doctor chooses to rotate through several disciplines rather than specializing immediately) is an introduction to reality. It is a year in which the doctor listens attentively, learns on the run and acts. The secret is to learn without revealing ignorance, to exude at least minimal confidence. It is not easy to be both receptive and guarded.

Diane Rahman is a first-year resident in Obstetrics-Gynecology. Fresh out of N.Y.U. Medical School, she will spend four years in OB-GYN at Bellevue before she is ready to take her chances in the outside world. She is one of six first-year residents who will divide their year between Bellevue's OB and GYN services, spending four months at University Hospital as well. Her second year will add a stint at Booth Memorial Hospital in Queens. In her third year, she'll be a senior resident, at both Bellevue and Booth, and in her final year she'll be a chief resident.

In OB-GYN, all six first-year residents will, if they survive, be chief residents in their final year. In some services, like Surgery, the pyramid structure is used; those residents who make it through—and a number of them do drop out, change specialties, move to other hospitals—are named chief residents. In other services, the designation is an honor awarded by the chairman of the department; it can be divided among several residents during their final year. In Medical services, the title is administrative; it connotes supervision of other residents. In Surgical services (including OB-GYN), it implies operating room privileges, making decisions to operate with the consent of an attending.

Rahman's schedule requires her to be out of her nearby Kips Bay apartment before 8 A.M. As a first-year resident, it means working some nights and weekends as well, on minimal sleep, and a vast number of menial tasks. At 25, she doesn't tire easily. She knew it would be like this when she first decided to go into medicine, because she "enjoyed working with people, caring for them, taking the responsibility." Later, as she progresses through her residency, each year will mean more patients to care for and fewer minor chores to deal with.

Rahman is five feet five inches tall, with short brown hair, light complexion. She wears glasses, no make-up. She has a high voice, girlish but not coy. She is pudgy but not fat; plodding the corridors at Bellevue helps her deal with that problem. She is single, but wears two rings on the third finger of her left hand.

She is self-protective, careful. In conversation, she tends to avoid nonmedical frivolity, preferring to stick to the jargon of Obstetrics. Her skirt and jacket are hospital white, her blouse simple.

She looks younger than 25, and her high soprano voice could reinforce the impression of inexperience, but she is well informed about medicine. The manner she's chosen is like that of the smartest girl in the class who doesn't want to be known as the smartest girl. Much of what goes on in her head is distilled before it is verbalized. She listens to senior residents and is patient, in turn, with medical students she escorts in introductory tours of Obstetrics.

Today, two male medical students have arrived at 8 A.M. to spend a few hours on the ward with her. They are third-year students; next year, they'll spend more time on the wards, making the transition from student to M.D. easier. At Bellevue, third-year medical students observe, listen, make notes, assist in doing paperwork. Fourth year students, termed subinterns, do more (e.g., blood tests) under the close supervision of interns and residents. These students are pleased to be in Obstetrics for two reasons: it is a happy service where few depressing events disturb the mood and Dr. Rahman is patient, bright, helpful.

The first patient she sees this morning is a 26-year-old Puerto Rican woman, a patient in the Methadone clinic, who is pregnant and in pain. She's come to Obstetrics for immediate care; this could be an emergency and she didn't want to wait in the clinic. As Rahman walks in, the woman points to her navel and grunts in pain. Rahman gets a Doptone, a device that includes both microphone and amplifier, to ascertain a fetal heartbeat. It is present and rapid, healthy.

Rahman asks the woman a series of questions, then decides that "she's not in labor and not going to abort." But she wants another opinion. She calls a senior resident on duty and he cheerfully checks the patient, too. Urine, stool and blood tests are ordered. He agrees with Rahman to give the woman Mylanta, an antacid, urge her to eat small meals and drink milk. Her complaint is a common one: the pressure of the growing fetus on the stomach during pregnancy causes discomfort.

The senior resident leaves and Rahman urges the woman to attend the Bellevue OB clinic. The two medical students have hovered on the periphery throughout the examination. Now one of them steps forward and asks, "Wouldn't it be wise to feed her, to get her to vomit in order to detect the presence of blood?"

Rahman, remembering her own years as a student, looks at him calmly and, without any change in the tone of her voice, says, "There are other ways of discovering that." To make her point, she takes a stool specimen down to the lab herself, the students rushing to keep up with her.

"When you work at Bellevue," she tells them, "you do a lot of footwork. I don't like to wait for test results." In the lab, the test is negative; there isn't any blood in the woman's stool. "I want to know *now*," Rahman says. As they leave the lab, one of the students notices a sign, hand-lettered, on the wall: "The Filth in This Laboratory Has Reached a Disgraceful Level. . . . I Know We Can Count on Your Help."

Rahman walks briskly back to the ward. She encourages the students to see patients. There are usually thirty-five to forty patients in Obstetrics, so the students can keep busy. They prefer to remain as her escort.

Rahman asks one of the medical students to take a blood sample. "My first blood," he sighs. Rahman checks several patients who are awaiting discharge.

A woman lies on an examining table as Rahman makes certain that postchildbirth healing is taking place, that there aren't any sponges left in her vagina (those gauze pads, inserted to absorb bleeding, can be forgotten). This woman can go home; she's been at Bellevue for four days, an average stay in OB (except for a Caesarean section, which doubles the stay).

The next woman speaks only Spanish. Rahman searches in vain for the word for "ice pack." Fortunately, one of the nurses speaks Spanish.

An overweight black woman tells Rahman that she assumed that her thyroid trouble was the reason she hadn't had her menstrual period. She came to Bellevue, discovered that she was pregnant and had a miscarriage on the ward.

"You can go home now," Rahman tells her. "And you're welcome to come to the Bellevue clinic." She manages to be both cheerful and formal.

Before the woman can dress and leave, however, one of the medical students seizes the opportunity to explain to her everything she wanted to know about her thyroid, her "energy regulator."

The next patient tells Rahman that she wants to stay at Belle-vue. She's urinating too frequently to go home, she says. Rah-man recalls that the birth was a tricky one and realizes the bladder may be tender. She gives the woman some medication and suggests that she go home. "If you want to stay, I'll have to get approval," she tells her.

She tells the woman to drink cranberry juice four times a day. She explains to the medical students that cranberry juice helps prevent the growth of bacteria in the urinary tract; it makes urine more acidic, less hospitable to bacteria. As she finishes her explanation, the senior resident strolls in. "She wants to stay here," Rahman says to him. "Why not? We have room here," he says. The patient smiles.

Obstetrics delivers babies. It also performs abortions. The patients are in adjoining rooms in OB, and while births outnum-ber abortions by two to one, moving a few feet down the hall can bring about a drastic change of mood, for doctors and pa-tients.

Beyond the corridor with the rooms of the ward is the deliv-ery area, a series of labor rooms and two small operating rooms. Rahman puts on a sterile gown, pushes through the heavy doors, and visits a 21-year-old woman who has requested an abortion. She is within the sixteen-to-twenty-week period that this abortion service works on; in shorter terms, GYN takes over. After twenty weeks, a woman cannot get an abortion at Bellevue; it is too late, and after twenty-four weeks illegal. In this case, the woman, who has never been pregnant before, is slated for a saline abortion, the introduction of saline solution into the uterus to induce abortion. Rahman talks to her about her health; it appears to be fine.

If this abortion technique is successful, Rahman tells her, she'll have the same labor she would in a normal pregnancy, then will expel the fetus within forty-eight hours.

The patient does not reveal any emotion. Rahman goes to work, as the medical students, in a corner, watch. She washes the woman's stomach with a cold, orange-colored solution (tinc-ture of Thimerosal).

"It'll come right off in the shower, or with alcohol," she says.

She then injects a painkiller into the woman's abdomen, be-low the navel. "You'll just feel the pressure now, not any pain," she says, as she begins the abortion procedure.

She pushes a long spinal needle down into the abdomen.

Blood oozes through the cap, then clear amniotic fluid, produced within the uterus during pregnancy. The needle passes through the abdominal wall, through the placenta, into the uterus. A nurse attaches a bottle of 20 percent sodium chloride solution (saline) to the needle cap and it begins to flow. It will take twenty minutes for the bottle to empty. Rahman waits, holds the woman's hand.

The patient seems calm. When Rahman asks, "How are you doing, dear?" she nods.

Rahman explains to the students that if the saline doesn't work, it might be repeated. She cannot leave the patient while the saline is dripping. Pitocin, a drug that causes the uterus to contract, can be tried. Finally, if everything else has failed, surgery can be performed to remove the fetus. It is done reluctantly, she says, because it makes Caesarean sections necessary in future deliveries.

After lunch in the basement cafeteria, Rahman greets another patient, a Puerto Rican woman who has several children, is pregnant, full-term, and doesn't want to be pregnant again. She asks Rahman for birth control pills while Rahman examines her.

"I'm Catholic," she says, "but I want those pills."

"You can have them," Rahman tells her. She has read the woman's chart, which reveals that the father of this pregnancy is not the same one who fathered the earlier children. Rahman does not mention that.

The examination does not reveal anything alarming, but the woman will have a Caesarean section. She has had one before, the last time around.

"Once you have one that way, we like to repeat it, unless it is a premature baby," Rahman tells the ubiquitous medical students. "And we like to deliver the Caesarean prior to labor, so it doesn't get tricky. The trouble is that many patients don't keep track of time, making predicting the onset of labor very, very difficult."

The patient is escorted to the ward, where she'll settle down to await delivery. The senior resident on duty walks in. He has been up all night and looks very tired. He sits down, heavily, and talks to the medical students while Rahman stands by and listens.

"Most deliveries are easy," he says. "What happens here in

Obstetrics is less important than what kind of prenatal care the patient has received. That's what counts. Correct and regular advice before and during the pregnancy."

The senior resident has an aura of confidence, which encourages one of the students to ask him about the disappearance of internships in favor of residencies throughout medicine. Good or bad? one of the students asks.

"Experience on many different services, teaching a doctor to spot many different kinds of diseases and conditions, is no longer available to many medical school graduates. They move right out of school into a residency in the specialty of their choice. That's the trend and has been for years. Specialize. It's a mistake. That year of internship is valuable. Apparently it's not expedient these days. Our residency is four years. It could be done in three, but it's stretched to keep the bodies around, to keep more doctors on duty." His weariness seems mixed with irritation.

An attending from Bellevue's abortion clinic walks in. He is well dressed, glib, arrogant. He tells the senior resident that he wants to talk about a case they've been debating. The patient is now in the room being examined by Rahman, while the attending and the senior resident debate.

She is a 15-year-old black girl who seems oblivious to everything. She's been through an unsuccessful saline abortion attempt. Labor hasn't taken place. The fetus appears to be dead, the placenta shrinking. The attending wants to use a vacuum aspirator, to extract the fetus. The resident thinks that the pregnancy is too far along for that.

They discuss, formally and antagonistically, the value of another saline abortion try, and, failing in that, surgery. They cannot agree. Rahman sends the girl back to her bed. The girl smiles, oblivious, as she walks past the two doctors confronting her fate.

The confrontation becomes a standoff. The resident is smart and the attending knows it. The latter chooses not to pull rank, which he could do. They agree to do more tests before making a decision and part. The attending struts off. The resident shuffles away.

When they're gone, Rahman turns to a medical student—the other has chosen to prowl the ward—and says, "The fetus *is* getting smaller. It must be dead." She speaks in a very literal way. "But it hasn't been expelled and that's the problem. We'll do a fibrinogen test, to determine her clotting factor and detect complications caused by a retained dead fetus. We'll need that if it gets to surgery." She does not take sides; she explains the case to the student in medical terms. She glances at her wristwatch; it is midafternoon and there is more to be done.

She escorts a black woman to the Ultrasound room. Ultrasound, an electronic device that resembles sonar, sends out sound waves and records the echoes. The waves are sent into the abdomen and they produce a graphlike portrait of the fetus on a screen. Differences in densities, measured by the waves, reveal the fetal skull surrounded by placenta, tissue and the abdominal wall. A Polaroid photo is taken of the image on the screen. The diameter of the skull is compared to a gestation chart, to determine the precise point of the pregnancy. The patient, who entered the room in fear of the large apparatus, leaves smiling. It was painless.

The tension of the activity on the ward is getting to Rahman, after a weekend away from it. And it has been a relatively quiet day on OB.

Robert Nachtigall is a 27-year-old first-year resident in Gynecology. A native New Yorker, Nachtigall attended Carleton College in Minnesota and got his bachelor's degree in engineering at N.Y.U. Although his father, who succumbed to cancer, had been a doctor, Nachtigall's plan did not call for medical school. He changed his mind, after considerable soul-searching, and went to N.Y.U. Medical School. He spent a year in a rotating internship, between Medicine and OB-GYN, to get a broader background before deciding to specialize in the latter, so this is his second year on the wards.

Nachtigall lives in a small apartment near Bellevue. He is divorced, the father of an 8-year-old son. He is tall, slim, with fashionably long hair and a thin mustache. He looks like an updated version of Errol Flynn. At Bellevue, he wears the white pants and white jacket of the resident, the uniform, modified only by blue-tinted aviator glasses.

On this morning, at 7:30 A.M., he complains to a fellow resident about a phone call that awakened him at 5 A.M., after he had been on duty all weekend. The call was from a resident in the Adult Emergency Service, in a panic because a woman had arrived and told him that she was pregnant and claimed to be bleeding from a kick in the stomach. He needed Nachtigall's help immediately. Nachtigall raced to the AES, to discover that the woman was not pregnant, was simply having her menstrual period.

He did not have time to pursue his grievance. After a hurried breakfast, he is in one of the eighth-floor operating rooms. Along with the chief resident and a third-year resident, he will be in on several operations today.

The sprint to the AES and the gobbled breakfast have wakened Nachtigall. He is ready. The first patient is wheeled into the OR and transferred from bed to table. She is a 35-year-old Puerto Rican scheduled for a vaginal hysterectomy (removal of the uterus through the vagina), one way of performing a hysterectomy. (An abdominal hysterectomy, done when the uterus is enlarged and would be difficult to remove through the vagina, or, for example, when cancer is present and the doctors must see precisely what they're removing, is the other procedure). When she reaches the operating table, the anesthetist has her unconscious in a matter of seconds. There are a nurse and a circulating nurse's aide present as well. All are in surgical green, with gowns, masks and caps. The three doctors and the nurses wear surgical gloves.

At 8:30, the operation begins. The patient's legs have been raised in stirrups; she has been draped so that all anyone can see is her vaginal area. The two residents, holding retractors, stand on either side of the chief resident, who is seated on a low stool at the foot of the table and will do the operation itself. While the chief works, the three talk.

The third-year resident describes his effort to help medical students learn about OB-GYN, but he is intimidated by their doggedness.

"They want to follow me into the bathroom," he says. "I have to tell them it's okay, it's all right, they won't learn much by going with me."

The chief asks for a specific clamp and the nurse, seated beside him and next to a tray full of instruments, tells him she doesn't have any. He looks at her for a moment, then accepts a substitute. She can hear him mutter "Shit." A few moments later she says, "Oh, here they are. I found them." The chief glares at her.

Part of the uterus is now visible, as it emerges under the pressure of the residents' retractors and the chief's careful cutting. Bloody sponges accumulate in a pan on the floor.

The chief sutures as he goes, cutting and sewing, exposing more and more of the uterus. The heads of the three doctors, huddled over the patient, are less than a foot apart. There is very little conversation. For minutes, the chief continues to snip and suture; the other residents retract and sponge. For Nachtigall, it is demanding labor.

"It takes two hours, minimum. You can't see much. The numbness spreads from your hands to your shoulders to your back. And I'm two years away from actually doing one, so I'm not turned on by it," he says.

A suture snaps, breaking the silence. The chief replaces it. As he works, he is humming "Lollipops and Roses." He reminds the nurse that he is left-handed, so she can hand him the instruments more expeditiously. The operation is moving along, but not quite as smoothly as the chief would like.

"Where are all the easy ones?" he asks, to no one in particular.

"They do them on videotape at the medical school," Nachtigall says.

"Never mind," the chief comments, "I'm just talking to myself."

The chief continues to cut, to sew. "It's the spirit of competitiveness that keeps me going," he says. "It's me against the uterus."

A patient screams in a nearby operating room, then is silent; the anesthetic has worked. The third-year resident begins to tell a story about a clinic patient who screamed when he entered the examining booth. The chief interrupts.

"I'm doing all sorts of right things," he says, "but somehow the uterus is tight, won't move forward." Then, as if by wish, it does emerge. At 9:35, Nachtigall carefully lifts it out of the vagina, hands it, with cervix attached, to the nurse's aide, who puts it in a plastic bag for Pathology. It is a small pear-shaped organ three to four inches long.

Now the threesome patch up what they've done. The patient is bleeding.

"The bleeding is supposed to go away, but it won't go away," the chief resident says. "Shit."

He sighs and searches for the source of the bleeding. It doesn't take long. He finds it, a small pumping artery on the edge of an area previously cut, and sutures it. For a moment, the dialogue resembles all the tense film scenes in operating rooms:

"Spongestick."

"Here, Doctor."

"Another clamp, please."

"Yes, Doctor."

"Finish your story," the chief says to the third-year resident.

"Oh, yeah. Well, this woman came into clinic yelling and screaming."

"Was she scared or obnoxious?"

"I thought obnoxious."

"So?"

"Well, sometimes I want to haul off and whack a patient like that. I don't, but I want to. This time, while she had her mouth open yelling as loud as she could, before I even touched her, I just stuck a Q-tip into her mouth, all the way back. She closed it fast and hummed. Hmmmmmm."

"That's assault with a Q-tip," Nachtigall says. The three doctors laugh, without disturbing the rhythm of the operation.

"How far are you?" the anesthetist asks.

"We're about two-thirds of the way done," the chief answers.

At 10 A.M., the two residents assisting the chief are numb. They take a quick break, move around the operating room, stretching, bending, flexing fingers. The chief passes most of the tools he's been holding in a tray on his lap back to the nurse.

"I've been here for the past sixty hours. It's okay with me to go home now," Nachtigall says. The chief isn't done yet, however.

"Oh, shit, what did I do now?" the chief asks. No answer, so he solves his own problem without announcing it. There is talk about the speed of various surgeons at Bellevue.

"One doctor I know just looks at the clock, smiles and digs in. Two bites. Seventeen minutes," Nachtigall says.

"I can do a D&C as fast as anyone," says the third-year resident. "One day I did fourteen from eight to five."

"In a private hospital, you could do ten D&Cs in two hours," Nachtigall says.

"Less than five minutes to go," the chief proclaims.

"Is the next patient here?" the nurse asks.

"I sent for her," answers the nurse's aide.

At 10:30, the chief arises for the first time from the low squat he's been in since the operation began two hours ago. He snaps off his gloves. The patient is wheeled out, still asleep.

The three doctors walk slowly down the immaculate corridor; the operating-room floors at Bellevue are not simply the cleanest part of the hospital. They are spotless, gleaming. Tucked away on this floor is a small pantry, a refuge between operations. The residents have peanut butter on white and milk. There isn't much time to rest, however. The trio is due back in the same OR, to perform a laparoscopic tubal ligation on a 35-year-old white woman with three children; she doesn't want any more children.

In this procedure, carbon dioxide is injected into the abdomen, to inflate it. A sharp spike is inserted slightly below the navel and a lighted tube is fed into the abdomen. Through the tube, the entire lower internal area can be viewed and assessed. An electrical instrument is passed through the tube, to cut and cauterize within, removing a section of the woman's Fallopian tubes and cauterizing blood vessels, sealing the area from which the cuts were made.

The woman is in the OR when the doctors return.

"She's fat," the third-year resident says, anticipating a problem.

"That's the word," the chief agrees. "You're going to have to angle it." He's referring to the large needle that must enter the abdomen first. The chief holds a large fold of flesh and the resident pushes the needle through it. The carbon dioxide is turned on, the spike in a sleeve inserted into the abdomen and the lighted tube is passed through the sleeve.

All the lights in the OR are turned off, so the light can illuminate the area to be worked on, and it can be seen through the scope attached to the tube.

"Cut, cut," the chief instructs the third-year resident. "Good work, I'm proud of you." Two sections of the tubes are removed and held as specimens. The resident cauterizes what remains.

"You can actually see the smoke in the peritoneum," Nachtigall says. "You have to wait for it to clear."

The operation is over and, again, there's a dash to the pantry. Nachtigall has a cigarette as two slices of toast are browning. When the toast is done, he covers it with what he thinks is butter. He takes a bite. "Yech, margarine," he moans. "I may have some complaints about my parents, but they always took me to *fine* restaurants, restaurants where they served butter." He discards the toast.

It is 12:35 P.M. and Nachtigall is to do a D&C (dilation and curettage) on a 38-year-old Finnish woman who looks to be much older. She has had persistent, troublesome vaginal bleeding and the D&C is an effort to correct it or find out why it's happening. This is a procedure Nachtigall knows well; he is quick and efficient. The patient is given general anesthesia. Within a few minutes, Nachtigall has scraped the uterus and gotten four cervical specimens for Pathology to mull over. At 1:15, he's ready for a second D&C, this one an abortion. By 1:45, he is on his way for a hasty lunch in the doctors' cafeteria.

Nachtigall plans to leave early today to visit his son. He's promised to take him roller skating tonight. He may succeed in doing so. The two GYN wards are not full today; only thirteen beds, out of fifty, are occupied. Two of the patients, however, have cancer and Nachtigall has special feelings about them, and about cancer. He talks to another resident about it.

"My father died of cancer. He was fifty-eight, a doctor with a successful practice. One day he went into the hospital and they found cancer of the pancreas, a tough one. One of the best surgeons in the world operated on him, took out his pancreas, his spleen, his stomach. He went home in three weeks, then six months to the day he had massive GI bleeding. He could have been rushed back into the hospital for more surgery or transfusions. Or he could have been allowed to die at home. My mother talked to me and she decided that he should be allowed to die. He did, within a half-hour of our talk. So I don't think about cancer in some kind of vacuum. We have those two old women on the ward now, and I know the risks of surgery. Even if it's only a ten percent risk, one out of ten won't make it through. Why gamble with the life of an old patient? Other doctors don't agree with me. But cancer is the one disease that makes any doctor vulnerable."

He ends the conversation, to go to the GYN clinic, where he sees a few patients. He is back on the ward, in the chief resident's office, at 3 P.M.

The chief's office is full. It is time for chart rounds, at which the residents discuss the cases on the ward. Five residents and two visiting medical students cram into the small office. The residents cover each case; the chief comments.

"I've got a twenty-two-year-old girl who is two months late and she wants an abortion," one resident says.

"Admit her," the chief says.

"Actually, she doesn't want *any* children. She wants a sex-change operation."

"Put a clamp on her clit and pull," another resident suggests.

The chief talks about the case of a patient who once had a tubal ligation, now wants children, and has re-entered Bellevue to have it repaired. It is a difficult task.

"Tell her that her chances are slim," the chief says. "Don't give her false hope. She's a very nice lady."

An old woman needs blood.

"Give her two units and get the results of the bone marrow from Hematology. I think that this lady is a chronic alcoholic with a poor liver, being stressed by cancer. Draw a bunch of liver chemistries on her, too. She refuses to get up, to get out of bed. She's either ornery or out of it."

A resident tells the chief that a retarded woman has asked for an abortion.

"Is she retarded?" the chief asks.

"*She* doesn't know," the resident answers.

The chief tells the residents that he wants to do surgery on the Finnish woman on whom Nachtigall performed the D&C this morning. She has a prolapsed bladder and may have cancer as well; the experts in Pathology should be able to answer the latter question. The woman does not speak English.

"Please get someone to translate for her that we want to take out her uterus," the chief says.

"We need informed consent," Nachtigall adds.

"She's Finnish," another resident comments, "and who speaks Finnish?"

"Find someone who does," the chief says. He adds that he would wait to operate on her until the Pathology report is in, but indicates that he can do the operation by the end of the week, if necessary.

"She does have a brother-in-law who speaks some English and he'll be visiting her. He's a meek guy and we can get tough with him for her sake if we have to," one of the residents notes.

The chief wants the resident to get the woman to put an "X"

on the permission form for surgery, and get two witnesses to it. Meanwhile, Nachtigall can help by finding someone to interpret.

Nachtigall is silent, his head bowed in weariness.

The phone rings. A resident picks it up. He turns to Nachtigall and in a falsetto voice says, "Dr. Robert Nachtigall, please. It's one of your women." Nachtigall takes the call in an adjoining office, returns a few minutes later.

"It was one of my *patients,*" he says.

A resident and the chief debate the fate of a woman who has five children, but may want more. She has been bleeding, but the resident cannot find anything abnormal in his examination of her.

"Perfect uterus, perfect ovaries," he says.

The chief feels that a hysterectomy is justified. The resident does not. They compromise. The chief will do a diagnostic D&C on her this week.

The chief reads the operating room schedule for tomorrow and the meeting ends. Nachtigall runs out of the office, to meet his son. After that, he can enjoy his first uninterrupted sleep in several days.

Bruce Mack, a 29-year-old Bostonian, is the chief resident in Neurology. A Harvard graduate, Mack attended N.Y.U. Medical School, spent a year interning in Medicine at Boston City Hospital and came to Bellevue for his residency in Neurology. This is his final year at Bellevue; when it's done, he's committed to a two-year tour of duty as an Air Force doctor.

Mack's wife is an administrator at University Hospital. His older brother is a doctor, too. They come from what Mack calls a "traditional Jewish family—immigrants who started saving money the minute they got to America, to pay for their kids' education."

Mack is tall (six feet two), slim. The horn-rimmed glasses he wears and the pipe he smokes do not negate the gangly, boyish quality in him. He is smart but not pedantic; he has a sense of humor and an ingratiating smile that he offers freely.

Mack's domain is on the fifth floor of the old L&M building at Bellevue. There are two wards, one male and one female, that Neurology shares with Neurosurgery. The patient census is now thirty-five. A Neuro Intensive Care Unit (ICU) has four patients in it (the ICU patients are usually Neurosurgery cases shifted to the ICU from the recovery room).

The cases that Mack and his staff confront include the range of neurological pathology: seizure disorders, head traumas, Parkinsonism, headaches, stroke (usually treated in Medicine, with Neurology consulting), spinal cord disease and traumatic and degenerative diseases of the central nervous system.

Mack's day begins early. He leaves his Chelsea apartment for an 8 A.M. meeting with the Neurology resident who has been on call from 4 P.M. the previous afternoon. Over coffee in the doctors' cafeteria, the resident will pass along anything he feels Mack should know: patients admitted during the night, consults he has made to other services, information on ward patients. From that meeting, Mack crosses the Bellevue complex, several times a week, for a morning meeting with Dr. Clark T. Randt, the chief of the Neurology Service, in Randt's office in the Psychiatry building. The meeting is friendly, but banter takes second place to cases of special interest to both men, cases beyond the ordinary, cases on which Mack benefits from Randt's experience.

After seeing Randt, Mack goes to the Neurology wards. Each day, an attending physician joins Mack and the residents in a conference to discuss specific ward cases. This, along with paperwork and phone calls, keeps Mack busy until lunch. In the afternoons, he attends conferences that examine cases in depth, and puts in time at the Neurology clinic. He finds time to analyze X-rays in Neuroradiology and to handle the problems of the wards. At 4 P.M. or, more often, 5 P.M., he is ready to go home.

Today, his day begins with the coffee conference at 8, the chat with Randt afterward. At 9 P.M., Mack, five Neurology residents and an attending gather in Mack's office.

At Bellevue, attendings are ubiquitous. Full-time attendings help run services, supervise the house staff, do research, see patients when their expertise is needed. They receive faculty appointments from N.Y.U. Medical School and are paid by Bellevue, N.Y.U. or a combination of the two.

Part-time attendings have their own private practices, but put in time at Bellevue on a scheduled basis, treating patients and teaching residents and interns in the practical atmosphere of the wards. For that effort, they receive patient privileges (for their private patients) at University Hospital, an appointment to the N Y U Medical School faculty Some get paid for their time (again, by Bellevue, N.Y.U. or a combination). Others donate it. The Neurology attending today is middle-aged, speaks slowly and authoritatively in a Middle European accent.

The first case is that of a Puerto Rican man who had to aban don his career as a mechanic because he had difficulty using his hands; he took a job as a kitchen helper in a restaurant, but the problem persisted and he came to Bellevue. The patient is invited into the room.

He is chubby and is wearing pajama bottoms, a white T-shirt and a tartan robe.

"Make a fist and hold it," the attending instructs

The patient obliges.

"Release your grip," the attending says.

The man has trouble doing it quickly; seconds pass as his hand opens.

"Walk on your toes."

The man gets up, walks slowly on his toes.

"On your heels."

He tries, but lurches, almost falls.

The attending takes off the man's T-shirt; his chest is almost hairless. The attending does several reflex tests, then dismisses the patient.

"Myotonia dystrophica," the attending announces (myotonia —muscle spasms; dystrophica—atrophy). "It can be seriously debilitating, but in this case I don't think so. This looks like a very mild case, not likely to get worse. In fact, he looks rather good for the long history he's exhibiting. He told us he's had this trouble for several years. I don't think you can do very much for him. He doesn't need much."

"What if he grabs a hot pan in the kitchen and can't let go?" one of the residents asks.

"So he'll toss salads," Mack answers.

"The man should be active. That's important," the attending says, "but he should not get involved in physiotherapy. Whirlpools, massages, electrical stimulation and the like. It would increase the myotonia and it won't help the dystrophica. Various drugs might help. Dilantin or Pronestyl."

A second patient is brought in, another Puerto Rican man. The first patient is invited back to translate; the new patient doesn't speak English. He is in his forties, short, thin, edgy. He seems uneasy surrounded by doctors. His eyes flick back and forth across the room, without settling anywhere. He mutters to the translator.

The meeting proceeds with the patient telling his story through the translator. "He says he was fine for years, then one day he fell down, slipped on a floor and hit his head. That's when he got headaches."

"Yes, he came onto the ward complaining of a headache in his entire skull," one of the residents says.

"Now he says he has a headache only on one side," the translator states.

"We half-cured him," a resident jokes.

"No," the attending says, taking it seriously, "it's a typical pattern." He puts the patient through several simple tests, uneventfully, then the patient leaves.

"Probably a case of post-trauma headaches. No sign of organic disease. Medication ought to do it. You can discharge him," the attending rules.

The meeting ends at 11 A.M., giving Mack a chance to pursue a case that both fascinates and troubles him.

A few days ago, a well-dressed, beautiful young woman was brought to the AES by her date. They had been at a party, drinking vodka, when she became nauseous, weak, had several seizures, developed trouble breathing. He drove her to Bellevue; he didn't feel sick at all. In the Emergency Ward, doctors determined that the woman had severe acidosis, an accumulation of acid in the blood and tissues. Unchecked, it can kill. Her metabolic functions were slowing down dramatically. In the EW, she fell into a coma. Her respiration failed; she had to be maintained on a respirator. She was a patient of Medicine's, technically, but a Neurology consult was requested. Doctors from both services were baffled by her condition; she has been unable to speak, to tell them anything, since she arrived.

Mack has kept in touch with the case. Extensive tests were done in search of the smallest clue to her condition: a complete blood count, an arterial blood-gas study, a urinalysis, a spinal tap, skull X-rays, chest films, an EKG (electrocardiogram), blood cultures, toxicology tests on both blood and urine for common toxins, including drugs. Vital signs—blood pressure, pulse, respiration and temperature—were being monitored frequently.

Now, she is in a Medical ICU. Mack and another Neurology resident visit her. They stand beside her bed, staring at her helplessly. She is still, her lovely face in false tranquillity.

"You know, many problems are ultimately unexplained in Neurology because of the mysteries of the brain, its complexity," Mack says to the resident. Mack is discouraged by the riddle the woman represents; it is insoluble, he suspects.

"She's going to die," he tells the resident, grimly. "There's no question about it, short of the intervention of God."

The cardiac monitor beeps. Technically, she is still alive, although she is absolutely motionless, comatose. "A terrible metabolic disturbance," Mack says. "If we took her off the respirator, she would die in five minutes." He looks sad, continues staring at her for several minutes. "Come on," the resident says to him, "let's go to lunch."

Mack sits at lunch with the Neurology resident, but he isn't hungry. The food looks unappetizing and his mind is on the woman in the Medical ICU. The two residents raise unanswered questions:

Why didn't her boyfriend get sick, too? Did she really drink the same vodka he drank? Was it vodka? Is the vodka irrelevant? Did she have some sort of brain mass that simply exploded? If she did, it was probably too late for surgery the moment it happened. "No, no. I don't think it was a mass," Mack says. "It's a diffuse swelling, perhaps, difficult to explain and difficult to deal with."

"Was she poisoned?" the resident asks.

"If she dies, and she will, we can find out," Mack says, "when the Medical Examiner does an autopsy." All cases involving traumas and crimes require a mandatory Medical Examiner's autopsy.

After lunch, Mack returns to the woman's bedside. Her name, Mary Rollins, is printed on a card at the foot of her bed.

She seems lifeless. IV fluids drip into her arms. A respirator clicks like a metronome. Her blue eyes are barely visible behind the slits of her eyelids. Mack lifts an eyelid, touches the cornea with a swab of cotton, peers at her eye with a small light. "No corneal blink. The pupils don't change," he says, as if stubbornly trying to obtain some sign of life.

He lifts each of her feet and scratches it lightly with a key. No response. The cardiac monitor, beeping, is the only overt sign that she is alive. Mack removes the respirator tube for a few seconds. She is not breathing on her own, so he replaces it quickly.

A Medical resident assigned to the case walks in, stands beside Mack and shrugs her shoulders. There are a few specialized tests left to be done, she tells Mack. Are they appropriate? She wants his opinion. Yes, perhaps they ought to be done, he tells her. Together, silently, they stare at the woman. She has long straight brunette hair and a tan that has begun to fade. Her facial features are classical American, the face from an ad for bath soap. The two doctors sigh, almost simultaneously.

A team of technicians arrives to do an electroencephalogram on her. Mack and the Medical resident watch. The EEG will define brain function. Mack doesn't wait for the results; for him, it seems to be a matter of waiting until she dies. Feeling helpless and distracted, he heads for the Neurology clinic.

At the clinic, Mack sees a procession of patients, some he's seen before. He calls the Medical ICU and tells the resident on duty to keep him informed on Mary Rollins. He returns to the wards, where all is quiet. "No head injuries, no jumpers, in fact nobody really sick," Mack tells another resident. "Just a bunch of alcoholics with seizures." Those cases Mack can deal with; there are symptoms to define, diagnoses to be made, treatment to be prescribed. The cases that taunt him are the ones that resist such analysis, like the beautiful woman dying in the ICU.

Kalmon D. Post is a senior resident in Neurosurgery. Post, 31, is one of the most experienced residents at Bellevue. A native of Brooklyn, he zipped through Columbia University in three years, then went to N.Y.U. Medical School, where he was named to Alpha Omega Alpha, the equivalent of Phi Beta Kappa. He spent two years at Bellevue, taking an internship and a first-year residency in general surgery. At that point, he met his armed services obligation by spending two years in Neurosurgery at the National Institutes of Health in Bethesda, Maryland. He returned to Bellevue to resume his work in Neurosurgery. With one year to go, during which he'll become chief resident, he's pondering his future, which he sees as a blend of academic medicine and private practice.

Post is short, with longish brown hair and a mustache. He is married; his wife has a master's degree in psychiatric nursing. They have two children, a daughter, 5, and a two-week-old son, born three months premature and weighing two pounds. Post's son is in Bellevue's Premature Care Unit, showing all the proper signs of growth. Post and his wife can visit him easily; they live a block away from the hospital.

Post's day begins before 8 A.M. Today he was at Bellevue at 7:30 and had to deal with a cardiac arrest on a ward and a man with liver lacerations and possible spinal injury who was taken to the operating room a few minutes after Post saw him. This morning, Post takes a peek into the Neuro ICU, then heads for the Pediatrics ICU, where he has an 8-year-old patient, a boy.

The boy had been hit by a car two weeks ago and suffered a fractured skull. He was treated in the ICU for a week; doctors examining him did not detect any dysfunction of the nervous system traceable to brain damage, or any other symptoms of serious concern, so the boy was sent home to recuperate. At home, he was irritable, then began vomiting. He was readmitted to the ICU, where a blood clot was found in his brain, and he became comatose. He was rushed to the operating room, where the clot was removed.

Post is worried. The clot was close to the area in the brain that controls speech. Now the boy has a slight fever and a stiff neck. He is sleeping when Post arrives. Post wakes him up, gently, and tries to get him to talk. The boy does not, or cannot. He simply whimpers. There is a tube in his nose and he picks at it, unhappily.

The problem, as Post sees it, is the potential speech deficit. What will it be? But when Post speaks to the boy, he is alert and seems to listen.

"He understands me," Post tells the ICU nurse beside him. "That's a very good sign. I'll know for sure when he starts talking."

A Pediatrics resident walks up and tells Post that the boy "is much more responsive than he had been."

"Let's try to get him out of bed soon," Post tells him.

He walks down the hall to visit his own baby in the Premature Care Unit. It is a very small boy, perfectly formed but tiny. Post stares at him proudly, checks with the head nurse, who tells him that all is going well. Post tells her, graciously, that he chose the Premature Unit for his son because he feels it is the best in the city.

He walks to the Neuro ICU and as he enters the phone rings. It is for him from a nurse at the Veterans Administration Hospital. She tells him that a terminal cancer patient he has been caring for has died suddenly, that she tried to reach Post earlier, but hadn't been successful. Post is depressed and irritated.

"He expired?" Post asks. "Jesus. That is remarkable. Didn't anyone check his vital signs? That's *terrible*. I *was* available. Why didn't they call me? I feel bad, although for him to die may be the best thing that could have happened. It's still disturbing to me. I'll call the family and tell them he stopped breathing. I really feel bad about it."

He is upset, but there is work to do.

In the Neuro ICU, a first-year resident is at work; he wants Post to assist him, to double-check his efficiency. A woman patient has had a blood clot removed, a subdural hematoma over her brain. She seems stabilized, but there is need to measure her intracranial pressure. It is done on a Ladd Intracranial Pressure Monitor (LICP), an electro-optical device that measures the pressure within the brain and makes a permanent record on a graph for use in treatment and evaluation.

The resident shaves the back of the woman's head. Then, using an instrument that resembles a conventional manual drill, he makes a hole in the woman's skull. A switch is inserted, a miniaturized device, and the skin is sutured and taped. Post and the resident, who have said very little to each other during the procedure, wheel the woman's bed into the special Head Trauma Unit, where specialists will study her to determine the recoverability of her brain after surgery.

"We just put it in," Post says to a nurse who has come along. "They play with it."

By 9:40, he is back on the wards, checking patients. That done, he visits a Medical ICU to see a young black man who has been seriously injured in an auto accident. The man has casts on his fractured arms and legs and huge retention stitches over a long incision that runs vertically on his abdomen. There has been little change in his condition, classified as poor, for days. He is not awake and is rigid.

"The chance of his regaining brain function is almost nil," Post tells the nurse on duty. "There has been serious brain-stem injury."

"What now?" she asks.

"We can sustain people artificially, but you have to make a decision when you know that the brain function is gone. It's not an easy decision to make," Post tells her.

At 10:45, he is due at the VA Hospital. Many residents in the Bellevue-N.Y.U. training system rotate during their residencies from University Hospital, the modern private voluntary hospital to the north, to Bellevue, in the middle of the East Side chain, to the VA. The VA was built in 1950 and, like University and Bellevue, is medically staffed by N.Y.U.

Post finds the nurse who is on the unit on which his patient died last night. They have a talk in a private office. Post tells her about the need for better communication. He is firm, not visibly angry. She understands. She crosses her attractive legs, her short white uniform creeping up her thighs. Post is not distracted. They work out a plan to correct the problem in the future. It is simple: they will find Post, wherever he is, when such trouble arises.

Post phones the wife of a patient on the VA Neurosurgery Service, to tell her about a procedure Post would like to use on the man. The patient has had seizures. Investigation has shown an abnormality, a congenital abnormal "extra" batch of blood vessels in the brain, draining blood from normal brain tissue. Post wants to do an embolization on her husband tomorrow at Bellevue, where the facilities exist.

He explains it to her. It is done under general anesthesia. A catheter (tube) is inserted into the femoral artery in the groin, manipulated through the aorta to the carotid artery in the neck, and small pellets impregnated with barium are passed through the catheter to the brain. If they work, they cling to and block the blood vessels, which solidify and become harmless. The process is watched by fluoroscopy and X-rays are taken.

"We hope to block off a fair amount of it, but there is a risk. You should know that. The pellets can go into areas other than the area needing them. He could come out weaker or without improvement or better. It's less difficult than surgery, however," Post tells the man's wife.

"It will take about four hours and then he'll be watched for four hours in the recovery room. You can be there with him. Fine. I'll call you when it's over, so you can be here when he awakes," Post says.

After the phone conversation, he makes rounds, seeing patients he is responsible for at the VA. One terminal patient, an aged black man, is reading a Jehovah's Witnesses tract when Post walks in. It bears the headline "You Can Be Happy That So Little Time Is Left." Post raises one eyebrow slightly, says nothing.

His last stop before lunch is in the office of the VA's chief of Surgery. They talk, intensely, about the death of Post's patient; he wants the chief to know what happened and to know Post's feelings about it. Satisfied that he's gotten his message across, Post moves on to a greasy hamburger at the Bellevue snack bar. After lunch he visits Neuroradiology to look at some X-rays. A normal week would involve less walking for him; it would mean three operations, neurosurgeons invading the brain. This week is quiet in the OR for him. He revisits the boy in the Pediatrics ICU. The boy is still alert, still whining, but not speaking. Post would welcome a word, any intelligible word, but he comforts himself with the thought that this is not "a life-threatening situation." He will wait.

It is almost time for a Neurology-Neurosurgery conference at the VA. Post makes one stop: to take another look at his own son, who is kicking and crying. Post smiles with pleasure.

The conference includes doctors in both services at Bellevue and the VA; it is designed to confront the mysteries of a single case.

Chiefs of services at Bellevue and the VA, residents and medical students, a total of more than fifty, fill the room. Two of the chiefs are smoking cigars, puffing happily. As the conference opens, a medical student asks if those smoking, particularly cigars, would stop smoking. Both chiefs put out their cigars, smiling reluctantly. One of the chiefs begins an explanation of the case to be considered. In the middle of his presentation, he stops and asks a pointed question to the medical student. The student doesn't know the answer. The chief triumphantly lights a cigarette and proceeds.

A Neurology resident provides the details of the case. The patient is a 43-year-old man from Central America. He has a flood of complaints and symptoms. He has suffered from impotence, urinary difficulties, somnolence, stiff neck, back pain and numbness of his hands. He has an unsteady gait. He says he had chicken pox as an adult. According to the resident, "There is diffuse dysfunction, not acute, but mysterious."

The patient, in a wheelchair, is summoned. He is a black man in blue pajamas and a yellow-and-white terrycloth robe. He is sullen.

The chief does a few tests on him, to appraise his motor skills and reactions, then allows the patient to leave. The resident resumes. All sorts of tests have been done on the man, he tells the group, including skull films, chest X-rays, angiogram, blood-cell counts, sugar and protein levels. There is no discernible mass, no aneurysm. It is, the resident says, either infectious or arteritic (arterial inflammation). For days, while various cultures were done, from TB to fungus, theories were considered. Then, the resident says, a spinal-fluid analysis provided the first clue.

Doctors in the audience are encouraged to guess. Several try, without success. "It is a rare and odd case," the resident says. The diagnosis: central-nervous-system syphilis, syphilis of the brain. It is in its tertiary stage and has affected the cerebellum and possibly the medulla. Penicillin therapy has been initiated; it can stabilize him, but the damage is permanent. The "chicken pox" the man thought he had probably was early syphilis. He had told the doctors that he had a "healthy sex life" with prostitutes.

"Syphilis can do *anything*," the chief of Neurology at the VA says. "Patients forget the chancre or don't have an obvious one and it can or cannot produce pain." As he goes on, explaining the curious ways that syphilis can attack the body, Post, who has been listening attentively, is interrupted by the sound of his beeper. He gets up quietly and goes to a nearby phone. A Chinese man has jumped out of a fifth-story window and has been brought to the Emergency Ward; they need a neurosurgeon. Post looks at his watch; it is almost time to make rounds at the VA with Bellevue's chief of Neurosurgery, Dr. Joseph Ransohoff. Post sends a junior resident, one he trusts, to answer the EW call, and, as the conference ends, Post rushes off to meet Ransohoff.

Known as "The Boss," Ransohoff is a widely respected neuro-surgeon, the volatile, colorful director of the service at Bellevue and the VA, as well as head of the Neurosurgery department at the N.Y.U. Medical School and an active neurosurgeon at University Hospital. His father and his grandfather were doctors, and his presence, firm and knowledgeable, reflects that tradition. He is a short man, thin, with a gray crew cut. He wears a white button-down shirt, a narrow conservative tie, and chukka boots under the tightest pant cuffs since the zoot suit. His hands are carefully manicured; he busies them smoking cigars and cigarettes. Post and the other residents who have arrived to participate in rounds with Ransohoff treat him reverentially. The group studies X-rays, while Ransohoff comments on them.

They stare at X-rays of a man with multiple lesions of the brain.

"There's more than one tumor in that head," Ransohoff says, his voice trailing off. He shakes his head. Radiation or chemotherapy may be worth trying, he says, but surgery is pointless.

Another set of X-rays reveal enlarged ventricles in the brain. Ransohoff asks what's been done for the patient. Not much yet, one of the residents tells him.

"You don't sit on a guy like that," he barks. "You can get into trouble at any time." Ransohoff is not one to be indecisive when a patient seems to need immediate treatment.

The group weaves through the VA's corridors, newer and more joyful than Bellevue's, visiting patients in private rooms, again a change from Bellevue and its bleak wards. Ransohoff speaks with patients, directly to them in simple language they can understand. They can sense his authority. "Anything you say, Doc," one old man says as Ransohoff leaves his room. The residents, too, are timid in the face of that authority. They know that Ransohoff can be entertaining and informative, but can be provoked by signs of bad medicine. Today he is calm or simply tired, not interested in teaching, which is what the rounds represent, by provocation. Even for a resident as experienced as Post, rounds with Ransohoff are valuable. Something can be learned, so Post listens to every word Ransohoff utters. When Ransohoff leaves, at 6 P.M., Post can relax. He walks back to Bellevue, to make a few last-minute checks on ward patients. It is a daily ritual. When it's done, he can go home. But this is not a week in which details can be overlooked or abundantly delegated. Without OR time, and with a two-day trip to Boston coming up this week, Post knows he'll be occupied with details, on the Bellevue wards and at the VA before he gets those two days at Massachusetts General Hospital, watching other neuro-surgeons at work.

A pathologist does not perform complex operations; the glory and the torment of the surgeon are not his. The pathologist does not treat patients; he doesn't even see them. He doesn't pre-scribe medication or listen to patient complaints. Yet without the pathologist hospital care would be at a standstill.

When disease invades the body, it may not be conspicuously visible, the way a knife wound or a badly broken bone can be seen. Disease can produce alterations that only a pathologist can detect, in blood, in serum, in urine, in spinal fluid, in tissue. A patient can have cancer, or syphilis, without anyone except a pathologist affirming it. As a result, Pathology's presence at Bellevue is ubiquitous. It has its own building, where studious doctors spend most of their time sitting and thinking, peering at slides. In addition, there are laboratories scattered through-out the general hospital, to keep up with the demand for Pa-thology's services.

Some examples: Disease can create an imbalance in normal body chemistry. The chemistry lab can determine levels of concentration in blood, urine and spinal fluid, looking for devia-tions from the normal range. The pathologists in Microbiology look for organisms, like bacteria and fungi, in blood and sputum. The nature and number of blood cells can reveal trouble, too, and the hematologist, in counting and analyzing the cells, can define signs of disease. Serology pathologists can spot infectious diseases, like syphilis, in serum samples. The Autopsy Service, allied to Pathology, examines several hundred bodies a year. Research Pathology, a small part of Bellevue's complex, gets funds for its projects, a study of tumor formation high on its list of priorities.

Pathology is a field for contemplative doctors. Eugene Faz-zini is such a doctor. Bellevue's chief of Surgical Pathology, dealing with diseases accessible to surgical investigation, Faz-zini is a 34-year-old New Yorker. He is single and still lives where he was born, in the Bronx. He was graduated, Phi Beta Kappa, from C.C.N.Y. in 1958 and from the Albert Einstein

College of Medicine four years later. He did an internship at Cincinnati General Hospital before coming to Bellevue to serve his residency in Pathology.

Fazzini served in the U.S. Air Force medical corps as a captain, at a USAF hospital in Vietnam and at the Armed Forces Institute of Pathology in Washington.

It was not difficult for him to choose Pathology.

"I'm in Pathology because it's interesting and it's interesting because it covers most fields of medicine, not just one. And I didn't enjoy patient contact that much when I was an intern. Now I have constant contact with the other services and time to read and keep up," he says.

Reading and keeping up are only two of his activities. His work may keep him linked to a desk; his life style does not. He has co-authored two books on pathology, and writes articles as well. He is an insatiable traveler; he has been to Russia, Italy, France, England, Egypt, Jordan, Lebanon, Japan, Australia and Greece. He's an expert in Chinese food, as a cook and at restaurants. He plays the clarinet and the recorder. He's a gardener. He's now studying Chinese because he wants to go to China.

Fazzini shares a cubicle-office in the crumbling Pathology building with another full-time attending. His desk is in a state of disarray. On it are: three plants, a bag of Baken-ets (fried pork rinds), a large gray American Optical Series 10 microscope, innumerable slides, batches of pathology reports, jars containing tissue samples and miscellaneous scraps of paper. Around him are maps of Moscow and Italy, one of his own abstract paintings (more than ten years old; he has stopped painting). A radio blares constantly behind his desk, a flow of classical music. His own travel photos line the glass door to his office.

Fazzini is a large, burly man with a black-gray beard and brown hair that touches the top of his ears. Although he has been on a diet that has helped him lose twenty-five pounds in six weeks, he is thick from the waist down. He carries seven pens and a pencil across his shirt pocket. He does not wear a tie. His round face often bears a smile; when his eyebrows arch, that smile can look satanic.

Although Fazzini gets from the Bronx to his office before 8 A.M., his day officially begins at 8, when he meets with the Pathology interns, residents and attendings to discuss current cases. In some services (e.g., Medicine), rounds involve moving from bed to bed, patient to patient, evaluating charts and patients simultaneously. In other services, the walking tour is replaced by chart rounds, a meeting of doctors to discuss the treatment of patients under their care. Rounds, the term used to denote a regular, systematic review of patients and their medical status, provide the basic diagnostic contact between medical staff and patient; since rounds are accomplished by a group of doctors, a collective judgment, usually formulated by an attending, is obtained. At Bellevue, such activity is supplemented by conferences and meetings, which can be formal—the detailed presentation of cases of special interest—or informal—a gathering of doctors to share insights into one case of immediate concern. Whatever the form, the teaching process is evident, whether it's at rounds on a ward or listening to a doctor analyze a case in a classroom setting.

Pathology's equivalent of making rounds is done in a large area outside Fazzini's office, around a long rectangular table studded with microscopes. It is an old room in an old building; the walls, white and yellow, are aged and the paint is peeling. The room resembles one in a condemned building of a bankrupt university. The doctors are oblivious to it. Their minds are on the slides in their microscopes, as Fazzini gives them the details of each case on the day's agenda. Each case is numbered.

Fazzini sits at a small, separate table, peering through a microscope, passing slides to the others at the larger table. During the course of a given session, he can lapse into moments of brooding quiet or be openly cheerful. His is introspective work and what goes on in his mind often makes its way to his face.

"Case 5788 is a biopsy from a lesion in the colon of a woman who has a history of diarrhea and blood-tinged stools. What does she have?" Fazzini asks, passing the slides around. He knows the answer: colitis, not ulcerative. He wants the others to discover it.

"Case 5787 is an unfortunate twenty-eight-year-old man who is hoarse and has had vocal cord surgery before. Papilloma?"

The reports that accompany the specimens to Pathology give a sketchy case history. That and the sample itself are what the pathologists have to go on.

"5777 is a curiosity. Plastic repair of a cleft in the earlobe." The specimen is a fragment of a grossly deformed earlobe.

Fazzini prods the others. It is early in the morning and several of them show little inclination to be investigative.

"They want to know. What would you look for? Acute inflammation? Tumor? Ulcer?"

He continues to pass out the slides. Slowly, the group perks up, like a hungry family opening the food at a picnic.

More slides.

A liver biopsy on a 75-year-old woman who does *not* drink.

A damaged liver from a car crash.

A young man with a history of carcinoma of the thyroid.

An uncommon wart.

Fazzini reports that a member of the house staff has granuloma of the septum. He asks a resident to look at the slide and tell him what it is.

"Well, it certainly isn't . . ." the resident begins.

"No negatives. Give me positives," Fazzini says. "This guy is a highly sensitive person. I'm amazed he hasn't been over to see us. For your information, it's an ulcer with granulation tissue underlying it. Chronic inflammation with ulceration. If this were anyone else, we'd say he had been picking his nose. In this case, we'll call it factitial, produced by artificial means."

It is time for the slide of the morning, the puzzle to be solved.

It is a slide of a section of skin from a 72-year-old woman. The report from Dermatology that accompanied the sample indicated that their diagnosis was psoriasis.

"Wrong," Fazzini proclaims. "They missed it."

The interns and residents study the slide. Minutes pass. Fazzini announces his verdict: a common fungus infection. The others concur; there are nods, murmurs of "yes" throughout the room.

It is after 10 A.M. now and Fazzini escorts several interns and residents to a Pathology conference room, where he projects slides and analyzes them. Today he talks about four lung cases, unusual cases from a seminar held in Michigan (pathologists exchange challenging cases), including one example of rare measles pneumonia. The residents listen attentively to Fazzini, whose presentations have the tone and content of an expert.

The morning is passing at a leisurely pace. Fazzini returns to his office to work on lectures he will be giving to medical students in a few weeks. He selects examples of lung tissue (which were thinly sliced, applied to paper when wet, then sprayed to hold) to illustrate the points he wants to make. He collects slides for a conference later in the week; the sources for his selection are vast, because there are slides on file at Bellevue from the turn of the century.

It is time for lunch. Fazzini has brought some chicken from home, along with the Baken-ets. He nibbles at the food and browses through the *New York Times*.

As he folds up the *Times*, a resident from the Chest Service comes in with a sputum sample. He tells Fazzini that he has a patient who has pneumonia. All medication tried so far has been unsuccessful, he says. He wants Fazzini to tell him what the patient has.

"It's not ordinary pneumonia," he tells Fazzini. "Whatever it is, it must be rare."

Fazzini takes the sample to a nearby lab, where it will be processed. Several tissue samples are already being worked on. Surgical Pathology gets eight thousand tissue samples each year. When they arrive, they are screened and documented by size and description, by a Pathology resident. Then they go to the lab upstairs, where they can be processed in from two to twenty-four hours.

A frozen section can be done in minutes on a cryostat, but the cell detail is less precise than with the standard method: processing with alcohol, then in a paraffin mold. That mold, enclosing the tissue firmly, is sliced in sections 6/1,000th of an inch thick, put on slides and stained, to make identification easier (there are many types of stains and many methods of staining, each designed to emphasize a particular aspect of the tissue).

Back in his office, Fazzini resumes sifting through slides. There is a Pathology report on his desk. He glances at it quickly, then puts it aside. It deals with a woman patient on Ward I–5.

Specimen: non-union left femoral neck. Femoral head and mature granulation from acetabulum.

Diagnosis: 1. Femoral head with fibrosis and chronic inflammation. 2. Chronic inflammation of synovium lined with fibrous tissue, clinically from acetabulum.

Fazzini prepared the report; he doesn't have to review it. He pushes other things across his desk. Almost everything on it relates to the diagnostic process. His role in that process is pivotal. More than 95 percent of diagnoses can be made on the basis of tissue specimens, he feels. In rare, difficult cases, outside consultations by leading pathologists are obtained. Fazzini's mail contains opinions by pathologists whose views have been solicited.

"It is true," Fazzini points out, "that in ten percent of the cases the clinical staff and the pathologists may disagree about a diagnosis, but in ninety-nine percent of those the pathologist rules."

In Surgical Pathology, Fazzini and another full-time pathologist, and two part-time pathologists, guide and teach the staff. Interns and residents make preliminary diagnoses, but the attendings see all the diagnoses, and check them, before reports are sent back to the service requesting the analysis. Residents in Pathology don't act on their own, as they do in other services at Bellevue.

As Fazzini searches for slides, reads his mail, checks reports, the afternoon evaporates. Residents and interns come into his office, to seek his advice. He signs forms brought to him by the department secretary. He assembles material for lectures. He studies slides, peering for long periods through the lens of his elaborate microscope.

The room is silent. Pathologists work in silence, much of the time, and those at work now look back and forth, from microscopes to their own notes.

Fazzini has not been idle for a moment since lunch, yet he has not moved from his desk. It is 3:30, time for him to travel over to the main hospital for a pathology conference he will conduct at the Chest Service. He collects the slides he'll need and walks off to meet the Chest Service's chief resident, Lanie Eagleton, and his staff. It is something Fazzini does regularly, bringing his skills and interpretations to the services he works with. At such conferences Fazzini applies his discipline to the cases the service has asked him to analyze; the doctors on the service share their knowledge with him. If it works, they combine on an accurate diagnosis.

When the Chest Service conference ends, it is after 5 P.M. Tomorrow, Fazzini has the day off. He can work on an article he's been researching, study Chinese, tend to his garden.

The Emergency Ward at Bellevue is the hospital's busiest room. It is where the truly acute cases are brought for immediate treatment. Patients are in and out within hours, usually, stabilized in the EW and transferred to a service that will provide long-term treatment, rushed to the operating room, or treated quickly, observed and released. Some of them die.

Often the EW staff does not have a great deal of time to deliberate; it must move expeditiously. It is trained to do just that. Residents from all major services find themselves in the EW every day. Trauma Service doctors—a subdivision of Surgery—find themselves there frequently. The nursing staff, Bellevue doctors say, is the best in the hospital. One of the best in the EW is Loretta Chiarelli.

Chiarelli is 30 and single. She is the head nurse on the day shift, from 8 A.M. to 4 P.M. A native of Queens, she is the daughter of parents born in Italy and she has spent her life in New York City. She was graduated from Bellevue's nursing school in 1963, then spent eighteen months as a nurse in Surgery at Bellevue, waiting for an opening in the EW. She got there in 1964 and a year later was promoted to head nurse.

Doctors say that her knowledge of medicine is comprehensive and her dedication to her job and to the EW cannot be matched by any nurse in the entire hospital.

Outwardly, she is cool, poised, attractive. She is five feet six inches tall, weighs 105 pounds. Her face is a beautiful one, vaguely Oriental in structure, with high cheekbones beneath dark brown eyes. She has long brown hair, swept back and clipped. She wears a white pant suit some of the time, conventional white uniform at others.

She moves gracefully. For six years, she's been studying ballet. She's been a consultant on one nursing textbook, is collaborating on another one now. She travels. She's been to Italy, Spain, England, Ireland, Switzerland, the Caribbean, the Mediterranean and Mexico. Her style, avoiding the insulation that work in a hospital can mean, is compatible with her reason for working in the EW. She'd rather be refreshed and challenged by what she finds each morning than bored by being able to predict it. The EW is the perfect place for such a nurse.

The ward itself is a long, narrow room; it stretches from an emergency entrance at one end to a high platform at the other, where doctors can fill out charts, oversee the patients. Midway between the two ends, there is a corridor connecting the EW to the Adult Emergency Service (AES), from which the EW gets many of its patients when their troubles are severe. The nursing station and clerk's desk are at that crossroad. Beds line both sides of the ward, with emergency equipment at each bedside.

Chiarelli's day begins at 7:30, before her shift goes on duty. As she enters, she passes a bulletin board displaying a declaration from Bellevue's Nursing Division:

In Our Culture the Public Has Come to Expect the Right:
1. To wellness.
2. To receive adequate and qualified health care.
3. To participate in decisions regarding their care.
4. To be helped to understand their health and illnesses as well as the treatments undertaken in their behalf.
5. To be cared for with concern when they are ill.
6. To be accepted in a state of dependence when they are unable or feel unable to care for themselves.
7. To be kept as comfortable as modern science permits.
8. To decline and die in reasonable dignity.
9. To feel that someone cares and that they are not alone in their illness or dying.

She gets a rundown from the night head nurse. This morning, eight beds are occupied. As Chiarelli arrives, a ninth patient is wheeled in. Medical residents are scattered around the ward, studying patients, making diagnoses. The low hum of voices and the continual beeping of cardiac monitors creates a contrapuntal pattern. Chiarelli, who conducts much of her work in silence, moves rapidly from one end of the ward to the other, checking patients' charts and medication orders. Her concentration is constant.

In the background, a resident is talking to a restless old woman, toothless and grimy, who was found in the street, curled up and sick. "Close your eyes, relax and go to sleep," the resident is chanting.

Another resident talks to a young Puerto Rican man. "Be patient, please. I'll take the tube out of your nose in a few minutes."

As Chiarelli takes stock of what she has inherited from the night shift, a staff nurse arrives, flashing an engagement ring. She's engaged to a doctor. Chiarelli smiles. She keeps to herself any thoughts about the advisability of marrying a doctor. A second nurse arrives for duty; she's just returned from her honeymoon with her doctor husband.

Another resident's voice cuts through the gaiety, reminding

the nurses that it's time to go to work. He is leaning over a bed, staring at a wooden old man. "Do you know where you are? Where are you now?" the resident is shouting. Nearby, a frightened old woman suddenly sits up in her bed, straining her IV tubes. Her eyes are wide as she babbles. A nurse runs over to her, calms her down.

A nurse from the night shift is on her way out with a colleague. "Let's get the hell out of here," she says. "I've had enough. Definitely enough."

Two residents peer at a patient's EKG.

At 8:30, Chiarelli leads the other nurses on rounds, going from bed to bed, checking vital signs, test results, drug orders, symptoms. It is important to Chiarelli that all the nurses understand the patients' problems, know what to do if anything goes wrong.

Today most of the patients are old. At 8:35, an 84-year-old black woman is wheeled in from the AES, accompanied by a resident. He interrupts rounds to tell Chiarelli, "Her family just brought her in. She's somebody's grandmother. Fell down in her bathroom. Probably a stroke." Her daughter and granddaughter, he tells Chiarelli, are waiting outside.

A new nurse shows up for duty. Chiarelli greets her, introduces her to the other nurses and gives her a short course in doing things the way Chiarelli wants them done. "If you're charting the way you should, I shouldn't have to communicate with you," Chiarelli tells her. When it gets busy in the EW, there's no time for instruction or clarification.

There are now ten patients in the EW; seven of them are old, two are young men and one is a woman in her thirties. The latter is having a seizure, moving jerkily in bed, and a Neurology resident is with her. He knows her; he's treated her before. Chiarelli asks him for information.

"She's been having seizures since she was one year old," he says. "Retarded." He looks at the patient, who, in her torment, seems to recognize him. "You're my little fat flower," he tells her, and begins singing "There is a Rose in Spanish Harlem." Then he turns to a nurse and whispers, "Pathetic. There's nothing we can do for a brain that's already damaged. We can control the seizures, but that's all."

At 9:15, rounds are done, the EW is quiet. Doctors and nurses are at work throughout the ward. No one is idle. Chiarelli keeps in motion, wordlessly, with a kind of elegance.

A woman patient is transferred to a Medical ward; the EW has done all it can for her. Chiarelli erases a block of information about her on the Board, a kind of floor plan–master chart that Chiarelli prepares at the beginning of her shift to keep it current. Her handwriting is almost microscopically small.

She paces, double-checking trays of supplies that will be needed during the course of the day. It is something she might assign to a staff nurse, but she doesn't want to spare one of the nurses to do it. Her own compulsions add to the efficiency of the EW.

An off-duty nurse shows up with a cake. She hands it to the ward clerk, a tough and experienced black woman, and leaves.

"Why did she do that?" one of the nurses asks.

"Because she loves us," the clerk says.

A Neurology resident arrives, having been paged, to check out the 84-year-old woman who fell in her bathroom. A spinal tap is clear, indicating the absence of hemorrhage. She does have a history of hypertension. The resident puts an instrument, an otoscope, into her ear and peers into it. As he does, a passing resident shouts, "If you see Forty-second Street, let me know."

The Neurology resident feels that the woman has had a stroke. He's baffled by the fact that there is no evidence of hemorrhage; many cases of head trauma have it. He prescribes steroids and orders immediate skull X-rays. He's opposed to an angiogram because the woman may be too old to bear up under that procedure; it involves injecting dye into the brain through a main artery and observing the state of the blood vessels through fluoroscopy. At 10 A.M., a young Puerto Rican man is transferred out of the EW to a Medical ward; he is a gastrointestinal bleeder and can get specific care in Medicine.

One of Bellevue's Roman Catholic chaplains walks through the EW and finds an old patient, a man, to talk to. Chiarelli looks around and concludes that things will be peaceful long enough for her to take a coffee break in the snack bar.

When she returns, she hears the voice of a woman patient moaning, "Oy, vey," over and over again.

"Don't move," a resident is yelling at her.

Chiarelli walks up. "Will you stop that," she says to the woman. "Stop it. Lie down. You're going to drive us up the wall." It is the old lady who wants to sit up in bed and babble. "Do you know how many times your bed has been changed?" Chiarelli asks her.

At 10:30, there's a new admission: an older man, staying at a Manhattan hotel, who awoke with chest pain and lung congestion. He's escorted from the AES into the EW, where he's placed in a bed.

"Let's get your pants off," a nurse says to him. "Then you can rest. We'll keep them for you, don't worry."

A resident examines the man. He is alert, but his heartbeat is rapid and there is fluid in his lungs. There is a discussion with another resident about the merits of electrical heart conversion-cardioversion versus the use of Digitalis. A first-year resident who has joined the two others hopes they'll try the former; he's never seen it done and he wants to learn. The decision is made, by consensus, to try morphine and diuretics; one of the residents will try to reach the patient's home-town doctor for more information, some history.

At 11:25, another old man is transferred out, to a ward. The 84-year-old woman is back from X-ray and is surrounded by an attending neurologist and several residents, who are discussing her case. An EEG technician arrives with her portable EEG machine. "When that's done," the attending announces to the residents, "we'll want to get a brain scan on her." A resident notes it, in a small, tattered black notebook he stuffs into his white jacket pocket.

It is noon. Chiarelli summons several other nurses to an early lunch at the snack bar. Over a hamburger, french fries and coffee she recounts stories from the past to nurses who haven't been at Bellevue as long as she has.

"I was supposed to be covering several wards in those days and one of the patients in one of them had a cardiac arrest, so I ran like mad to get to him and started pounding his chest. As I was doing it, I looked out the window and there was another patient of mine, stark-naked, strolling around the parking lot. I screamed for an aide to get out there and bring back that wild man while I kept pounding the guy's chest."

She remembers making rounds with student nurses. During rounds, supervised by a nursing instructor not known for her sense of humor, a male patient walked up to the group and with giddy deliberation proceeded to take off all his clothes.

"Well, the nursing instructor thought it was an opportunity to make a point. You know, what do you do when the unexpected happens? So she turned to the students, while this guy is standing there grinning, and she asked, 'What should you do under these circumstances?' One of the students stepped forward and said, 'Well, you could just tell him, "Later, later." ' The instructor didn't quite know how to deal with that suggestion. She got red in the face and just stuck her arm out with her thumb down and led the students out of the ward."

When Chiarelli and the other nurses get back from lunch, there are six patients in the EW. A man from Housekeeping is mopping the floor. The only voice is that of a resident grumbling to another resident:

"This guy had just shot and killed four people and now he's in Bellevue, the armpit of mankind, and he has lower-back pain and I'm supposed to examine him and ask him, politely, how he's feeling. It's dehumanizing. It bugs my ass. Doctors are dreamers, man. They believe that if you pound on the chest of a ninety-year-old man, you'll save his fucking life."

Chiarelli slides past the resident, to resume her chores.

At 2 P.M., a bearded black man, 62, is wheeled in. He was found drunk on a park bench in the rain and complains of being cold. He is blind in one eye from an untreated cataract.

A resident rushes up to help. A nurse takes the man's temperature: 80. Three doctors and a nurse move in to help. They discover that the patient has an irregular heartbeat. They cover him with blankets. Slowly, his temperature begins to rise, from 80 to 84, from 84 to 88 within an hour. They want a urine specimen. A nurse asks the man for one.

"Can you urinate?"

The man just stares at her with his one good eye.

"Can you pass water?" she asks.

He says nothing.

A resident leans over the bed, hands the man a steel container and shouts, "Piss, man."

"Yeah, baby," the patient mutters.

Lanie Eagleton, the Chest Service's chief resident, walks by, looking at patients' charts. Eagleton, who looks for interesting cases in the EW, likes to know who's down there and likes to check them out in person, to find out if the Chest Service can adopt the patient. He finds one to his liking.

"Shopping?" a resident asks Eagleton.

"I bought," Eagleton says, smiling.

Chiarelli waves at Eagleton as he leaves, but has no time to talk to him. She continues to pace relentlessly, from one end of the ward to the other. She checks supplies, checks the narcotics cabinet, kept locked. She looks at patients and their charts, gives medication. When she sees doctors or nurses in need of help, she helps. She does not intrude. She rarely speaks, preferring to keep moving, like a puppetmaster, through the ward.

At 3:30, the ward is quiet again; two groups of doctors are talking, informally, about their day at Bellevue, as the new nurses begin to arrive for the evening shift.

A new admission is in and out of the EW rapidly. He is the Chinese man, brought in by police, who jumped out of a fifth-story window trying to escape from them. At the EW, he is quickly surrounded by doctors and nurses, and a Neurosurgery resident who's come running over from a conference at the VA, then rushed to the operating room. His internal bleeding is more than the EW can handle; only surgery can possibly help him now.

At 3:45, Chiarelli meets with her successor and the staff nurses on the four-to-midnight shift. They go over the Board, so the evening head nurse now has her own updated version. When that's done, Chiarelli can head for home. Tonight she hopes to practice her dancing and do some work on the nursing textbook.

George Feldman is the son of a general practitioner in Rockland County, New York. He will be an internist when he leaves Bellevue. Now he's a first-year resident in Internal Medicine.

He was born in Pilsen, Czechoslovakia, in November, 1946. The family left Czechoslovakia when Feldman was a child, to escape Russian domination. They moved to England, then to Australia, before coming to America, settling in New York, in 1952. Feldman went to Trinity College in Connecticut, graduating in 1968, and to N.Y.U. Medical School, finishing in 1972.

He spent his year of internship, in Pediatrics (with two months in Medicine), at Los Angeles County Hospital. After that, he decided to leave Pediatrics for a residency in Medicine, and Los Angeles County for Bellevue.

Feldman is five feet eight inches tall, weighs 154 pounds. He is a quiet man with an angelic face, an almost perpetual expression of serenity on it. He has brown hair that covers his ears. His manner is calm, serious, without being intense. He speaks softly. He seems in control, like a wise cherub.

This year he will spend most of his time on the Medical wards, supervising the work of interns, teaching medical students. In his second year he will rotate through subspecialties of his choice, and in his third year he hopes to land a subspecialty fellowship. Right now, he doesn't know what that will be. It is too early.

He lives in Manhattan, near Bellevue, and his day, which usually begins before 8 A.M., can extend into the night and often does.

Feldman arrives for the day's eye-opener, the 8 A.M. X-ray conference, bearing a brown bag with coffee and a Danish. He is one of ten interns, residents and medical students who begin the day by listening to a radiologist discuss several cases. The first three sets of X-rays show patients free of symptoms that might show up in X-rays. The fourth set deals with a black man with malignant lymphoma, one of Feldman's ward patients. The X-rays show that the man is developing pneumonia. More important, they reveal an enlarged splenic mass.

When the X-ray conference ends, at 8:30, Feldman leads his staff of nine, interns and medical students, on rounds. They make rounds of patients Feldman is responsible for; several are now in the Medical ICU, today's first stop. The ICU looks like other wards, but it isn't. Intensive care is evident in the number of doctors and nurses scurrying around, and the equipment available to them. ICU patients need constant attention.

Feldman stops at the bed of an old woman who has had a stroke. She has been intubated—that is, a tube has been inserted into her trachea to assure the passage of oxygen to her lungs—and is now on a respirator. Feldman notices water in the respirator and turns to the intern assigned to the case.

"Empty that," he says, firmly, "so she doesn't aspirate it."

A nurse, poised nearby, empties it.

The interns debate what the woman might have. Feldman

knows that one thing she does have is a pulmonary embolism.

"We need a lung scan," he says, "but we can't get one until she's weaned off the respirator. And we can treat the pulmonary embolus. We don't know yet what else she has. It's another one of our diagnostic problems."

He moves to a second old woman, thin and wrinkled, who is sitting up, looking spent, slumped over, her chin touching her chest. There are irregularities in her blood chemistry and she has chest congestion.

"Talk to a hematologist. Make sure we're not missing something," Feldman tells an intern. "And call Chest, to find out what's going on there."

He visits an old Jewish woman who has been suffering from chest pain, a symptom of cardiac trouble. Nitroglycerin seems to be keeping the cardiac symptoms in check, but Feldman feels she needs a sedative.

"What are you sedating her with?" he asks an intern.

"Really nothing," the intern says.

"Sedate her."

"Okay. I'll give her thirty phenobarb."

Feldman moves on, and the others follow him, to the bed of another old woman. The ICU seems filled with them. This one has come to Bellevue from a nursing home, suffering from respiratory distress. Feldman instructs an intern to call the nursing home, to get a medical history on her.

The group moves out of the ICU to C–2, a two-room Medical ward, one room for women, one for men; during the day Feldman covers it. At night, he is responsible for a second ward, as well. The interns do much of the bedside work, but Feldman must supervise their work. It is their first year out of medical school and they learn by doing and by being taught. Their workload is heavy, their free time minimal.

In the ward, he stops a few paces from a young woman covered by a sheet up to her frightened face.

"She's had everything but a barium enema," the intern tells Feldman.

"So?" Feldman asks.

"I talked to her for an hour about it. She refuses."

Feldman is irritated. He leads the intern out into the corridor, away from the patient.

"She has a lesion. We have to know all we can about it. I'll talk to her, if I have to, because she could have cancer and we can't play games," he tells the intern.

"I'll do it. I'll do it," the intern says. "Don't worry about it."

The intern and Feldman return to the room, where the intern introduces Feldman to a new patient, a middle-aged woman from the South.

"Because she has the good fortune to have very rare symptoms, she is getting all of our esoteric lab studies," the intern tells Feldman.

"Ah want ta know whut's wrong with me, too," she tells Feldman. "Ah've nevuh be-yun ta the tropics, so ah jus' couldn't have gotten this down theah."

The group moves on, to look at an aged ninety-pound Puerto Rican woman; she's lost eight pounds in a few days.

"The stigmata of liver disease are very obvious in this woman," the intern proclaims pedantically.

"Let's set her up for a biopsy," Feldman suggests.

"It might be a dangerous procedure, a disservice to her," the intern replies. "We can attack her chronic active hepatitis now, but I don't think we should do much else." Feldman does not debate the matter. In this instance, the intern can have his way. The woman is old and frail; a liver biopsy is not a totally benign procedure.

An old Puerto Rican woman is sitting in a chair watching the doctors. An intern points her out to Feldman and says, "Her blood pressure is down to 90 and I'd like to send her home and follow her in the clinic."

"Okay. But the most important thing is to speak to her family and tell them what she must do to take care of herself," Feldman says.

In the male room, the group stops at the bedside of the man with malignant lymphoma. A nurse reports to Feldman that the man's stomach, once distended grotesquely, is down and his bowels seem to be functioning normally.

"Hey, that's the best news yet," Feldman says to the patient. The man lies listlessly in bed, manages a slight smile.

"He wants soup," the nurse says.

"No, give him some water," Feldman tells her.

The next patient is a man in his forties. He is sitting up in bed, seemingly healthy. Feldman picks up the man's chart and asks an intern, "What do you think of this temperature of 100 last night?"

The intern smiles. "I think it's hot in this room."

"Right," Feldman says. "Remember, this guy needs limitations set for him. I don't want him out of bed. He walks around all night smoking cigarettes. He had a heart attack and he's crazy. One night he got up and smoked twelve cigarettes in an hour."

As the doctors leave the room, the patient hungrily picks up a copy of *True Story* magazine. The cover line reads "A Minister's Wife Rents Me Every Saturday Night."

At 10 A.M., Feldman has finished rounds and heads for the snack bar to have coffee with three interns. The conversation is all medicine. Then, back on the ward, he visits a new patient, a black woman in her fifties. Her elaborate wig is askew, giving her a demented look. She complains to Feldman of headaches, vomiting, high blood pressure, kidney pain, most of them secondary, Feldman suspects, to diabetes.

"Are you a diabetic?" Feldman asks her.

"Yes. It's right there on my chart," she says, briskly.

"I know it is, but we don't want to miss anything, so I ask questions." He is not provoked by her attitude; he is here to care for her, not necessarily to like her.

The woman mumbles angrily to Feldman as he examines her. Nearby, a TV set is blasting a game show: "Here's twenty dollars for you and twenty dollars for Sally," the giddy emcee is shouting. A man from Housekeeping has entered to mop the floor. Feldman stops examining the woman, walks to the TV set, turns down the volume and returns to the patient.

When he's done, he meets with a group of medical students to work out an improved method for them to draw blood from patients early in the morning. Then he walks over to the ICU again, to check a patient. He adjusts the patient's respirator, tells an intern that the rate was "intolerable" and should have been adjusted earlier. The intern apologizes. Feldman is concerned about such details; they consume much of his time.

As he leaves the ICU, Feldman turns to the intern and says, "One good thing about working here is that you don't have time to find out what's going on outside. That way, you don't get mad about society being in a bad way."

He walks out of the ICU, passing a handwritten sign taped to the door: "When You're Down and Out Lift Up Your Head and Shout I'm Down and Out."

He has taken a specimen for a blood-gas test from the old

woman on the respirator and is hand-carrying it to the lab. The intern tags along.

"It's not reliable to wait on these; you need quick results," Feldman tells him.

Blood gases are only one of many tests that are an integral part of the vocabulary of Medicine. BUN analyzes kidney function. CRIT indicates the number of red cells in the blood, a test for anemia. The SED rate is a nonspecific test to diagnose the presence of inflammation. CBC is the complete blood count. Electrolytes give a chemical picture of the body, its chemical balance or imbalance, acid level, metabolic changes. LFT tests liver function. Blood-gas tests reflects lung function, the oxygen intake, the adequacy of the lungs, and the acid-base status.

As they walk toward the lab, the intern reminds Feldman of a woman whose white count, 270,000 when she was admitted, raced to 600,000 on the ward. She died.

"Leukemia," Feldman sighs. He doesn't want to talk about it.

The intern changes the subject, to a film he's seen about World War II.

"My parents met each other in Nazi concentration camps," Feldman says. "They were both at Auschwitz. When the war ended, they got married. The Russians wanted both of them to remain in Czechoslovakia. My father was a doctor and my mother was from a wealthy family that owned several textile mills. The Russians wanted them to stay, to legitimatize their takeover. There was some trouble, but they managed to get out. The quota for Czech immigrants here was low in those days, so they went to England and Australia on temporary visas. My mother became a seamstress and my father did odd jobs. Finally, their application to come to America was approved in 1952. I don't remember much before that, but I hope to visit Prague someday. My mother has told me it is a beautiful city."

"I've never been there," the intern says. Feldman drops off the specimen at the lab and rushes off to Medicine's Journal Club meeting, a conference of residents who assemble to listen to an attending analyze a medical article. It is noon. Feldman is at the conference until 1 P.M. There isn't time for lunch today; he's due to report to Home Care shortly after 1.

Feldman works for the Home Care Service one day a week. It was begun at Bellevue in 1948 and provides medical and social service care to homebound patients. From Fifty-ninth

Street south to the Battery, river to river, Bellevue covers such patients.

The Home Care station wagon and driver take Feldman down to Mulberry Street, where an 80-year-old man, Aaron Greenberg, has lived for almost twenty years. The neighborhood is largely Chinese. The man's wife has broken her leg and is in Bellevue; he is home alone. He has diabetes, heart disease, high blood pressure. He has had a stroke. His legs have been amputated; he is in a wheelchair. He welcomes Feldman, one of the few visitors who come to see him.

Greenberg has a gray fringe of hair, glasses, and is wearing a T-shirt and has draped a towel across his lap. The paint on the apartment walls is peeling everywhere. Bare bulbs glow in the ceiling. Copies of the *Daily Forward* are scattered around.

The apartment consists of two rooms and a small kitchen. The rooms are full of threadbare old furniture, worn-out linoleum, piles of clothes, papers, food. Boxes of Uneeda Biscuits are everywhere, opened and unopened. A TV set gleams on a stand. There are two calendars nailed to the wall: one from the Rabbinical Seminary of America and another from Bankers Trust.

Greenberg's face seems to express eternal pain. He tells Feldman about his wife. "She fell down. She fell down three times and I couldn't help her. I had to call the Emergency."

They talk about the assortment of medication the man must take.

"If that one gives you ringing in your ears, Mr. Greenberg, stop taking it," Feldman tells him, pointing to a pill on the table.

"It didn't ring in mine ears," Greenberg says. "My problem, Doc, is aggravation, something like that."

"I've got a flu shot for you," Feldman says. "It's important, worthwhile."

"I leave it to you, Doc, whatever you say."

Feldman takes Greenberg's blood pressure, checks his pulse, listens to his chest.

"Ay. Ay. Ay. It hurts me terrible," Greenberg grunts suddenly, clutching his stumps. Feldman takes out a brown bag and extracts five new bottles of pills and two bottles of liquid medication.

"I got to take a pill," Greenberg moans.

"Chest pain? Take one."

"It takes a minute sometimes, sometimes a little more for me to feel better. It doesn't stop right away."

Feldman gives him the flu vaccine and takes a blood sample. Greenberg seems unaware of what is going on; he stares emptily at a wall.

"For more than nineteen years I've lived here," he tells Feldman. "I should get out of here altogether. But I'm sick and my wife is now sick too."

Feldman produces a form for Greenberg to sign, to confirm the fact that he's received the flu shot.

"You have to sign this," Feldman tells him.

"For what?"

"The shot."

"It's maybe an experiment? I'll die from it?"

"No. Just to say you got it, that's all."

"I got it. I'll sign. Okay."

He picks up a pen. "I can't write with this hand. It moves away on me," he says. He signs.

"Ay, it hurts me terrible. The legs."

Feldman makes notes in Greenberg's chart, while Greenberg stares at him silently, as if he now realizes that Feldman's visit is almost over. Feldman moves slightly, as if to get up.

"When I feel very tired to close my eyes, I feel like I pass out," Greenberg says. "I open my eyes and feel better, but then I can't sleep."

"Take a Librium before you go to bed," Feldman says, remaining in his chair, understanding the man's need for his concern.

"For how long?"

"Until your wife comes home."

"Also, why when I pass water it takes so much time?" Greenberg is leaning out of his wheelchair, his face close to Feldman's. "I should be scared of it?"

"Don't worry. It's age and being a man. The prostate. If it gets worse, we'll do something about it."

"If I'll have more trouble, I'll tell you," Greenberg says, the grimace of accumulated loss frozen on his face. It is 2:30 and Feldman must leave for his next stop. He shakes Greenberg's hand, walks down the stairs of the shabby slum building, mumbling, "What happens to people in this city . . ."

The next stop is in the East Village. In a crumbling, neglected tenement, Feldman finds Maria Diaz, a 78-year-old woman who has lung and heart trouble and high blood pressure. Feldman is greeted by her dog and a man; he may be her husband, her brother, her son. Feldman doesn't know. Mrs. Diaz, in a baggy, pale-blue housedress, is all bones and wrinkled skin, a tiny, emaciated creature. Her hair is multicolored, as if the subject of a hairdresser's experiment. Her face, the skin tightened, the features exaggerated, is like a caricature. She is very happy to see Feldman and she smiles and waves at him when he walks in. She has a bowl of stew beside her.

"Ah, you're eating. That's good," Feldman says, smiling. "You weren't eating when I saw you two weeks ago."

Mrs. Diaz gurgles in laughter. Feldman speaks to her in minimal Spanish, which he learned treating Chicanos at Los Angeles County Hospital clinic. He takes her blood pressure, checks her pulse.

The apartment is very small, two claustrophobic rooms connected by a narrow doorway; one room is the kitchen, with a dining table; and the other, slightly larger, contains two large chairs and a sofa, all covered in different floral patterns. Mrs. Diaz has three radios and two television sets in the larger room. The walls are pink. On them hang a photo of John F. Kennedy and his wife, several travel pictures and a calendar from a local Latin grocery store.

Feldman has brought a bag containing several bottles of Gelusil and several bottles of pills. He asks Mrs. Diaz if she wants a flu shot.

"*Sí,*" she says, smiling.

"*Un poquito de dolor,*" Feldman warns her, just before she feels the sting of the injection. He takes a blood sample, then she signs the form for the flu shot. While Feldman makes notes on her chart, she resumes eating her stew, her quivering hand making the spoon clatter against the plastic dish.

A few minutes before 4 P.M., Feldman leaves. The driver has waited for him outside in the station wagon. When Feldman gets into the car, he is grim.

"Slums a few blocks away from luxury," he says. The driver continues to drive, humming a private tune.

"These people can't help where they are," Feldman says, "and unless this society changes . . ." His voice trails off, as the car pulls up to Mrs. Hearn's apartment, near Bellevue.

For some patients, there is a special bond to Bellevue. For a few, it is their primary contact with the world. For at least one, it is crucial.

Margaret Hearn is 99 years old and every time she enters Bellevue the residents wonder if she'll be discharged again. She lives alone, a few blocks from the hospital in a renovated small apartment her friends at Bellevue helped her find. She is hard of hearing and her vision is fading. She has been treated for TB and heart trouble and has undergone surgery.

Miraculously, she is not visibly senile. She greets Feldman in a floor-length red-flannel robe, white socks and pink slippers. Her face is freshly powdered, and she wears a short gray wig. She holds a glass of sherry, places a second on a table for Feldman. He does not examine her. Instead, he sits and listens.

She entered Bellevue, she tells him, for the first time twenty years ago. She remembers every moment of it. She found friends there. She has no relatives and only one friend outside the hospital; that friend is entrusted with her possessions and their distribution after her death. Her friends at Bellevue are her support, her audience, her aides. They treat her ailments, sip tea or sherry with her, take her shopping, send her postcards, give her presents.

"When I first came to Bellevue twenty years ago, I was living on Seventy-third Street and I was a dressmaker. I was working very hard and then one day I felt I couldn't work any more. I called my doctor at nine o'clock at night and at ten I was at Bellevue," she remembers.

"They really didn't think I would live, but here I am. I was there for five months that first time, then released, but Bellevue never dropped me. I've been in and out of there many times and they've always been perfectly wonderful to me. It's really beyond expression."

She gets up, shuffles slowly across the room, returns with a greeting card, a photograph of four cheerful children in a Christmas setting. On the back is a message from a doctor who treated her years ago; he is no longer at Bellevue, but he keeps in touch.

"The doctors are my friends, my good friends, my personal friends," Mrs. Hearn says. "I remember once I was on the Chest Service and it was Christmas Eve. I asked the doctor if I could go home. I lived alone and he told me he didn't want me to go out there in the cold by myself. A friend of mine came to visit me, with a present, and offered to take me home. Then the doctor agreed. It was a bitter, bitter night, don't you know. But the doctor took us both in a cab, with my medicine, and got us home. It was very cold out and it took him a long time to find a cab, but he did it. I didn't even know his name and I thought, 'That was a wonderful man.' Super service I'd say. I've found many doctors like that at Bellevue, who gave me service beyond what you'd expect."

She wonders if Feldman believes her. She is conscious of the lavish nature of her praise. He smiles at her, without interrupting.

"I speak of them all as being remarkable and they *are.* You know, I just can't understand why Bellevue has had such a black eye. Even I wouldn't have gone there all those years ago if I had a choice. But I've been saved there, a couple of times, from passing on. Once, I remember, I was in bed, flat, and my doctor was just sitting beside the bed in a chair, watching me, and I almost think I passed on then. I don't know why, but I think the doctor knew it too. He just sat there and sort of helped me through it. Another time I was in Bellevue and my rent was due and my doctor sent his personal check for it."

She sips her sherry deliberately, her head bent forward. Around her apartment, pictures of cats and landscapes are scattered over the walls and ancient furniture sits on the bare floors, in varying degrees of disrepair.

She points to an old beach lounge chair she found on the street and explains how she repaired it, bought new webbing for it and sewed it in. A Bellevue nurse helped her carry the lounge from a pile on the street into her apartment.

"Outstanding people, that's what they are," Mrs. Hearn continues. "Some of the doctors I've known have retired, of course. But always, they attend to you medically and personally; if you've got a problem, they try to eradicate it. The nurses, too. I never met a nurse who was anything but nice. Never. I couldn't mention one disservice. Not one. I loved every one of them and they loved me."

She still cooks for herself, still serves visitors, still sews. The details of her past are vague. A husband who died when she was very young, no remarriage, a career to keep her busy ("Without that," she says to Feldman, "it is hard to live"). Yet without the friends at Bellevue, she insists, and their medicine, she would be lost.

"To me, there's nothing more wonderful than Bellevue," she says, affirming it with a shake of her wrinkled face, a slight motion of her aged and leathery arms. "The people there have gone to the greatest lengths to help me, outside of what they're supposed to do. I've never seen anything like it. Even in a gilded atmosphere, I couldn't have more.

"One last thing. I used to live on the ground floor of what you'd have to call a tenement. The doctors at Bellevue thought I needed fresh air and sunshine and they worked with a social worker there to find me this place. Amazing, I'd say. It just isn't the usual sort of treatment, don't you know."

Feldman thanks her for the sherry, which he hasn't finished, gently clasps her hand and leaves.

When patients in Pediatrics are sick, they're often too young to talk about it. They suffer in silence. When they get better, they may not be able to express that either, but they may smile or want to play with the doctor. For Sol Zimmerman, those rewards are more than enough.

Zimmerman, born in the Bronx in 1948, went to Columbia and N.Y.U. Medical School. He is now in his second year in Pediatrics. He did not go into the field to be a father figure.

"I was an only child," he says, "and when you are, you look for other children. What better way to find them than in Pediatrics? It's a field in which the prognosis is better. I don't usually have to deal with degenerative diseases. And I get the satisfaction of doing something for a child, from premature infants to kids nineteen years old. At their best when they're very young, when they get better, they want to play with you. That's when this is the most fun for me."

Zimmerman is short (five feet seven) and stocky (170 pounds). He dresses in vivid shirts and ties, along with the standard white pants. He is smart and confident, a combination of scholarly and diagnostic skills. He is married to a high school English teacher, and they live near Bellevue. His salary is $14,700 a year, in the mid-range of residents' pay.

For Zimmerman, the day begins at 7:30 A.M., with rounds in

the Pediatrics ICU on G–8, the top floor of one of Bellevue's old buildings. Pediatrics has space on several floors; Zimmerman's zone of duty keeps him pounding the corridor between the ICU and the Premature Care Unit not far away.

Zimmerman joins the chief resident, a senior resident and another first-year resident in the ICU. It is a small, orderly, immaculate room, extremely well equipped. Most of the small babies are in the main area itself; two isolation rooms are held in readiness at the far end of the ICU. A nursing station, as spotless as the kitchen in a model home, dominates the room.

Today the group of doctors tours the ICU, going from infant to infant. The first to be seen are premature twins, a boy and a girl, who were born four to five weeks before the normal gestation period of forty weeks (thirty-eight to forty-two is the range). There were complications and, as Zimmerman tells the others, "they have been chugging along for twenty-eight days, a long time to be on a respirator." Both infants are on respirators, their link to life. Without the respirators, they might die; with them, damage can be done, exposing them to the risk of chronic pulmonary disease. Both have trach tubes, another risk, prolonged use can lead to erosion of the trachea. Both are being monitored closely, twenty-four hours a day. Nurses keep in motion in the ICU. In fact, what ICU means, as far as Zimmerman is concerned, is intensive nursing care.

Zimmerman, who was on duty last night, reports that the parents of the twins came to visit the babies, not long after the boy had begun to have respiratory distress. The mother seemed oblivious to their condition. She kept repeating to Zimmerman how lovely the girl's hair looked, how pink the boy's skin was, how strong and filled out he seemed. Zimmerman knew that the boy was not filling out, but was edematous. He felt obliged to explain to the parents and took them to an empty isolation room. It took him forty-five minutes, and when it was over, Zimmerman wasn't certain he had penetrated the mother's tenaciously maintained façade. The father seemed to understand. Zimmerman told them that based on his experience babies on respirators for weeks rarely survive. The girl, he told them, was born essentially dead, without a supply of oxygen to the brain. "If we can feed her, make her stronger, she might get off the respirator," he told the parents, "but it isn't likely." The boy had shown early improvement, but then cardiac failure intervened, changing the prognosis. The boy was too sick, too weak, for diagnostic tests so the type of cardiac problem remained undiagnosed. The father was depressed, but did not debate Zimmerman's findings. The mother was unwilling to accept them.

"I'm worried about my babies and feeling guilty and can't sleep," she told Zimmerman. "Isn't there something you can do?"

"All I could say to her was that there was nothing for her to feel guilty about," Zimmerman said.

His report to the other doctors concluded, the group glides over to another baby: a three-month-old girl, at Bellevue since birth, suffering from a thoracic deformity, a cleft palate and enlarged tongue, impairing breathing, as well as orthopedic difficulties and possible chromosome abnormality. In some cases of severe deformity, Zimmerman tells the others, the parents don't want the child to survive. Zimmerman won't give up on her. She is on a trach tube, so she can breathe by bypassing that troublesome tongue and, as he puts it, "If she can breathe, she can live." In Zimmerman's opinion, if she can be kept alive, surgery can be done to correct some of her problems.

The next patient is a beautiful 10-month-old girl with a Gerber baby food face. She weighs seventeen pounds. She was brought to the hospital by her parents; she had second-degree burns on the lower part of her body, additional burns on her legs and feet. The parents insisted that when they gave her a bath, patches of skin fell off. In a variation on that story, the father said he was bathing her with lukewarm water when the cold water suddenly went off, scalding her. Her temperature when she was admitted was 94; she had no palpable pulse, was not urinating, was moribund.

Zimmerman, unconvinced by the parents' explanation, had little time to refute it, because the child demanded his attention. Now, after several days of treatment in the ICU, the child's vital signs are stable. She's been sedated with paregoric. She is alert at times. Antibiotics have been employed, but she remains septic, vulnerable to an undiagnosed infection that plagues her, and the medical staff has been at work on that riddle, often tough to solve in small children. As the doctors look at her, she clutches a molded yellow plastic cat, and whimpers.

In one of the isolation rooms, Kal Post, from Neurosurgery, is examining an 8-year-old boy who has had a clot removed from his brain. He is Neurosurgery's case, but the Pediatrics ICU is where he can get the best care. Zimmerman and the other doctors nod to Post and move on from the ICU to the Premature Care Unit (and high-risk nursery).

Bellevue's Premature Care Unit is one of the best in the country and hospitals throughout the city refer cases to it. There are two interns on duty (they report to Zimmerman) and eighteen babies, most of them in incubators. There are two sets of twins, growing slowly, and the son of a heroin-addict mother who admitted taking a dose shortly before giving birth. This means a withdrawal problem for the baby, who has been vomiting and suffering from the characteristic symptom, the jitters, a relentless shaking of arms and legs. Another patient is Kal Post's premature son, his weight is up, he's doing well and he may go home this week. As Zimmerman and the others stroll through, Post pops in, quickly, to smile at his son.

When Zimmerman has covered each child in his running explanation, the other doctors scatter; they have work to do elsewhere in Pediatrics and Zimmerman will take care of the ICU and the Premature Care Unit, summoning help only if he truly needs it.

At 8:45 A.M., he checks the delivery schedule in Obstetrics. The two services collaborate; at every birth having possible complications, someone from Pediatrics is on hand to inherit the baby. Then he visits the nursery, to look at the newborn infants, in search of any problem children who may arrive in the ICU or the Premature Unit later.

The nursery is a bright, neat and cheerful place. From the nursing station at the entrance, to the examining area nearby, to the four connected rooms filled with babies, it is the world of the newborn. They are not made to wait for affection; the nurses and the doctors provide it constantly, picking up the babies, fondling them, feeding them, washing them. Often, the only sound is the gentle one of babies sleeping. Hunger and sickness make them cry. There are thirteen infants in the nursery today, including two nervously flailing babies who may be in withdrawal. At 9:30, Zimmerman is back at the ICU, where five nurses are quietly busy, caring for the patients.

Although Zimmerman devotes most of his day to the Premature Unit, which is his primary responsibility, and the ICU, he cannot resist the temptation to visit babies he's cared for in both places after they're transferred to a ward. He checks the wards, occasionally, to see how they're doing.

Today, he sees an 18-month-old boy who was in the ICU with pneumonia, had to have a collapsed lobe in one lung removed surgically. When Zimmerman walks up to his bed, the baby smiles. Zimmerman caresses his face, says, "You look good, nudnick," and gives him a loud kiss on the cheek.

A nurse is holding a 2-year-old boy and Zimmerman spots him. The boy was normal until one night a year ago when, suddenly, his temperature shot up to 106 and he began having seizures. Rushed to Bellevue, he was found to have a herniated brain (part of the brain had expanded into the available space around it) and a large, rock-hard liver. Most of the tests done were negative, but the boy remained retarded and spastic. His parents, shocked by what had happened and in despair, signed all the forms required to delegate the boy's care to Bellevue. Then they moved out of the city. This made the boy a ward of the city. It was not a move that Zimmerman urged or endorsed; he doesn't feel that Bellevue should serve as caretaker.

Throughout the ward, student nurses are holding, fondling, playing with the children. Without the presence of charts and beds it would pass for a day care center run by a group of particularly loving women. Zimmerman pauses at the bed of a small boy, 16 months old, who is yellow-green in color and has a conspicuously protruding abdomen. He suffers from a bile duct obstruction and has had ten massive GI (gastrointestinal) bleeds within a few months. His mother had been bringing him into the clinic every day, finally gave up and brought him in to stay. She has told Zimmerman that she can't endure it any more, that she assumes the boy will die at Bellevue. Zimmerman knows that she is probably correct. Further transfusions are futile, so the boy is being kept comfortable, on morphine and Demerol.

As Zimmerman walks through the ward, looking for familiar faces, he sees a small girl smiling at him. "Ah, that's one of our ICU saves," he says to a student nurse. The girl had been in the ICU near death, but was pulled through. She is now a spastic paraplegic; she can't move her legs. But she is alive.

In a room near the entrance to the ward, Zimmerman notices

a new admission, a newborn baby found in a shopping bag in the dress racks at Klein's department store. The baby, fully clothed and with its umbilical cord tied with a piece of string, was found by a nurse who was looking at dresses and was brought to Bellevue by police. The baby was jittery, a possible indication that an addict-mother had abandoned it. The baby is now doing well, a nurse reports to Zimmerman; the case has been turned over to the Bureau of Child Welfare. On the baby's bed, the sign reads "Baby Klein."

Most of the babies that Zimmerman deals with survive and most of those prosper. But the work in Pediatrics makes demands on a doctor who loves children, as Zimmerman does.

"We can have a baby die suddenly, without a sign of infection, so we're quick to completely culture a child, including a spinal tap," Zimmerman tells a medical student who has joined him.

"Mothers can have infections and this is one of those areas where we're in conflict with OB. It would help us if they would get cultures on the mothers, too, instead of simply giving an antibiotic which might mask the infection when we examine the baby. It's a matter of extra care, better communication and good judgment."

It is 10:15 now, time for Zimmerman to make rounds with one of the attendings who rotate in Pediatrics. In the ICU, the attending looks at the small girl with multiple problems and says that he thinks she should remain breathing through the trach tube for a year, until she's old enough for surgery. Zimmerman tells him that the baby's father isn't willing. He told Zimmerman that he expects the baby to die or get better and can't seem to deal with an in-between status.

In the Premature Unit, the attending sees several infants, confers with interns. As he leaves, he passes a bulletin board completely covered by photos of Premature Unit graduates, babies who got through the crises of the first harrowing days of life and have thrived.

At 11:45, Zimmerman meets with the Premature Unit's nursing supervisor, who tells him that one of the interns is sluggish; according to her, he resists the nurses' calls for aid. "There's no question," Zimmerman says. "You don't have to elaborate." He pages the doctor in question, gets him on the phone, tells him to shape up.

In the background, one of the senior residents, a jolly, chubby woman, is examining a rash on the bottom of a tiny, active baby. She picks it up, hugs it gently, kisses it and says, "You're the one I want to keep."

After a quick lunch, Zimmerman stops off at the nursery, where an intern is giving a newborn a spinal tap. The baby is suspected of being in withdrawal; it is irritable, shaking. "They can be very irritable," the intern says to a nurse. "And they can easily cry all night, even despite phenobarb. Often, when we let them go home, they're the victims of abuse by mothers who are annoyed because the baby is so irritable."

Zimmerman tours the nursery quickly, then heads back to the Premature Unit. There is a problem to greet him. A premature black baby seems to be failing. A stool specimen is suspicious, full of mucus and blood, and Zimmerman fears that it may be a case of the bowel lining peeling away. The baby has an infection, despite doses of antibiotics, and Zimmerman is worried. He checks a recent X-ray, which shows a normal bowel. He takes the picture to Pediatrics Radiology, where the radiologist finds nothing alarming. Zimmerman, still concerned, returns to the Premature Unit. "You'd hate to miss it," he tells an intern, explaining why he wanted another opinion. "And in a medical center like this, you ought to take advantage of whatever services you've got."

A resident from Surgery arrives to take a look at the baby. He finds the abdomen benign, doesn't see anything that might demand his services later.

"In case something happens, you've seen the baby," Zimmerman says to him. "And we won't have to waste time explaining the case."

The surgeon lingers and Zimmerman tells him a story about a child he treated recently.

"She was a six-year-old girl and she was inseparable from her doll. She wouldn't do anything for us unless we did it to her doll first. The doll had an IV taped to its arm and an oxygen mask on its face. And when the girl got better, we had to make the doll better, too, or she wouldn't leave the hospital. It was a game, sure, but a fun game for all of us."

The surgeon's beeper goes off and he leaves. Kal Post, who has checked the 8-year-old boy with possible brain damage in the ICU again, drifts in to take another look at his own son. Zimmerman waves at him, resumes his conversation, with an intern replacing the surgeon.

"It isn't always a game. Babies who were pink and healthy and alert and kicking have turned blue and died on us in seconds. Many of the deaths are anticipated. You've told the parents that the patient is not good, so it isn't a complete shock, even if they're unwilling to accept it, which can be the case.

"One father whose daughter had been in here fourteen times in nine months didn't want her to go home again. Then she came in for what I knew would be the last time. The father and the mother came in and I tried to tell them that this would probably be her last visit. Then I had to tell them that the baby had died. The mother wouldn't believe me. 'Surely, there are plenty of things you can do,' she said to me. I had to convince them both that the child was gone. And the mother kept saying, 'Certainly there is something you will do.'

"I once told a father, on the phone, that his baby was doing well. The guy was an older man and his wife was in her forties, too, and they had waited for years to have this baby and the baby was premature and, at first, not doing very well.

"Then things improved and I told the father about it on the phone. I hung up and walked over to the baby to take a look at it. It was dead. God, how could I call back the father? It was an instantaneous death. Very rare and very horrible."

It is now 3:30 and time for Zimmerman to join the other residents in sign-off rounds, to acquaint the new staff coming on duty with the acute problems present.

As they begin the rounds in the ICU, where new nurses are arriving for the evening shift, an intern informs Zimmerman that one of the babies in the nursery will be coming up to the Premature Unit. The baby, the intern says, is suffering from a calcium deficiency, heroin withdrawal and congenital syphilis.

"That's an unlucky kid," Zimmerman says.

Tonight, Zimmerman will be on ICU duty. Although the walking may be limited to the one room, there are monitors to check, oxygen to regulate, drugs to administer, babies to observe closely.

Mary Anne Williamson is unique at Bellevue. She would be unique at almost any hospital. She is a woman, a surgeon and a nun.

A short, green-eyed blonde with a cheerful, round face and

an accent that confirms her Brooklyn-Queens upbringing, she is one of the chief residents in Surgery. Born in Brooklyn in 1937, she moved to Queens, went to high school at St. Mary's Academy in Providence, Rhode Island, and to college at Emmanuel College in Boston. It was at Emmanuel that she realized she wanted to be a nun. She became Sister Mary of the Franciscan Missionaries of Mary. She continued her studies as well, in chemistry at Fordham and in medical school at St. Louis University. She got her M.D. in 1969 and became an intern in Surgery at Bellevue.

She is now in her final year of the five-year program in surgery at Bellevue. She is known as Doctor, Sister Mary or simply Mary. She wears the white skirt and jacket of the doctor on rounds, the surgeon's green scrub suit in the operating room, her nun's habit out in the world. The money she earns goes to the order, to educate younger sisters, just as the order provided the money for her education.

Her aim is to work in a missionary hospital in Africa; her order maintains such a hospital in Ghana. She visited it in 1971 and became convinced. After Bellevue, she'll be in West Africa indefinitely.

Her day begins in prayer at the order's residence on East Forty-fifth Street. Then, at 6:15, she is at Bellevue, to make rounds. After rounds, she manages to eat breakfast in fifteen minutes, enabling her to arrive at the OR by 8 A.M. Her day from that moment on takes place largely in the OR. As one of the chief residents, she operates steadily, making rounds and being on call at night as well.

Two floors, eight and nine, house Surgery's operating rooms. The daily operating schedules are posted the previous afternoon, based on requests surgeons make for the ORs. The ORs themselves are germ-free green and steel constructions, brightly lit.

In a five-day week, there may be more than 150 operations performed. The general Surgery group, which includes Williamson, may be doing—to sample a week's schedule—operations including: cholecystectomy, bilateral stripping and ligation, below-knee amputation, repair of incisional hernia, excision of lipoma, skin grafts, biopsies, hemorrhoidectomy, gastrectomy, resection of great toe and surgical treatment of an abscess.

The subspecialties are busy in the ORs, too, including GYN, cardiology, plastic surgery, neurosurgery, eye surgery, oral surgery, ENT (Ear-Nose-Throat), among others. The schedules do not include the constant flow of emergency surgery cases at Bellevue.

Williamson can find herself in the OR, for procedures that take from minutes to as long as twelve hours, more than twenty times a week. She thrives on it. She is very happy she chose surgery.

"There may be a group personality about surgeons, I suppose," she says. "The sort of people who are surgeons are oriented to doing or getting involved rather than reflecting or directing. A surgeon has to have some aggressive drive, a determination. But he *must* have it to make decisions quickly without having time to reflect. I think you need this sort of quality to go into the field, to deal with patients in a physical way, maybe even sacrificing human interaction. But you really don't have to be impersonal. When you do interact with patients, you sometimes become a kind of life-giving figure. We wear ourselves out, without enough sleep, for hours in the OR so someone else may live and be healthy. That's a very real, very warm thing. To slave over others and pull them through as if they were your own children."

She hopes that, in addition to being a skilled surgeon, she is a good doctor, as she defines it: "A sincere devotion to patients, however you can express it. Intelligence. The willingness to work intellectually to find the answers you need. Humility. Being humble enough to realize what you don't know."

Her beliefs are tested daily. Today, after 6:15 rounds and her fifteen-minute breakfast, she's on the ninth-floor OR labyrinth at 8 A.M., ready for her first operation: to repair a hernia in the incision of a previous gastrectomy, on a 45-year-old Puerto Rican man. She will remove scar tissue and repair the abdominal wall, to correct the hernia.

At 8:15, two Oriental nurse-anesthetists are at work on the patient, who is conspicuously overweight. He is calm. Once he seems unconscious, an anesthetist intubates him. He moves. One of the residents who has joined Williamson for the operation stares at the anesthetist and says, "The patient is awake. Give him some more."

The anesthetist obliges and completes the intubation, which

enables oxygen to flow into the patient's lungs during the operation.

Williamson cleanses the patient's abdomen from chest to pelvis; the flesh moves in waves as she swabs. A third-year resident will do much of the actual work in this case; he bathes the patient's abdomen in Betadine. The patient is then draped with green sterile cloth, leaving exposed only a strip of flesh running vertically down the abdomen.

The resident sees a stray hair on the patient's abdomen; he picks it off with a clamp and throws the hair and the clamp on the floor. A nurse picks up the clamp and scowls. Williamson has gotten into a long surgical gown and gloves and steps up on a stool for a better view of the patient.

The resident opens, running a scalpel lightly along the route of the earlier incision. The resident and Williamson are forehead to forehead above the patient. The incision, now oozing blood which is quickly sponged, is almost a foot long. The resident carefully trims, stretches and removes a long strip of scar tissue and cauterizes blood vessels. A black scrub nurse at the foot of the table masterminds the instrument tray, passing them on command. The resident moves his scalpel delicately and the incision deepens. Except for an occasional request for an instrument, no one speaks.

At 8:50, the team is into the man's abdomen. Using surgical scissors and snipping tissue bit by bit, the resident exposes the man's intestines, which seem to be groping for air, protruding like a large, pink snake. At 9:15, Williamson breaks the silence. "We're getting there," she says.

A nurse repositions the large light above the table; it is shaped like a searchlight. She does it with a sterile cloth, so she won't contaminate her gloves, then the instruments. The two anesthetists peer over the green drape shielding the patient's head from the surgeons, watching intently. The tissue on one side of the incision has been clamped, trimmed, pulled over in a flap. Tissue samples are sent to Pathology for analysis. Williamson asks for "warm saline, please."

The saline is squirted into the incision, then the area is suctioned. Permanent stainless-steel wire sutures are used to close the primary incision.

"This is a tedious operation," Williamson says, as the resident labors with a large curved needle and the steel sutures. He inserts the sutures and Williamson pulls them taut.

She tells the nurse to get the next patient ready. It will be the same operation, basically, but with a smaller incision. It is 10 A.M. and the suturing proceeds. Williamson puts on a second pair of gloves over the first, which have become too slippery. A retractor holds down the intestines while the suturing goes on, so the procedure, when completed, will guarantee that the intestines remain in place and do not herniate again.

"Is the next patient here?" Williamson asks.

"Outside," says the nurse.

Williamson notes, with pleasure, that a nun, two Orientals, a black nurse and a Jewish resident have been operating on a Puerto Rican.

The newly sewn incision is flushed with saline; the outer edges of the skin above it are sewn, too. Williamson and the resident work at it simultaneously, silently, using straight needles, sutures and an Adson forceps (resembling a large tweezer) for neater skin closure. At 10:50, the incision is almost closed and Williamson leaves the rest to the resident, who finishes within ten minutes. The incision is taped down. The patient, slowly waking up, is wheeled out of the OR at 11:15, to make way for the next hernia case, a 43 year old man.

At 11:30, the patient is on the table; the operating room has been cleaned, new instruments brought in and a new resident has joined Williamson. They peer at the patient.

"What are your plans?" she asks.

He answers by pointing to an old incision on the patient's abdomen, drawing a line down it with his scalpel. Three medical students have scrubbed in, to observe. The patient still has a few old stitches in him; the resident removes them. This is a smaller incision than the previous one, not much longer than four inches. There is more bleeding, however. Suction is used. Blood vessels are tied off. Tissue is sliced away.

Williamson looks at the cardiac monitor, supposedly watched by the nurse-anesthetist. It shows signs of cardiac arrest.

"Give him one hundred mg. of Xylocaine and ventilate him," Williamson shouts at the anesthetist. "He won't die of this," she says, pointing to the incision, "but he could die of that," pointing to the monitor. "Why didn't you tell us?" she says. "We could be fixing a hernia on a dead patient."

The anesthetist is rattled. "I call for my attending," she says.

"We can't wait," Williamson insists.

A second anesthetist puts the Xylocaine into the IV line. Williamson glares at the cardiac monitor. The operation resumes and is done, quickly. "When he gets to the recovery room, one of you do a cardiogram on him," Williamson tells a medical student.

At that moment, the resident announces that there may be a needle missing.

"Oh, no. Stop. Count them," Williamson says.

"We've got three," the scrub nurse says.

"How many did we have?" Williamson asks.

"Three," the nurse answers.

The three relax, momentarily.

"Call the ICU for the next patient and get him ready," Williamson tells a nurse.

A Housekeeping aide, a middle-aged black man, mops the floor of the operating room.

Williamson hasn't time for lunch. She finds an apple and devours it, waiting for the next patient to arrive.

Williamson's next patient is an 18-year-old boy who suffered burns on 80 percent of his body in a gasoline fire. He was cleaning a stove with it when it ignited. If he had not been young and healthy, he might have died, from loss of fluid leading to shock or from infection. As it is, he is in bad shape. Today's operation, the first of several Williamson plans to do, will débride him, remove dead tissue, and put pigskin on the burned area débrided.

She has not quite forgotten about the possible cardiac arrest during the last operation. "If you know something's wrong, you stop, you wait," she says to a resident. "You know that the risk of anesthesia can be greater than the risk of surgery."

She is distracted from that thought by the arrival of the burned boy. She talks to a resident about the use of pigskin. Once the dead tissue is removed, the pigskin is applied. It will "take" temporarily, before the body rejects it within five or six days. It protects the burned area, holding down the bacteria count. If the pigskin does take, the surgeon can assume that the patient's own skin, when it is ready for grafting, will take, too. In second-degree burns, the patient's own skin can regenerate, creating his own graft supply. The pigskin is essential and is flown in from Arizona; it is costly, almost $20 per square foot.

Before the procedure begins, Williamson makes several phone calls, about pending cases. "It's a two-out-of-ten chance," she tells another doctor on the phone. "That's the best we can offer this man."

The burned boy is in bed. At the foot of the bed is a plastic mailing bucket with the pigskin in it. The patient himself looks like something out of a horror film.

His face is disfigured and multicolored, with skin hardened and flaking away. He tells Williamson that he wants to "feel" water in his mouth. He knows he cannot drink it. She doesn't want to take the chance. They talk about the procedure itself.

"I won't feel nuthin', right, Mrs. Williamson?" he asks.

"You'll be asleep," she says, "and we'll give you pain medicine afterward."

His eyes seem burned shut and he is quivering. "I'm freezin'," he says, "and I can't breathe too good. You give me some water. I'll clean my mouth and I'll spit it out, I promise."

Williamson avoids the request; it is not one she can grant. She turns to tell a nurse, "We'll work very quickly on this, as fast as we can. After an hour, the patient deteriorates and if we have to do this two or three times a week, with anesthesia, he'll risk other problems."

It is 1:15 and the patient is now in the OR. "Let's go," Williamson says. "Every minute counts." Two residents, three medical students, two anesthetists and two nurses are with her.

The operation is done in the bed the patient arrived in, to make it easier on him. There are very few areas of his body that are not burned. It is as if he wore fireproof shorts and shoes and nothing else.

One of the medical students begins trimming the patient's hair, first with a scissors, then with a razor. Williamson announces, "We want to get off the superficial layer and get it oozing."

The patient is anesthetized with Ketamine, IV, putting him in a trancelike state.

Two residents, using a Brown dermatome, an electrical instrument that looks like a large razor, start shaving away dead skin from the patient's calves. Dr. Williamson, with scalpel and forceps, begins scraping his forehead and face. The dermatome delicately carves away thin layers of skin, like papyrus. The residents move on, to thighs, arms, chest. The patient is covered with drops and rivulets of blood. He sticks out his tongue, slowly, runs it over his lips. Williamson and the residents apply strips of pigskin to the areas they've débrided.

"We'll leave them on for four or five days," she says. "We'll see how he does."

Now the patient's mouth is wide open, in an almost hallucinatory way. He does not utter a sound. Then, he closes his mouth, again very slowly, and moans, in his tortured dream, rhythmically.

A medical student asks about the advantage of using pigskin.

"There is some adhesion," Williamson tells him. "You'll see, the pigskin will stick."

The residents, helped by the students, wrap the patient in dressings. Sulfamylon cream is applied to all exposed areas. The patient, slowly coming out of the anesthesia, begins to quiver again within his cocoon of bandages. Several residents lift him from his bed to the operating table, where his back is worked on, while Williamson and a nurse make his bed. More dressings, more cream, and the patient is back in his bed. It is 2:40, almost time for Williamson to make rounds on the Surgery wards.

"That was pretty good, I'd say," she tells the others. "Thank you very much, everybody."

She turns to the patient, who is trembling, then to the resident who will be on the case. "Watch him tonight," she tells the resident. "He may be febrile and septic." The resident nods.

Williamson is weary, more from the exhaustion of concentration than from any drama inherent in what she's done. And her day is not over. After rounds, she'll be on duty tonight.

Tom Spencer is the assistant head nurse on the 4 P.M.-to-midnight shift in the Adult Emergency Service. Spencer is 37, tall and muscular, with short, prematurely gray hair and glasses. He followed a circuitous route to Bellevue. Born in Toledo, Ohio, he was 11 when his father died. He finished high school, went on to a medical laboratory school, which bored him. He spent four years as a Medical Corpsman in the Air Force, worked as a fireman on a railroad, as a worker in a glass factory. For two years, he worked with emotionally disturbed children; that experience convinced him that nursing would be a fruitful career. He came to Bellevue after being graduated from the Kings County Hospital Nursing School, in Brooklyn, in 1970.

Spencer, who is single, lives a spartan life. He pays $20 a month for his room at Bellevue; it will be adequate, he says, until he gets married.

"It's like the YMCA, with a bed, desk, all I really need."

His life keeps him within the confines of Bellevue most of the time, between the silence of his room and the bustle of the AES, one of the busiest places in Bellevue. The AES is a walk-in clinic until midafternoon, but is an emergency facility twenty-four hours a day. It is a one-story building, an architectural after-thought attached to the body of the Bellevue labyrinth, without style, strictly functional. It is where ambulances wait and where ambulances arrive. It is where the most serious cases, those in immediate need, are brought. It is a unique facility in the city in that it combines a clinic, emergency treatment area, an emergency ward, observation unit, laboratories and X-ray in one area.

When an ambulance screeches into the driveway to the AES double doors with its siren on, that is a signal to the doctors and nurses inside to rush forward. They must be ready.

From the central desk, where patients register, to a series of small examining rooms, to a shabby waiting room for the friends and relatives of those brought in, the AES is a work choreographed by a madman. Patients often lie on beds in the corridors, awaiting their turns at treatment.

Stab wounds, bullet wounds, suicide attempts, heart attacks, trauma cases, drug overdoses, all make their way from the streets of the city to the AES. The worst cases, demanding in-hospital care, bypass the AES to the Emergency Ward that adjoins it. Many of those who walk through the door are treated and sent home. Others are referred to an outpatient clinic. Some go to the wards of Bellevue. It is motion with progress and Spencer keeps in motion. His movements and his words are expeditious; he doesn't waste either.

When Spencer, dressed in white pants and white shirt, gets to the AES at 3:30, it is already crowded. There are patients on stretcher-beds—high, narrow, stretcher-sized mattresses on wheels—in the corridors. The triage nurse has begun to do her job: to screen patients, assigning priorities to their complaints, directing some to doctors immediately, telling others to wait.

"Triage" is the French military term for doing exactly that, with casualties of war.

Spencer's first move is to check out the equipment in the resuscitation room, which resembles a small operating room. The supply of Narcan, to counteract heroin or methadone overdoses, is adequate. "It wakes them up right away," Spencer says. "Great stuff." The staples include epinephrine, used for cardiac arrests, concentrated dextrose (50 percent solution) for diabetics in insulin shock, padded tongue blades for seizure victims. IV poles are ready, along with an EKG machine and several suction units.

Spencer makes a last-minute tour. Room 8b is called "the dirty room." It is used for the treatment of drug abscesses, Bowery bums, people suffering from bites (animal and human). Body lice can be troublesome. "So many doctors and nurses hate bugs," he says. There's a supply of Cuprex to delouse Bowery types and a nearby shower room in which to do it.

When Spencer pokes his head into 8b, there's a Puerto Rican woman in it, bathing her finger in a small basin. She tells Spencer that another woman bit her when they had a fight and she waited two days to have it looked at.

"A human bite is more dangerous than a dog bite," he tells her. "The human mouth is dirtier. Next time, come right in."

"Eef I gonna get in a fight, I don' want no bite. Ees bery painfool," she says. Spencer takes her blood pressure and notes it on her chart. A doctor will be in shortly to examine her. Spencer resumes his tour and is walking down the corridor when there is a loud voice from the front door of the AES. The triage nurse is shouting, "Gunshot!"

Spencer, another nurse and several doctors run to the door, where they surround a young Puerto Rican woman, her husband and some of their friends.

The husband explains, nervously, that he and his wife had gone to their neighborhood grocery store when two men, in a fight, began shooting. One of the bullets struck his wife in the right arm. Her blood streaks the floor, through a crude tourniquet someone had wisely tied to her arm. She is in pain, terrified, groaning and shrieking.

Spencer stays calm. He helps the woman into the resuscitation room. Pressure is applied to the wound, a small round opening in her arm. There are eight doctors and nurses working on the woman, who continues to scream. One of the doctors yells at a nurse, "Big syringe. Big syringe. Big syringe." A splint is put on the woman's arm. A male nurse's aide speaks to her in Spanish. Spencer checks her blood pressure and pulse. "Blood pressure 120 over 80, pulse 80. She's stable," he says.

Throughout this, another patient has been reclining on a bed in a corner of the room, watching. He is catatonic, destined for a trip to Psychiatry, and seems unaware of the excitement around him.

"Sorry we haven't gotten to you yet," Spencer says to him. The man doesn't seem to hear him.

The bullet is still in the woman's arm, but the bleeding has been controlled. She is taken to have an X-ray, to pinpoint the location of the bullet. Spencer thanks the doctor who supervised. "It's his first day here," he says to another nurse. Residents rotate through the AES as part of their Bellevue training, and it takes a while for many of them to get used to the pace, the sudden demands on their skills that the AES makes.

The other nurse asks Spencer what happened.

"She had a pumper, an arterial that was spurting. Good thing she had that tourniquet when she got here. They'll tie off that bleeder and the X-ray will show where the bullet is, so they can get it out. A minimal case for us. She could be home by tomorrow."

Spencer remembers the psychiatric patient and turns to talk to him. The man won't talk to Spencer, so he checks his chart. It reveals that he was brought in today by his parents, after he had lost the job he had held for ten years and fell into depression and succumbed to insomnia.

As Spencer is reading the chart, another nurse stops in the doorway and says, "Tom, get ready. There's a prisoner coming in. He could be dangerous."

Spencer resumes his walk around the AES. On his shift, all emergencies, real and imagined, come tumbling into the AES; after 5 P.M., most Bellevue clinics are closed.

In the Ear-Nose-Throat examining room, Spencer sees a resident from the ENT Service examining a young man, a black aged 18.

"Wow, Doctor, I mean this is really something," the man is saying. "It's that scratching. I ain't ever had nothing like that. I can't stop it." He points to his right ear.

The doctor probes with a thin instrument and extracts a cockroach, still flailing.

Spencer sees three patients in the Observation Unit. It is a ward in which patients stay who should be watched overnight, without having to be admitted to the hospital: asthma attacks, certain kinds of head traumas, Bowery drunks who can be seen by social workers in the morning.

At the long desk at the back of the AES, doctors assemble to get patient charts which have flowed to the desk from up front, where five clerks process patients rapidly. When patients arrive at the AES, they are given a number and a time of arrival. It is now 4:45 and thirteen patients have checked in since Spencer's shift began. Near the front desk, two hospital policemen keep an eye on the desk. Unarmed, they must anticipate trouble; they can't allow themselves to be surprised by it.

There are 124 members of the Bellevue Hospital police, chosen by civil service exams, as an arm of the Health and Hospitals Corporation. Fifty are on duty during the day, fewer on the evening and night shifts. They cover posts throughout the hospital, including the AES, the PAO and, during the day, the clinics. They patrol unarmed—guns frighten patients—the entire hospital, making rounds of all the hospital buildings, including basement and offices, and at night around the outside of the hospital.

The two on duty at the AES keep an eye on the front desk. If there is to be trouble, it can be spotted there. Anger, in some patients, can become threatening.

The triage nurse, an assignment that is rotated nightly among the AES evening staff, screens the patients at the front desk, sending them to one of the examining rooms inside. The doctors, first-year residents for the most part, work twelve-hour shifts. Spencer walks around, greeting them, so he knows who is on duty and they know that he is there if they need him.

In one of the examining rooms, he finds a young man who has been mugged. "They got three dollars," he says, "three fucking dollars. And I think they broke my nose."

"A doctor will be in in a minute," Spencer tells him.

The mother of the psychiatric patient stops Spencer in the hall. "My son is just nervous and exhausted, that's all. He should rest. He needs rest," she says.

"He should talk to a specialist in Psychiatry," Spencer tells her. "You can go with him. I'll get a messenger to take you both." The Psychiatry building, three blocks away, can be reached through a desolate underground passage; patients en route are accompanied by a messenger and a hospital policeman. For patients still in touch with reality their companionship in the tunnel is reassuring. The Bellevue basement is dark and menacing. Light bulbs glow ominously; steam pipes hiss. Cats chase mice. Puddles of unidentifiable ooze and grit-covered walls sustain a depressing mood.

"He's only thirty-four," the mother says, "and he's been over-worked."

Her husband, smaller than she, has crept up beside her, silently. He stares at Spencer, helplessly. A few feet away, a doctor is talking to a woman on a bed; she fainted and came to the AES alarmed.

"Let's talk for a second," the doctor says to her. "You can go home right now if you want to. But you should see a doctor. Your blood pressure is out of control. See your own doctor if that's what you want to do, but do it tomorrow. Passing out is not a good thing."

"Okay, I'll see my doctor tomorrow," she says, edging off the bed.

"Promise?"

"Promise."

She leaves, and as she does Spencer turns to the doctor and says, "She's a nice lady and she understands, but for every one we get with some sense, we get ten who don't have any."

"You're telling me?" the doctor asks, laughing.

Spencer gets a blanket for the psychiatric patient, drapes it over him, announcing that it is one of Bellevue's Civil War relics. The patient does not speak, but does smile at Spencer. The patient's parents stand vigilantly beside their son's bed. Spencer moves on.

A prisoner brought over from jail has swallowed a spoon to get out of jail and into Bellevue. He has done it before and Spencer recognizes him. The man is black, husky, surly; he is guarded by two policemen. "Here we go again," Spencer says. "We'll X-ray it as usual." As he goes to arrange the X-ray, he mutters, "Psychotic."

A few minutes later, he's back, going from patient to patient. A young pregnant woman with asthma needs medication.

Spencer summons a resident to see her. Two Orientals, one very old, one young, sit solemnly in an examining room. A grandfather and grandson. The old man has been complaining of abdominal pain and insomnia. His grandson, translating, tells Spencer that the old man has cancer, but he is afraid to tell him. The old man clutches his stomach. Spencer finds a hospital gown for the man, lifts him onto a bed in the room and signals for a doctor.

The AES at its busiest is like Lourdes, without the blessings, the rituals, the faith. Ambulances roll up to the front door. Patients walk in, on their own or with help. The flow is constant.

In the next room, Spencer sees a diabetic old Puerto Rican man with a gangrenous toe. He is in a wheelchair and Spencer bends over to remove his shoes. On one foot, the supposedly good one, there are only four toes. On the other, the conspicuously diseased toe is almost totally rotted. The old man's daughter tells Spencer that it happened "little by little."

"How? How? How?" Spencer asks, incredulous. "Diabetics have to be so careful with their feet as they get older. Sometimes just a little scratch will become infected and a diabetic's circulation may be poor. Do you understand that?"

The woman smiles and flaps her arms. A doctor enters and, with Spencer's aid, examines the man. He must be admitted to Surgery; the toe must be amputated.

It is now 6 P.M., time for Spencer to have dinner in the snack bar, more expensive but quieter than the doctors' cafeteria, with another male nurse, one who is new to the AES.

"For the first time in my life, I'm doing something that gives me a good feeling," Spencer says, in response to the other nurse's question about life in the AES.

"I don't have to tell you that in the old days there was a stigma attached to being a male nurse. You know, if you were one, everybody thought you were gay. That's vanishing.

"I remember once I thought I wanted to be on the police force, because my father had been in law enforcement and my brother is a policeman, but when I was rejected because I had a heart murmur, I was very happy to consider being a nurse."

Spencer tells the male nurse that he was one of three children in a lower-middle-class family. When his father was killed in an auto crash, his mother "did a super job of keeping the family together. My mother and baseball kept me out of trouble when my dad was killed. She was wonderful to me, and when I wasn't with her, I kept busy playing ball."

Spencer gets back from dinner in time to join four nurses and a doctor who have pinned an OD—a patient who has taken an overdose of drugs—to a table in the resuscitation room. The addict, who is young with dirty long hair, is thrashing.

"What did you take?" the doctor is screaming.

The addict refuses to answer.

"We don't know what he took," one of the nurses tells Spencer.

"Any pills on him?"

"No."

Spencer injects Narcan intramuscularly. The resident is trying to put an IV line in the addict's arm, to provide sodium bicarb in saline to flush out any poisons that may have reached the kidneys. The resident has missed the vein several times and the sheet underneath the patient is turning increasingly red.

The addict, now in a panic, urinates in his pants and moves wildly. A nurse holds his head down.

"Take it easy," the resident says to him. "Come on now, take it easy."

The addict vomits.

"Hold him on his side so he doesn't aspirate it," Spencer says.

"There aren't any pill fragments in it," a nurse comments.

"Okay, then let's give him more Narcan to stay on the safe side," the resident orders. A nurse injects it.

"He's groggy but fairly alert," Spencer says. "I don't think there's reason to worry."

The resident moves to another case.

"Frankly, I think he could have gotten along fine without that IV," one of the nurses, an older woman, says to Spencer.

"Some of these things just aren't necessary," Spencer agrees. The patient is washed, covered with a clean sheet and wheeled out. He is still now. Spencer will keep an eye on him.

The mother of the psychiatric patient comes in search of Spencer.

"I've decided to take him home. My son," she says. "It's been two hours now and there's no messenger and we're all nervous and exhausted and I want him to go home with us," she says.

"Okay, okay. We can't keep him here if you don't want him to be here. But you see to it that he sees his family doctor,"

Spencer tells the mother. As the trio leaves, he turns to the triage nurse and says, "If he had gone to Psych quickly, at least they could have talked to him. It annoys me."

Spencer is not easily irritated. He expresses his wrath simply, calmly. It takes extreme provocation to inspire him to curse.

In the Plastic Surgery room, an Oriental resident is putting a cast on the right arm of a black man, tall, skinny, with goatee, guarded by two policemen. The doctor works slowly, carefully, while the prisoner recites a monologue. Spencer stands in the doorway and listens.

"I'm Humphrey Bogart's bodyguard. I am. Indeed. Also, it is important for you to know that I am Jesus Christ, too. In fact, it is indisputable that I am the best people on earth. I am the king of the President. I can fire the President's ass, man. You can't hurt *me* with no bombs, baby."

At 8 P.M., a new crew of residents reports to the AES, relieving the previous group. A one-legged man, drunk, is wheeled in hallucinating. On his chart there is a familiar designation: AOB. Alcohol on breath.

A young woman, neatly dressed, has come to Bellevue from a restaurant in Greenwich Village. While munching a barbecued rib, she thinks she got a bone sliver in her throat.

An old woman went to the dedication of a new church and as she was going forward for communion, she tripped and fell, breaking her left arm.

The father of one of the drug overdose cases finds Spencer, who tells him that his son will be sent on to Psychiatry.

"You know, when he got off dope, he went on pills," the father says. "He started at fifteen or sixteen, then cut the heroin habit himself. So now it's pills."

"Here's the phone number in Psychiatry where you can check on how he's doing," Spencer tells the father, handing him a slip of paper. "It's important that he be detoxified slowly and carefully, because he could go into convulsions from abrupt withdrawal."

A well-dressed musician from Caracas, on tour in America, has come to Bellevue with an infected eye. He's gotten medication from a resident, but doesn't understand how to take it. Using a Spanish-speaking clerk as translator, Spencer conscientiously explains.

It is 9 P.M. and Spencer has not sat down since dinner. He

goes to the kitchen in the Observation Unit, where he finds a friend who works in the Blood Bank. They have a cup of coffee together.

"What's it like out there tonight?" the friend asks.

"It seems like a quiet one to me," Spencer says, "but I've never really been able to find a pattern."

After his coffee, Spencer walks up to the front desk, where an angry black man is arguing with one of the clerks. "Baby, you can just go fuck yourself," he screams at her. It is a cue for two hospital policemen to edge closer to him.

"I don't want to stay here," a black woman with a red Afro is shouting at the triage nurse.

"She should stay," one of the residents is arguing, "but we can't strap her down if she doesn't want to."

On a bed in the corridor, an old man, hoarse, wheezes, "I want my methadone. My methadone."

It is 9:40 and forty-one patients have come in since Spencer went on duty. The forty-second is another OD, also young.

The resident summoned injects Narcan, looks at the patient and says, "John, I saw you here just two weeks ago and a month before that. You're on downers again and you've been drinking." Spencer asks him what should be done.

"Not much now. He's in withdrawal. The symptoms are there. He'll be restless, then he'll sleep," the resident says. "You know that one night I had fourteen ODs. One ODed in the afternoon and we got him out of here by 8. He was back at 3 A.M."

The OD is wheeled out into the corridor, beside his predecessor. Both are snoring. Passing nurses will prod them periodically, to keep them conscious. It is a ritual.

At 10:10, Spencer checks the drug and narcotics supplies. They are kept in two locked rooms. A few minutes later, he hears a police-car siren getting louder and louder until its sound is pulsating through the front door of the AES. Spencer, several other nurses and two doctors rush to the driveway.

It is a stabbing victim, found by police on Bleecker Street. The man is a mass of blood. His throat has been cut and he has been stabbed in the stomach. He is wheeled directly into the Emergency Ward. Within seconds, he is surrounded by thirteen doctors and nurses, each one performing a separate, vital task. His clothes are cut away and discarded: his personal possessions collected. His intestines are protruding through a deep gash in his stomach.

A priest arrives. Blood transfusions are begun. Four IV units are going at once. The action around the man approaches controlled frenzy. One of the policemen who brought him in talks to a nurse about it.

"We got the call and raced over. Usually, when you get there you can see the body on the street. I didn't see one. I just saw this guy standing there, and when we pulled up, I could see that he had been slashed badly. He couldn't speak, but there he was standing there pointing down the street. Two of our plain-clothesmen went to chase a suspect, so we put this guy into our car, held a roll of toilet paper, which was all we had, against his throat and got him here."

"Who is he?" the nurse asks.

"I don't really know," the policeman answers. "I think he may be a merchant seaman, because we think he was staying at a hotel better than most of those on the Bowery. But he had only $2.55 in his pocket."

Around the table in the Emergency Ward, the EW staff has taken over. Shouts are heard:

"Venous or arterial?"

"Arterial."

"Second unit of blood. Fast."

"Blood pressure 70. It was 11 a few minutes ago."

"Steroids. Antibiotics. Blood."

"He aspirated some blood."

"Slashed trachea. External jugular cut."

A catheter is inserted into the man's penis, to drain his bladder. An X-ray machine is wheeled in. The patient begins to move.

"Take it easy. Don't move around. You're going to be all right," one of the Trauma doctors says to him. Everything has happened rapidly, with the Trauma team, surgeons especially trained for such emergencies, dominating the action. At 10:55, the patient is rushed up to the operating room, his condition stabilized for surgery. As he is pushed out of the EW, one of the policemen says, "Man, this place is the best. I mean the *best*. I thought he was fucking *gone*."

In the hallway outside the EW, two plainclothesmen are guarding the suspect. He is middle-aged, black, potbellied and calm. He is handcuffed, but he is not resisting. The police found a bloody knife on him, but no blood on his clothing. They wanted the victim to identify him, but he was too weak to do so. The plainclothesmen take him away.

Spencer, who has lingered in the EW to help out, walks back to the AES. A young man is soaking an infected finger in one room. In the hall, an OD awakens and tries to punch a nurse. A resident rushes up. "Cut it out, buddy," he says. "Just tell us what pills you took, that's all you have to do."

"It's none of your fucking business," the addict answers.

"Well, then take your fucking business somewhere else," the resident shouts at him.

A second resident, watching it all, tells the other, "You really do hate junkies, don't you?"

The first resident simply grunts.

"Let him sleep," Spencer intervenes. "If he gets active again, we'll tie him down." Spencer towers over the two residents, who look up at him and go their separate ways.

In the background, a resident is looking at a young attractive nurse. "Will you stop being so sexy?" he implores. She smiles at him, wiggles seductively.

It is 11:00 P.M. and the seventieth patient of the shift is registering. But the pace is beginning to slow down. A woman who slipped and fell in the subway is having her forehead stitched by a doctor, with Spencer's help.

At 11:25, a 16-year-old Puerto Rican girl is brought in by her agitated husband.

"She took some pills and she left me a paper," he tells the triage nurse.

"Let me out of here," his wife screams.

"What did you take?" Spencer asks her. "Tell us or we'll have to wash out your stomach."

"They were black," she says.

"What do you use them for?" Spencer asks her.

"My husband he uses them, to soak his hand. I took six of them at five o'clock and three more at nine."

One of the nurses standing nearby whispers, "Potassium permanganate."

The Puerto Rican girl begins to cry. In seconds, the nurse who guessed the nature of the pills has checked on remedies and is back. "Milk, fluids, activated charcoal. Looks to me like she took

45 grains and the lethal dose is 150," she says to Spencer.

Spencer pours Ipecac into a paper cup. "We have some syrup to give you," he tells the girl. "Don't sip it. Drink it down, like whiskey. We'll give you water, too."

She drinks the Ipecac. The others leave. The girl and Spencer are alone.

He holds her hand.

"You must have been very upset to take those pills," he says, softly.

She nods.

"Angry, too?"

She nods again.

"Well, I guess it all can get pretty complicated sometimes," he says. "But if I were you, I sure wouldn't try that again."

She smiles at him.

"That syrup may make you nauseous. You may want to throw up. Don't hold back. Let it go. You're going to be okay. We're here to help you, that's all."

He waves at her and walks out of the room; a nurse's aide takes his place, to watch the girl.

"Not a serious overdose," Spencer says to the nurse's aide as they exchange places. "But stay with her."

Spencer stands in the corridor. There is little activity; most of the examining rooms are empty. Several residents huddle together at the back desk; only four hours into a twelve-hour shift, they seem ready to collapse. Spencer notices that several other nurses have put on their coats and are leaving. He looks at his watch for the first time all night. It is midnight.

Mary Williamson is in the Surgical ICU at 5 P.M. A senior resident who had been waiting for her tells her that a patient she operated on is having trouble, a GI bleeder who is bleeding again. He also tells her that an attending told him that he felt one of the operations Williamson had performed was an example of "unnecessary surgery." Williamson tells the resident, calmly, that she doesn't agree. They drop the subject.

Another resident and a nurse are working on the GI bleeder, an old man, draining blood from his nasogastric tube, which winds its way through his nose into his stomach. The resident, frustrated, stops and runs out to the Blood Bank, to order units of blood for transfusions.

Williamson walks over to the bedside. Now there are three residents and two nurses around the bed. The old man is awake, in distress, frightened. He has a fringe of white hair and a face full of prominent features, out of Dickens. There are large, rubber retention stitches down his abdomen, from the previous operation Williamson performed in search of the source of the bleeding. He trembles as Williamson irrigates his esophagus with saline solution, through the tube. What returns is bloody. A nurse, suctioning his trach tube, comes up with blood, too. The patient's gown is spotted with it.

"He could be bleeding from everywhere," the senior resident comments.

"I think it is a localized lesion," Williamson says.

"Look at this!" the senior resident says, pointing to a large bottle of bloody fluid already suctioned. Williamson stares at it intently, then orders one of the residents to get eight more units of blood ready. The patient is crying, silently, distorting his face without emitting a sound. Williamson decides to have an angiogram done, sending dye through the femoral artery into the stomach, in an attempt to pinpoint the bleeding.

"Mac, we need an X-ray," the senior resident says to the patient. "You're bleeding again. We need your consent." The resident talks as if he were speaking into a cave.

The old man trembles but seems to understand. As he is gripping the pen, the resident waits impatiently. In a nearby bed, an old black man seems aroused. A nurse runs over to him.

"James, what are you doing?" she says to him. "Are you playing with yourself again?" She lifts the sheet, peers, says "yech" and walks away. The old black man has a demented smile on his face.

The senior resident waves the form in front of the old man again. The man makes an illegible scrawl across it, like an EKG graph gone berserk.

"Okay, Mac, it's the right thing. You understand," the senior resident says.

"I want the bedpan," the old man gargles.

Williamson studies the man, looks into space. "Suture-line bleeding is correctable. If that's what it is. Big varices? Well, we'll try to find out."

"Angio's ready," a resident shouts from the entrance to the ICU.

The crew around the bed mobilizes. They change the patient from his respirator to a hand-bagged air supply. They take a unit of oxygen along, to connect to a respirator in the Radiology room. It is a few steps down the hall. They are there in seconds.

A respiratory therapist is there, to monitor the patient's breathing. The radiologist is ready. Units of blood have arrived. The patient is bleeding from his trach tube; the plastic pipe from his neck to the respirator is starting to turn pink.

Incongruously, a small angel doll on a coiled wire spring dances from the ceiling in an arc over the table.

"What we need is a diagnosis for that bleeding, that terrible bleeding," Williamson says to the radiologist.

The angiogram begins.

At 6:50, Williamson rushes to dinner before the doctors' cafeteria closes. She races through it: fried liver, mashed potatoes, peas, a piece of bread with peanut butter and jelly on it, tea. As she's eating, smoke fills the cafeteria and a fire alarm goes off. She keeps eating. "Would you believe this?" she says to a resident at the same table. Slowly, the smoke vanishes.

She is conscious of the pace she sets. It deprives her of opportunities she wants. "You can get close to patients. You can laugh with them, meet their families. But it is a luxury in terms of time. There never seems to be enough time."

She returns to the ICU, to check the young boy she had done skin grafts on earlier in the day. A resident tells her that the boy is being investigated by the police, who suspect that he was attempting arson. The boy's story, that he was cleaning a stove, may be only partially correct, according to the police. They assert that he wanted the insurance money. If so, they say, he made two mistakes. The first was when he allowed his insurance to lapse.

Williamson talks to the resident about the old man undergoing the angiogram. "This man has been alert and awake for days. If he had been comatose and his chances were slim, you might call our effort meaningless. He *is* an old man and he *is* very sick. I think it is meaningful, however, if we can buy time for a terminal patient. You can buy time to die."

The patient is still in the angiogram room. Williamson walks over to it. The radiologist tells her that he thinks, tentatively, that he detects bleeding in the stomach. He tells her he'll know more soon.

With another resident, Williamson visits several ward patients, but she is preoccupied with the old man. "If he doesn't stop bleeding, we'll have to operate tonight," she says. She phones the attending who was present when she first operated on the man. "Our GI bleeder is bleeding again," she tells him. "It was bright, could have been arterial. They're doing a selective left gastric now. It could be an erosion. I just thought I'd tell you. He is jaundiced. His liver is decompensating and his portal pressure is rising."

The attending offers his opinion. Williamson walks over to a woman she operated on a few days ago, a woman who underwent a subtotal gastrectomy and breast biopsies.

The woman is awake. There is a nurse beside her bed. Williamson walks over to the bedside and says, "You know those biopsies we did on your breasts? It was cancer and we're going to have to remove your breasts." The woman, old but alert, listens without any sign of emotion. "We'll give you medicine to try to stop it from spreading. So far you're doing fine," Williamson says.

"What about my stomach?" the woman asks.

"You had two big ulcers blocking off your stomach. We took out most of your stomach, but we saw no malignancy there. You'll be able to eat again very soon, but small meals, because your stomach is smaller. We're going to set up the operation for your breasts. You'll feel better after the operation than you did after the stomach operation. Then we'll help you get into a convalescent home."

The woman has no reply. Williamson walks away with a resident, who has been listening to the conversation. "You don't always tell the whole truth," she says to him. "What I told her was true. She already suspected *that*. What she doesn't know yet is that she has a lesion on her hip, too."

She walks over to see a middle-aged black woman, a new admission to Surgery. She has a lump behind one ear. "There's no way to tell the bad lumps from the not-so-bad lumps without operating," Williamson tells her. "We can take it out and find out this week."

By 8:15, she's back in Radiology. While she was gone, one of the residents gave the old man epinephrine when his blood pressure dropped.

"He doesn't need epinephrine, he needs blood," Williamson snaps. "He needs blood."

"We've given him six units already," the resident says.

"Maybe he lost seven," Williamson says, her face reddening. It is the closest she gets to anger.

The angiogram is still in progress. She is restless and goes back to the ICU. She talks on the phone to an attending about the OR schedule for the week. It is hard for her to hear, because a policeman guarding a comatose patient is listening to a *Gunsmoke* rerun on television.

A resident interrupts her.

"He's still actively bleeding," he tells her.

"It *must* be arterial," she says.

"His blood numbers are still okay."

"We must be keeping up with him. But we will have to go to the OR."

They return to Radiology. The patient is still bleeding. Seven more units of blood are ordered. Blood is oozing through the retention stitches on his abdomen. He is streaked with red and yellow from his jaundice. Suddenly, four big clots, like cherry Jello in large portions, come out of his mouth when the nurse attempts to suction him. She reaches in with her hand and pulls out more clots. She is distressed.

"He's full," she says. "He's got a whole pot in there."

The blood gushes from his nose.

"I've never seen anyone bleed like this," the nurse says. "It's pouring. Unbelievable."

The patient's hair and face are bloody now. Williamson is alarmed. She runs out to get a Blakemore tube, a device that is inserted into the stomach and then inflated, compressing bleeding varices. When she returns, the radiologist, who has been studying X-rays, tells her, "It's an arterial bleed in the stomach. You won't control it with a Blakemore."

"What's his blood pressure?" she asks a nurse.

"Seventy."

"Pump the blood, please," Williamson urges.

She is puzzled, as she has been since she first operated on the man and found almost nothing to contribute to a diagnosis. He bled and stopped. Now, tonight, he's bleeding again, badly. She tries to phone the attending who is familiar with the case. His line is busy.

"Oh, busy. Busy. Busy," she mumbles, pacing with the phone in her hand.

She pages one of the residents, to help out. He arrives a few seconds later, ready.

The radiologist offers to inject Pitressin, to stop the bleeding.

"If you can get it in the right spot," Williamson says.

He isn't certain he can.

Williamson calls the nurse in charge of the OR tonight.

"We have a GI bleeder to go to the OR. How fast can you set up? We'll need an arterial monitor. We'll be up shortly," she says.

She looks at the old man. He is dripping blood, twitching fearfully, his eyes wide open in fright.

"You're bleeding again," she says to him. "We have to do an operation. I've talked to your son before and I'll call him again about it. You've got to sign another paper. Make a mark on this paper, please."

She holds up the consent form. He makes a mark on it with the pen and leaves a bloody smudge on the form as well.

The newly arrived resident asks, "Are we going to the OR, Mary?"

"Yes."

"Okay. We've got seven more units of blood in the bank."

"Let's get him on a stretcher," Williamson says. "We better get him up there before he bleeds to death."

They lift the old man from the table to a stretcher. The resident picks up the phone and alerts the elevator operator to be ready for an emergency, an express trip to the OR.

It is 9:45 and for Williamson the day is far from over.

The elevator ascends rapidly to the OR floor and Williamson rushes the patient into an OR waiting for him. Several residents are scrubbed and ready; Williamson prepares rapidly, too. In minutes, the doctors and an anesthetist are working on the patient.

It is a search for the bleeding point. The anesthetist is monitoring the patient, supplying units of blood to try to keep up with the loss. Five doctors surround the patient. Within an hour, the man's stomach is visible, the bleeding point discovered. The elation is momentary. The patient's heart rate and blood pressure descend; the anesthetist makes the announcement with a sense of urgency in her voice. Suddenly, the bleeding resumes, in other locations, beyond control.

For two hours, the team has tried to solve the problem. It is too late. At 1 A.M., the patient dies.

"Pulmonary edema," Williamson sighs. "Probably based on a myocardial infarction." The man's heart simply gave out. "That bleeding. *Everywhere,*" Williamson tells the other doctors. "And his clotting factor was gone. We couldn't correct the blood pressure or the heart rate whatever we did."

The other doctors trudge off. Williamson walks very slowly to a phone, to notify the patient's son.

TUESDAY

Nursing Service Report

A&B—A pipe is leaking in the Ground A corridor—has been reported to engineering.

B-4—Refrigerator out of order—icing—reported to engineering.

L&M—No elevators yesterday or last night—reported to engineering.

G-5—Maria Perez, 9 year old, possible battered child—all agencies notified.

The Premature Bus went out on a call to St. John's Hospital—while there the resuscitator was stolen from the ambulance. Statements from the nurse to Mr. Porter.

F-4—Edward Martinson, 8 year old, with pneumonia and retarded —mother had given permission for a kidney donation. Patient died at 6:15 A.M., was taken to OR, and kidney removed. The kidney was picked up by Montefiore.

Bernard Weinstein arrives at his office in the Administration building at 9:15 A.M. Today he is dressed in a conservative blue suit, for an appearance he must make before the New York City Health and Hospitals Corporation's capital committee. Since 1970, that public corporation has operated the municipal hospitals; it is the bureaucracy Weinstein must master, and now must appeal to for funds to remodel an interim location for the medical prison unit. The building it is presently in is slated to be evacuated. The eventual location will be in the new hospital, but the space won't be ready for three years.

The administrative resident walks in to discuss with Weinstein a project he's working on, a kind of standard operating procedure manual for inpatient services in the new hospital, a who-does-what kind of study. He shows a sample of what he's done to Weinstein.

"The format is fine, but it doesn't answer all the questions," Weinstein tells him. He explains what he wants: a longer, more comprehensive report. It is an example of the sort of delegation of responsibility that enables Weinstein to remain generally unfrazzled. He runs Bellevue like the mayor of a small city, by such delegation.

Weinstein's approach is appropriate. Bellevue *is* a small city. As its chief, Weinstein must understand its intricacies. He must know its components: medical, clerical, cashiers, medical records, nursing, personnel, mail, accounting, telephones, admitting, chaplains, elevator service, engineering and maintenance, food service, laundry, housekeeping, libraries, medical and surgical stores, payroll, pharmacy, two public schools, arts and crafts and recreation among them.

Bellevue is massive and complicated. He keeps in touch with it, as much as possible, through personal contact. His basic view of the hospital, however, is gained by phone.

The telephone operators at Bellevue think of themselves as "the forgotten people." In a cramped office just off the main lobby, seven or eight operators, out of a total of thirty who man the phones around the clock, can be seen during the day (three others work at the nurses' residence). To help them, the phone company has permanent repairmen at Bellevue during the week, and enough equipment to cover a small city.

Phone operators at Bellevue deal with an incoming call every fifteen seconds. The page operator, responsible for finding doctors, gets a page request almost every second; two Bellevue operators do nothing else. A third covers pages for doctors who can be reached by their electronic beepers, the small unit they carry with them that beeps, then gives a voice message, the number the doctor should dial. Operators at Bellevue have to master a system that covers more than three thousand instruments in the old and new hospitals.

In many situations, the phone operator is crucial. Cardiac arrests are reported to them and they alert the staff to respond. Disaster calls from the ambulance dispatcher come to them and they, in turn, have to contact the medical-surgical team and notify the hospital administrators. Fire alarms are set off manually, but the phone operators have to interpret the code and call for firemen. A "stat" page, calling for immediate action, means that the operator must move speedily, to get oxygen, a doctor for a critical patient, police help.

Most calls are routine, some are not. Cranks call to page names that don't exist at Bellevue; if the operator is busy, she doesn't have time to check the name against the hospital directory.

Suicide calls are transferred to the Psychiatric Admitting Office; the operator tries to trace the call, if there's time. Many callers simply recite their symptoms.

One young man has been haunting the lives of the operators for months. He has figured out which hospital phone line is used when doctors accept outside calls. He calls that line and holds on until he receives an "answer" from a doctor who has been paged. When he gets the doctor on the line, he tells him that he likes old women, particularly nurses. The operators have been unable to trace the caller; he may be inside or outside of Bellevue. They treat his presence in their lives with tolerance.

At 9:45, Weinstein walks speedily over to Psychiatry, where a renovated courtroom, for sanity hearings on mental patients, is being dedicated.

When he arrives, the room is packed. The courtroom itself and the adjoining rooms, for judges, lawyers and their clients, seem to sparkle. It is a small favor; most New York courts are a shambles. The renovation cost Bellevue $30,000. It included a new paint job, varnish, curtains, air-conditioning, new plastic chairs to replace the old rock-hard wooden benches.

Weinstein presents an engraved gavel to one of the presiding judges and several judges speak glowingly of this "important new facility." A *Daily News* photographer clicks away. Judges, lawyers and Bellevue staff mingle for a few minutes, then disperse. As Weinstein gets into the elevator, he greets a judge he knows. "This court is beautiful," the judge says to him. "Where we bring the *sane* people is really crazy."

Back in his office, Weinstein finds a memo from his chief engineer, with the eight grievances about the new Bellevue that Weinstein requested. There are references to "Forced Hot-Water System," "Steam Station," "Roll-a-Matic Filters," "Domestic Hot Water," "Secondary Water" and "Openings in Perimeter Walls." He doesn't understand all the references, but he'll see the chief engineer later about it.

His secretary hands him a HHC cost analysis for Bellevue, newly delivered but for a period more than a year ago. The pace of the bureaucracy is not Weinstein's; he tries to be current and keeps his own accounting to accomplish that.

"I have my own reporting system for the hospital," he says to his secretary, Rose LaMarca. "I can't understand these figures." He thumbs through the HHC report. "We come in at around 95 percent of our budget. Unless you're reckless, you can anticipate unspent dollars. I have brought in budgets at 99.8 percent, but never over 100. It is possible to make ends meet, even in a hospital this size."

He sorts through some papers, preparing for the afternoon meeting with the executive committee of Bellevue's Employee Advisory Council. The group is an invention of Weinstein's, a way he devised to keep in touch with hospital employees on all levels, in all areas, from Nursing to Housekeeping to libraries to elevators. It wasn't easy to set up because the labor unions—and there are fourteen unions and nineteen locals at Bellevue—suspected he was trying to bypass them to court their members. He told them that he wasn't and, in fact, endorsed a set of bylaws that specifically excluded it.

At 11:20, the administrator for Psychiatry, Ed Stolzenberg, and Weinstein's deputy, Madeline Bohman, join him in his office. They talk about the use of gates in the prison ward when it finally gets moved into the new hospital.

"What we'll need up there," Weinstein tells them facetiously, "is an electrified fence. Dogs. Whips. Something nice and homey."

Weinstein refers to the meeting with the HHC capital committee. He tests his arguments for funds on the two administrators. One of them asks, "Are we asking them for $65,000 to do D-2?" referring to the ward Weinstein has chosen for the interim site.

"Damned right," Weinstein replies.

The conversation drifts away from the interim prison ward. Stolzenberg tells Weinstein that a new man interviewed for a job may not be a high school graduate, that another interview has been set up to find out. A phone call interrupts. The HHC committee will see the Bellevue delegation earlier than planned. Weinstein arranges for a car to take him downtown, to the HHC main office on Worth Street.

He chats about the evacuation and demolition of building L&M, nearly sixty years old, and timing it with the move of its patients, many of them surgical cases, into the new building, in nine months. He scans a memo from the HHC, suggesting the demolition of part of L&M earlier. He will deal with that later.

After being made to wait in an anteroom at the HHC offices downtown, Weinstein and his two administrators are invited into the HHC's capital committee meeting. Weinstein walks briskly into the conference room, which is enormous, yet almost filled by a massive conference table, heavy wood which is matched by wood paneling on all the surrounding walls. Around the table are some of the heavies from the public corporation.

He presents his plan for the interim prison ward, carefully, factually, free of jargon. He pauses, anticipating objections to his request for $65,000 to do the job. There is none. Weinstein's plan is approved, the money allocated. He knows there will be bureaucratic obstacles to overcome later, but now he knows the job will be done. Pleased and smiling, he escorts his two aides out of the room.

Back in his office, Weinstein browses through a series of memos regarding Bellevue's affiliation contract with the N.Y.U. Medical School. Bellevue pays N.Y.U. more than $9 million a year to provide medical services, so it is not something he takes lightly, or for granted. An N.Y.U. administrator has asked him for additional funds and Weinstein is resisting.

He recapitulates in his own mind what happened at the HHC meeting, collating a batch of earlier memos on the subject over many months. The matter has a cluttered history. Weinstein's position had been to use the present Adult Emergency Service building, relatively new and self-contained on ground level, for the prison ward, keeping it out of the new hospital. His assumption was that the hospital staff and the Department of Correction would not want to transport prisoners through the hospital to a unit on a high floor.

The AES, he felt, provided direct access from the prison bus, inpatient and outpatient and emergency-treatment facilities, lab and X-ray services. The Urban Coalition and the hospital's community board objected to what they felt were separate and unequal facilities for prisoners, violating their rights. The *Village Voice*, in several articles, agreed.

"I thought it was a medical-care issue," Weinstein remembers, "but it turned out to be a civil rights issue."

The libertarians prevailed, which meant that a new location had to be found for the prison unit in the new hospital. The only available space was on the eighteenth floor. Although his present problem, now seemingly solved, is to remodel a ward for interim use, Weinstein worries about getting prisoners in and out of the eighteenth floor in the new hospital, once it is ready for occupancy, getting them to clinics on the lower floors and back again.

His thoughts are cut short by the arrival of his administrative assistant, Susan Wick, to discuss matters Weinstein must deal with for the community board. They go through them, one by one, and she makes notes, to dig out information the board wants, to send memos, to check files. By the time they're done, he must go to the Employee Advisory Council executive committee meeting.

It is held in the Administration building's conference room, the same one where the medical board and the community board meet. The medical board, the directors of services at Bellevue, is a collection of experts whose collective presence can be imposing. The community board is a collection of latent radicals, vigorously seeking answers to questions about the quality of care at Bellevue and satisfaction for complaints about the hospital. The employee group, in contrast, is placid. Seven employee councils are represented today, along with members of Weinstein's staff. A total of nineteen are present.

The employee delegates raise various issues. A handful of the seven hundred methadone addicts who come to Bellevue for maintenance and are causing trouble by provoking staff and visitors must be dealt with by the hospital police. The quality of the food in the staff cafeteria must be improved. There is a perpetual parking problem. Security patrols at night are inadequate, muggings in the neighborhood continue and brighter street lights are needed. Weinstein tells the group that he has informed the 13th Police Precinct and the hospital police and has requested high-intensity lamps for the nearby streets. Then he introduces an assistant director who discusses patient clothing, an issue of significance to those who care about patient morale. They all seem to care; several of them have pleaded for more colorful patient clothing.

The present slippers given to a patient, the assistant director points out, are nylon and washable and Bellevue gets 15,000 pairs for $29,000 each year. He shows a pair of all-foam slippers, sized by colors, and notes that he can get 100,000 pairs for the same money now spent on the old model. He can get rubberish tong slippers for 48 cents a pair. He passes samples around.

Currently, he points out, Bellevue spends $60,000 a year on robes, or $3.95 per robe, and $48,000 or $4.04 (he speaks deliberately) per pair of pajamas. He can't do much better than that, he asserts. To get more colors would raise the price. Nightgowns, he announces, can be bought for $2.21 each, an annual outlay of $33,000, and he can get prints or patterns for less than that.

Around the table, a spirit of encouragement rises. He responds by saying that he'll consult with Nursing, for that department's advice (will the nightgown fit too snugly for proper care?).

Weinstein puts in a plug for the hospital's sports activities (it fields competitive teams in several sports), and the meeting ends at 5:30 P.M.

He returns to his office, to see how many phone messages have accumulated. Not many. He signs his mail, makes notes about two meetings he will have tomorrow with the medical board. The first, at 8 A.M., is to discuss an Antioch College proposal to train Physicians' Associates, a relatively new category in the medical-care field, for Bellevue to employ. The board has been studying the proposal. Tomorrow Weinstein will know what the board thinks of it.

Dirk Berger confesses to his secretary that he wasn't feeling well yesterday, but managed to conceal it and get through the day. On the drive home, he almost fell asleep at the wheel and that frightened him. He went to bed at 9:30, missing a television program he had hoped to watch, and woke up feeling better. It was, he says, the earliest he had gone to bed since he was a perpetually tired intern.

The staff assembles for rounds, filling the conference room. The chairs are hand-me-downs from old school classrooms and squeaky folding chairs donated instead of being discarded. The room is full, chairs arranged in a large oval. Berger nods and the head nurse, reading from notes kept by the evening and night shifts, informs the day staff.

The ward is full, she tells them; it will be difficult to find space for any more patients. She refers to her notes.

One patient was "verbally abusive to the staff." Another was "confused and rigid" most of the night. A third, seemingly alert and oriented, requested visiting rights for his dog.

There were two new admissions. A 22-year-old man had jumped from a second-story window and was complaining of backache. He was coherent and cooperative, but depressed. A 33-year-old woman was depressed, agitated, withdrawn, suffering from hallucinations; she had been at Bellevue three years ago. The black alcoholic pleaded for his release and persisted in talking about killing the policeman who brought him to Bellevue. A female patient, young and attractive, was being seduced by two male patients. She is scheduled to be discharged, solving her problem and compounding theirs. A male patient went out to buy food for the staff, a gesture of friendship. Another returned from a pass because he felt people were staring at him. One nubile female was found in bed with one of the horny men, with another man guarding the door.

One of the residents interrupts, to suggest giving Thorazine to a patient with a history of seizures.

"Give him that and he'll seize for sure," Berger says.

The head nurse resumes. The fat black woman is showing signs of progress. Instead of reading the poetry of Keats aloud at the top of her voice, she is now writing her own poetry. A patient complained because his glasses are too tight. A restless man watches the ward door from a chair he's placed nearby. Berger warns the staff that the guy might try to make a run for it when the door is opened.

The rounds end at 9 A.M. and Berger walks the few steps to his office, to meet a patient he sees privately, a student whose problems are neurotic rather than psychotic. The student leaves, and at 10 Berger can read the charts on the new admissions.

A patient's chart at Bellevue embodies the oppressive amount of paperwork the staff must face. As he flips through the forms for a single patient, Berger finds:

An admitting slip

A Face Sheet, with facts about the patient, diagnosis and disposition of the case

A computer admission form

An admission report which contains the initial interview with the patient

A Physical Examination form

A Continuation Record, a log of the patient's condition

A Medical History

A Doctor's Order Sheet, which lists drugs prescribed

A Medication Record, listing daily dosages

Pathology and X-Ray reports

A Record of Vital Signs, which records blood pressure, temperature, pulse and respiration

Nurse's Notes, indicating behavior as observed by the nursing staff

A temperature chart in graph form

A clothing and property record

A Voluntary Request for Hospitalization form, signed by the patient

A Note of Legal Rights for Patients, which is given to all incoming patients

A Nursing Patient Care Plan Card, for daily use in the master file at the nursing station

Berger scans each sheet, looking for clues he can develop in treating the new patients. At 10:30, the woman resident arrives, with Charlie Johnson, the alcoholic Berger had seen yesterday. The ward cat, Charlene, slinks in and sits on an empty chair.

Johnson, manhandled by the police when he was brought in, wants to kill one of them.

"You were pissed, right?" Berger asks.

"Hell yes, man," Johnson says. "But now I don't want to kill that mother. I just want to get his ass into court."

He recites his story for Berger. He was trying to catch a train, had too much to drink, and his behavior attracted the attention of the police. Berger has concluded that the man was drunk, not psychotic, but he listens to the story.

"The cops, man, they really didn't want to bust my ass, because that would make them have to be in court one day and that's a day without pay. So they took me here. If you believe in God, man, believe me now. I've lost $90 pay in two days here. I'm not sick. I don't belong here, man. I just want to get out and take that cat to court."

"Fine," Berger says. "Get yourself a lawyer and do it." He explains the man's rights to him, then shakes his hand. As Johnson walks out, Berger tells the resident to discharge him soon.

The phone rings. A former patient, one of the ward's regulars now living at the Aberdeen, must be readmitted. Berger knows the ward is full, at thirty-two, but he is fond of this patient, an old, frail, eccentric woman, who chain-smokes. He finds an extra bed.

"She's got a lot of charm for such a crazy lady," he says to the resident, who has lingered outside Berger's office. "When she's well, she's fine, but when she starts giving history orations, she's in trouble. She starts on World War II, then goes back to Rasputin. When she gets to Napoleon, watch out. And when she starts lecturing about Mary, Queen of Scots, she's ready to come back to the ward."

When the resident leaves, a patient is standing in his doorway. It is Sarah Morgan, a sad, prematurely old woman. A crumbling version of American Gothic, she had come to New York from her rural home in the South when many of her contemporaries would have done exactly the opposite. Poor and frightened, she succumbed to the terrors of the city. Her health failed. Her psyche was not prepared, either, for what she would find in the city. Her skin is pasty white; her blond hair hangs straight down to her shoulders, clumpy and unwashed. She is on medication and she stares straight ahead, never moving her head. She walks with a shuffle, the side effect of Thorazine. She had been admitted to Bellevue when she cut herself with a knife. Taken to Medicine to treat the wounds, she was later transferred to Psychiatry; before the transfer, an X-ray revealed an ominous cloud on her lung. Berger is concerned about her. She looks 65. She is twenty years younger than that.

She shuffles into his office and slowly sits down. She is a country woman talking to a big-city doctor, and across the gulf that separates them she tries to make the one point she came to make.

"I want to get out. I'd like to get out," she says, without moving her head or changing the solemn expression on her gaunt, bony face.

"Where will you go?" Berger asks, more like a relative who cares about her than a doctor interested in a case.

"Back to the South."

"Why?"

"That's where my sister lives."

"How many sisters do you have?"

"Four."

"Do you have children?"

"Two. One is twenty-five and the other is twelve. They live with my sister."

"Do you see them?"

"I couldn't tell you when I saw them last." She is wistful, apparent in the sigh with which she answers the question. Her face remains impassive.

"If you get out of here, where will you live?"

"In my own home down South."

"Who takes care of it now?"

"Nobody. But I own it and an acre of land."

"Why did you come to New York?"

"I answered an ad for a job. But when I got it, I just couldn't make it and I quit. I get very nervous now, very nervous."

"Does that happen often?"

"Yes."

"You lived here, in New York?"

"Yes. On welfare. In an apartment."

"Where did you eat?"

"I just got hot dogs, chicken, stuff to eat in my room."

"That must be a tight budget."

"It is."

"How did you get here? To Bellevue?"

"I cut my leg. I just wanted to go home afterward, but I couldn't."

"Did you ever do that before? Cut yourself?"

"No."

"Have you ever felt like killing yourself?"

Mrs. Morgan stares at Berger and begins to rise, very slowly, from her chair, moving toward the door. Berger gets up and puts his arms around her, gently, and leads her back to the chair. She is crying, quietly. Berger repeats the question.

"Yes."

"Is it hard to talk about?"

"Well, my sister's son is dead. My mother and father are dead. It is awful that people have to die," she says.

"Are you religious?"

"Well, I have no religion. I was baptized, all right, all that talking about the Holy Ghost."

"Why are you crying?"

"I don't know."

"It can be scary here. It's rough, I know. But I believe you can handle it. What can we do to make you feel better?"

"You can give me a job."

"Where?"

"Anywhere. I don't mind sweeping and mopping."

"We can get you into a work program. If you can take care of yourself. You should try to build yourself up."

"All right. Okay. Thanks for talking to me," she says, expressionless. She rises, again very slowly, and shuffles away. As she leaves, Berger thanks her.

Within the next fifteen minutes, she returns three times, like an apparition at Berger's door, to tell him she would like to find some work to do. Finally, she shuffles off to her room.

Berger talks to one of the residents about her.

"Look at her. She spent three weeks on the Chest Service with a spot on her lung they couldn't figure out. With test after test and tubes into her, not sure what she had. She was cooperative. She's psychotic, and someone psychotic with a spot on a lung is touchy about the subject of death. She's got cancer, no doubt, and they're debating about what to do for her.

"These pathetic ones stay in my head. I see them disintegrate. I see them ravaged by disease, the kind we can't see and the kind we can see. This woman's got both. I think about them when I'm at home, at night. We don't know much about cancer and we don't know much about schizophrenia either." Just as he finishes, Mrs. Morgan returns.

"I'll take any kind of job," she says to Berger.

"Keep yourself in shape. Go to our meetings on the ward. I believe you."

"Fair enough for me," she says and leaves.

As she does, another patient is waiting to enter. She is a neat, composed, hands-folded-in-lap, Southern woman in her forties, who has known better times. Before coming to Bellevue, she lived on welfare, in a cheap hotel. When she went berserk, she was brought to Bellevue by the police. Her history shows mental hospitals from Texas to Manhattan State. Berger has watched her improve for several weeks; he feels she may be ready to return to the outside.

"We have a hotel called the Aberdeen," he tells her. "It's a safe place. Our ex-patients go there. Would you like to live there?"

"I guess so," she says in a soft drawl. "I tried to get a room there once."

"We can arrange it. We have hospital people there to help you. You can go out to dinner when you live there. And I'm there during the week, too, if you need me. Interested?"

"I guess so."

"I'll work on it."

"Are you a doctor?" she asks.

"Yes, I'm Dr Berger. I thought you knew. By the way, have you ever had a drinking problem?"

"No."

"Ever try to kill yourself?"

"No."

"You know, when people are ready to get out of here, as you are now, they can lose contact with us. We want to be in touch. Where have you lived?"

"In many states. I was married then and we lived everywhere. We liked Minnesota, and we were going to stay there, but a doctor said the climate was bad for me."

"How are you now? Ill?"

"No. I don't take medicine."

"How old were you the first time you got sick, psychiatrically?"

"About ten years ago. My husband and I had troubles. We didn't have any friends. We lived out in the country. I thought it was a lonely place, a real lonely place, and I got to thinking about it too much. I didn't want to live then, I remember, but I wasn't going to kill myself. I don't feel so good right now, but I sure want to live."

"Some days you won't feel good, but you can always talk to the staff at the hotel. And to me."

"When can I leave the hospital?"

"That's up to your doctor here," Berger says, deferring to the resident on the case. "Maybe you need more time. But I'll talk to him about it."

She leaves and within minutes Berger talks to the resident,

phones the Aberdeen and gets her a room.

He rushes out of his office to attend a staff meeting at the Aberdeen, stopping at a delicatessen to pick up his lunch, a can of Tab.

There are more than four hundred SROs (Single Room Occupancy hotels) in New York City, with more than forty thousand people living in them. Each tenant gets a room, a bed, a closet, a chest of drawers and a weekly linen change, paid for, in most cases, by welfare funds. Most of the tenants are men, middle-aged, and most are black. The SRO was born during World War II, to house single servicemen and workers. In the fifties, the Welfare Department began to send persons released from jails, hospitals and mental institutions to them. In 1965, a law prohibited the renting of them to tenants with children. Most of the SROs are in a state of decay, as infested with problems as are the drug addicts, prostitutes, alcoholics and psychotics who reside in them. The Aberdeen is one of the best and it cannot be compared favorably to any comfortable hotel.

Bellevue's psychiatric staff has joined forces with several social agencies to make the Aberdeen workable. Drug addicts are forbidden. Health service and psychiatric counseling are available to all of the tenants of the two-hundred-room, thirteen-floor hotel. The Aberdeen is tucked away amid the bustle of the garment district, west of Fifth Avenue on Thirty-second Street. Outside, a few former Bellevue inpatients linger, contemplating their own torments quietly or simply wondering how they'll spend another day. The lobby is tidy, uncluttered. Dirk Berger makes his way through it, waving to the desk clerk as he passes, to attend today's meeting.

Nine men and nine women sit around the oval table in the cramped meeting room, which doubles as recreation area for tenants. Most of them have brought lunch in brown bags and the table is packed with cole slaw, pickles, salami on rye, coffee, Cokes. There are delegates from the Waverly Welfare Center, a visiting nurse on duty at the Aberdeen, medical personnel, social workers, two doctors from Manhattan State Hospital (another source of tenants) and the hotel manager.

Berger is concerned about former NO-6 patients now at the Aberdeen. He wants to know how they're doing, if he ought to see any of them while he's there. One patient, Nathan Rothberg, he's told, insists on singing loudly in public. Berger knows about that. One of the staff aides adds, "He can sing all day as

far as I'm concerned, as long as he keeps his hands to himself."
Berger knows about that, too.

One of the patients seems pleasantly tranquilized most of the
time. "What's she on and where can I get some?" asks one of
the social workers, a woman who manages to be cheerful and
serious at the same time.

There is some abrasive interplay about tenant admissions,
whom to admit, whom to turn down. The debate seems to
center more on the personalities of the debaters—a prim, well-
educated white woman and a soulful, earthy black woman—
than on the merits of the cases. Berger smiles and avoids taking
sides.

There is an apparent thief among the tenants. A doctor wants
a suspect evicted. Another tenant, just released from a private
hospital after intestinal surgery, arrived at the Aberdeen with
just a bandage over the incision, which was draining through
her dress. She'd been given bandages to change her own dressing by the private hospital staff. Outraged, a social worker demands medical care for the tenant. Berger guarantees it. The
activity therapist reports on her dining-out program for Aberdeen tenants. Berger suggests she do a study of it, titled *The
Psychotic Gourmet*. She offers the subtitle, *All the Thorazine
You Can Drink*.

The meeting rambles its way to a close at 1:30. Berger remains at the Aberdeen, to accompany the visiting nurse to the
room of a middle-aged man, a former NO-6 patient, who is not
well, according to the word from a friend. In the halls, Berger
passes tenants sitting around, staring into space. Some of the
walls are peeling away. The furnishings are spare, simple, old,
but the place is clean.

Johnny Rogers is in his room. Berger can hear him coughing
badly when he knocks on his door. Rogers is tall, shaggy-haired,
with a craggy Western face. Dressed in denim, he looks like a
cross between a cowboy and a recluse. He greets Berger amia-
bly, tells him he's taken an old family remedy: aspirin, sugar and
lighter fluid. Berger quivers.

In the room there are tubes of paint and paintings the man
has done, taped to the wall, an empty bottle of cheap sangría,
a pair of drumsticks, several photos of Bruce Lee in kung fu
action and a small candid photo of the entrance to the Grand
Ole Opry House in Nashville.

Berger's primary worry is that Rogers is a potential suicide.

He notices that Rogers has placed his bed directly in front of a large window, which has been opened wide.

Rogers anticipates Berger's question.

"I like to sit close to the open window," he says. "To remind myself not to jump. Hell, I'm ten floors up."

Berger is not convinced. The man is a drifter in search of a real or imaginary ex-wife and has been in trouble in several states. Rogers sees the skepticism on Berger's face.

"I like to back myself into a corner," he says, "and battle my way out."

Berger doesn't respond.

"You know, I walk over to the Hudson in the middle of the night. I know it's not smart, but I do it."

Berger asks him if he's taking his medication.

"It gives me bad dreams. It makes me dopey and it makes the sunlight hurt my eyes."

"True. But it helps you beat your other problems."

They continue the exchange. Rogers tells Berger, elaborately, about his quest for his ex-wife, about seeing women who look like her, being disappointed. Once he threw himself in front of a moving truck.

"I've stopped making phone calls looking for her," he says. "But I'm still depressed. Now I got a headache after talking to you, and I want a Coca-Cola. My mouth feels like a dust storm in Texas. And I want to go back to bed."

Rogers has not shaved in several days; he scratches his stubble.

"What else?" Berger asks.

"Well, I panic when I'm short of money, and when I have it, I spend it fast as hell."

"What about a job?"

"I can't get a job without my doctor's approval, and I don't want to go for a job and have them check on me, call Psychiatry about me."

"Look, if you have a bad time, let me know. Call the desk here or the hospital or just phone the police, if you feel troubled."

Rogers shakes his head equivocally. Maybe he'll call. Maybe he won't. Maybe he'll see the resident who's been treating him at the Bellevue clinic. Maybe he won't. Right now, all he wants is a Coke. Berger and the nurse, who has remained in a corner silently throughout the conversation, escort Rogers to the lobby and the Coke machine. As they leave him there, Berger sees an old, misshapen woman watching him. Obviously disturbed, she pushes another woman aside rudely, roughly, bellowing, "Let me by."

Berger looks at her and says, "Say 'please.' "

"I don't say 'please,' " she shouts.

"You're a stinker."

"I am and I always will be."

"You'll make me crazy, Bertha," Berger says.

"Sometimes you gotta be fresh to get somewhere." She tugs at Berger's hair, mumbling that she's surrounded by nuts.

Berger laughs as she rushes past him.

He leaves the Aberdeen and hails a cab.

"Where ya goin'?" the cab driver asks.

"First Avenue and Thirtieth Street," Berger answers.

"Bellevue? Oh, ya mean Murder Incorporated," the driver says. "Ya know they sterilize people there by da thousands? You know they lock you up there when they say ya crazy? An' you can't get out."

Berger's placid expression is not shattered. The driver talks himself out, without any encouragement, by the time they reach Bellevue.

It is 2:30, time for the third ward-team meeting of the week. Resident, nurse, social worker and activity therapist file into Berger's office and review cases.

One case particularly intrigues Berger. A man in his fifties says he's been a biology professor and has been lobotomized. Berger has seen him.

"Most lobotomized patients just sit there and smile," Berger tells the resident. "He doesn't." Berger suggests that the resident try to check out his story, somehow.

A 21-year-old drug addict is back, a chronic problem case. The resident says he's prescribed Thorazine, to combat withdrawal symptoms.

"Get him on methadone. Thorazine has more serious side effects," Berger tells him.

The cases are discussed, recommendations made, then the team scatters.

The wife of a young suicidal patient is waiting to see Berger. She has brought her three children with her; she couldn't find a baby-sitter. She is both sad and angry about her plight and her husband's presence on NO–6. She remembers all his suicide attempts, but she feels betrayed and abandoned by him. Berger tries to calm her, to assure her that her husband is making progress and should be back home with her soon.

A new admission, found catatonic in a hotel lobby, has come, cautiously, to see Berger. He can't remember how he got to Bellevue, but he remembers facts about his life. They talk, factually, for a few minutes, then Berger asks him if he has a drinking problem.

The patient, a young, unshaven, overweight Italian, glares at Berger. He stalks off, enraged. Berger lets him go.

In the corridor, a resident and a lawyer debate the merits of releasing a patient.

"He's not suicidal, not homicidal, I admit," the resident says. "But he won't function out there."

"He called me to come up here and help him," the lawyer snaps back, "and you haven't convinced me that he belongs in here."

In the background, the jolly black poetess is overwrought. She wants to join a group of patients going swimming in the pool in the nurses' residence, but she can't find a bathing suit to fit her. An aide joins the search.

Berger's friend from the Aberdeen, the skinny, chain-smoking old deluded history lecturer, comes rushing up to Berger, who is standing in his doorway watching the activity. She is screaming incoherently, but relaxes when Berger puts his arm around her. "Don't worry," he tells her, "you've always got me." She gives him a crooked smile and asks him for a cigarette.

It is almost 6 P.M. Berger walks down the corridor to confer with a resident who's asked for his advice whenever Berger has a few minutes. He has a few minutes now. He'll deliver them to the resident, then drive home.

At 9 A.M., Ken Kirshbaum attends a lecture, along with a few other conscientious residents. There is an epidemic of yawns to greet the professor from N.Y.U. He is an expert on interviewing techniques and the author of a two-volume work on psychiatry. He is a man in his sixties, with thinning gray hair and glasses. Dressed conservatively, he is the prototypical academician. He has ninety minutes, he tells the residents, and in that time he hopes to summarize his own theory of therapy. It is a race against time and he doesn't hesitate.

"There are neurotic facets in most people, but they adjust, adapt to their environment through neurotic defenses. They function in society. If stresses arise, however, the signs are evident.

"There is increasing tension, not necessarily understood by the patient, and accompanying physiological changes. If the tension can't be dealt with, it leads to anxiety, which is evidenced in physical ways. Nausea. Increased pulse rate. Anxiety leads to a psychosomatic preoccupation with the body, the heartbeat, hypertension, headaches, spasms, gastrointestinal symptoms, and actual organic damage where a constitutional weakness exists."

One of the residents closes his eyes and picks his nose. Kirshbaum concentrates on the words; it is difficult to regress to the classroom once you think you've finished with it forever.

"The therapist is responsible for mastering, or helping to master, the anxiety attack immediately, with medication, but that's less valuable than getting the patient to talk, to reveal conflicts. If the doctor can connect the symptoms with personality distortions, it starts a chain reaction. If the patient acts upon it, a massive change can result."

He is well into his ninety minutes now, racing through his notes. One of the residents, with a folded *New York Times* on his lap, shifts it so he can read it. Another, his eyelids almost closed, sips his coffee. The professor hasn't time to notice.

Kirshbaum sustains his attention. Unlike several other residents, who seem to be there to be seen there or to avoid being elsewhere, he listens loyally.

"Patients shift between defenses," the professor says, "but the last type of defense is the manipulation of inner physiology, massive metabolic disturbances that can lead to a psychotic attack and to something organic—affecting the enzyme system, for instance—basic to all psychoses. There will be distortions of reality, hallucinations, when all other defenses fail. And sensory disorders, defects in memory, hostile impulses, paranoia, schizophrenia, suicide."

One of the women residents studies the backs of her hands.

"The symptom is just one fragment of the Gestalt," he continues, peering for a split second around the room, then at his wristwatch. "You need more than that. Show empathy and other parts of the Gestalt will emerge. Develop relationships. Get the patient to talk about his past, his behavior, his dreams. Disengage your own feelings about the patient, your own problems.

"Then get the patient to utilize his own insights to change. He'll resist. His illness may be thought of as providing gains for him. He may have a stake in being ill. People are sorry for him. Not to be normal may be a distinction. And the patient wants the doctor to make decisions for him. Patients resist making mistakes and the therapist must push him to practice vital activities.

"Don't give up until the patient can master his abilities. Don't resent the patient's inability to act. Don't push too hard, too fast. Respect the uniqueness of each patient. Be directive or nondirective as the patient requires."

It is 10:29 A.M. The professor, on the verge of being out of breath, concludes with some advice about terminating therapy.

"Prepare the patient by breaking up the dependency over a period of time, encouraging the patient to make his own decisions and be prepared to deal with relapses."

It is 10:30. The professor has succeeded in getting it all into ninety minutes. "Any questions?" None. Kirshbaum returns to the clinic for another day.

As he arrives, he sees a cluster of patients waiting. Each one will pay from $2 to $36 per session, depending on family size and income. No one needs an appointment in the walk-in clinic, an attempt to serve the community, an innovation just four years old.

Kirshbaum plucks a chart from the stack on the clerk's desk and takes it to his office. He has not seen this patient before, although the man has been coming to the clinic for three years, sporadically. He is a sad, introspective Puerto Rican in his fifties. When Kirshbaum invites him in, he sits brooding.

"I have no problem," he says. "Just the hotel where I live. The noise. The vandalism."

He wants medication and he wants Kirshbaum to complete a welfare form for him. Kirshbaum checks the medication previously prescribed and issues a new prescription for it. "How often do you take this?" he asks.

The man raises four fingers and says, "Three times every day."

Kirshbaum smiles, completes the welfare form and hands it to the man.

" 'Sokay," the man says.

The flow of patients continues; they walk down the hall to residents' offices every few minutes. When one leaves, another replaces him. The agonies of New York keep the waiting room well stocked with troubles.

Kirshbaum has his own distraction. His wife has been plagued by a neurological disorder that doctors can't seem to diagnose. She is staying with her parents during the day, because she can't stay alone. He picks her up at night and delivers her in the morning.

He cannot think about her for too long. The next patient arrives. She is a 40-year-old Puerto Rican woman he's never seen before. She is neat, wears glasses, has an Afro. She comes into his office glaring, hostile. She's been in and out of Bellevue, on the wards and in the clinic. Divorced, she has six children, from 3 to 18; a grandchild and a cousin live with her, too. She can't work because she has a seizure disorder; she goes to Neurology clinic, as well. She tells Kirshbaum that she's had two seizures in three days and is both tense and unnerved. He listens to her story, intently. "It seems to me that your problems are genuine," he says, "and I'd like you to come in to see me again." He gives her a prescription for Valium.

It is time for the morning staff meeting with other residents, social workers and the attending psychiatrist on duty. Today's meeting is devoted to Marvin Hoppe, a young, long-haired, former pusher of LSD who has spent two years in jail. He is on welfare now. He came to the clinic complaining of blackouts, a suffocating feeling, insomnia. He's invited into the meeting and struts in tensely, smiling incongruously. He doesn't think he needs care or medication, but he's delighted to talk about himself.

The attending psychiatrist asks him to describe his attacks.

"I get confused, man. I can't see clearly. I lose what I'm thinking."

"What is it like afterward?"

"There's physical pain and depression. Very deep. Very tight.

Very upsetting. I can't relate to the world. I feel out of touch. I can hear, but I can't respond."

"For how long?"

"From minutes to a half-hour. I get out of it by being quiet."

"And the next day?"

"I feel terrible, physically. Anxiety."

He seems to enjoy the audience, as if he were in an off-Off Broadway play.

"How are you today?"

"Nervous. But I can talk to you and understand you."

"Were you different before you ever took drugs?" the psychiatrist asks.

"Well, I was more balanced, I suppose, but LSD enlightened me spiritually. I was calmer, maybe. I had daydreams then, but now I've got fantasies."

"What does this proverb mean to you? 'When the cat is away, the mice will play.' "

"Adultery. Like when a cat is away, his old lady will make it with someone else. Any questions?" He laughs.

The social worker asks him how he feels now.

"Sort of amused and nervous. I'd like to be calm to talk like this. But so it goes." He gets up and walks out of the room.

"He's subjective, but not crazy or bizarre," the social worker says after he's gone.

"Organic flair. Thinking disorder. Interesting," the attending psychiatrist, in his forties and confidant, suggests. "He's almost within normal range. I don't think he's schizophrenic. He can't think consistently, which is secondary to his drug experience.

"The sort of blackout he's experiencing is like the flashback, the *déjà vu* feeling, former LSD users do experience, but not exactly so, because this patient's experiences are not really physiochemical. According to you"—the attending turns to one of the residents—"he came here because he needed a doctor's approval to enroll in a film course. Fine. Give him medication, low dosage, fill out his form and send him on his merry way. He's in a relatively stable state. He's rationalized his state."

Kirshbaum thinks about something the professor said at the morning lecture, links it to this case. "He's rationalized his state for now, a viable defense mechanism."

After a fifteen-minute lunch in the basement cafeteria, Kirshbaum is back in his clinic office. Rachel Miller, a 64-year-old woman on welfare, awaits him.

She smiles benevolently at Kirshbaum, revealing that several front teeth are missing. She tells him that she lives in a Catholic residence for women, has had a drinking problem, but hasn't had a drink in a year.

"I drank—you know, socially—for years. But I worked, too, and raised my two daughters. My husband was long gone, who knows where? But then, when one of my daughters got pregnant, I flipped out on alcohol.

"After school, my daughter went to this boy's house and they played house together," she says. Kirshbaum realizes she is not being ironic, just euphemistic.

She tells him that at that point in her life she sought psychiatric aid. It wasn't very helpful. Since then, she's tried to keep in touch with her daughters, but feels that they don't want to keep in touch with her.

"I don't know why. We were very close. The Three Musketeers. Then she got pregnant and everything split up. Now I sit around and I'm very bored. I guess I'll go back to work when my dental work is done."

"It's a good idea to work, not to be bored and lonely," Kirshbaum says.

"When my kids grew up, it was just too much. I had made their confirmation dresses. I loved them so much. We were so happy together. I took them on trips. I never had a boyfriend. Maybe that was my problem."

Kirshbaum raises his eyebrows, smiles wistfully.

"Now, can you believe it, they won't even send me money for cigarettes. It hurts. It makes me blue sometimes." She seems to be on the verge of tears, but she does not cry.

"Life doesn't have to be a void," Kirshbaum tells her. "Don't make excuses. Work part-time if you have to."

"Yeah. Maybe I'll try it. I know how to work. I've been working since I was sixteen, for God's sake."

"Don't let anything get you down. Don't harp on the past. You can help yourself. And get your kids back as friends."

She wants pills.

"There's more to emotional health than a bunch of pills," he says. He doesn't know this woman well enough to send her out with a bottle of pills. She leaves without them.

Kirshbaum walks her to the desk, picks up another chart, reads the name aloud, "Veronica Lincoln." A middle-aged black woman rises, without speaking, and follows him to his office.

She is 43, a nurse at a hospital in the Bronx. She is clearly depressed, almost catatonic. She enters Kirshbaum's office, sits beside his desk, her hands folded in her lap. She stares at them.

Kirshbaum reads her records. She has a small amount of impaired brain function, some history of schizophrenia and has come to Bellevue before. He asks her what is bothering her.

"My attention span is averted. I'm staring into space," she says, very softly.

"For how long?"

"A week. Since I started on my vacation."

"Can you tell me what you're feeling now?"

She does not answer.

"Can you tell me what you're feeling now?"

She does not answer.

"Can you hear anything?"

She does not respond.

"Can you look at me?"

"Yes." She does.

"What is going on?"

"Names. I hear names from outside," she says.

"Has this happened before?"

"A year or two ago."

"Did it go away?"

"I thought it did. Now it came back, making me miserable."

"Have you ever thought about hurting yourself?"

"Yes, recently."

"Today?"

"Yes." Her voice is barely audible.

"Do you live alone?"

"Yes. But the neighbors make a lot of noise. It annoys me."

"Do you think they're doing it to annoy you?"

She stares at her hands and does not answer.

"Have you ever been in the hospital before?"

"Twice."

"Have you seen a doctor since then?"

"Yes. Two years ago."

Her face reflects a growing pain within her, as if she is fighting to withhold it, struggling to combat it. She does not speak. Kirshbaum doesn't either. The room is silent. He stares at her for several minutes. She doesn't seem to notice.

"I think it would be a good idea for you to come into the hospital," he says to her. "Would you be willing to do that at this time?"

She says nothing.

"Is it all right with you? I think you should. You need some help. I'll get some papers for your hospitalization." She shows no reaction to what he has said. He leaves his office, returns with a batch of forms. It takes him ten minutes to complete them. While he does, she sits motionless. She has barely moved since she first entered his office.

"This is an application for you to come in voluntarily. Please read it and sign it." She signs it. Kirshbaum escorts her to the admitting office, where another resident takes over the case. She will be on a ward within minutes.

When Kirshbaum returns to his office, another patient is waiting. Kirshbaum checks out her chart, what other doctors have noted about her: She is possessive, angry, overpowering in relationships. She has seen a string of doctors after suffering menopausal depression. Her name is Becky Finklestein; she is 58. She comes charging into his office. She is wrinkled, gnarled, but carefully groomed, with plenty of make-up. She isn't interested in what he might say. She has things to tell him.

"Listen, Doctor, it's my family that aggravates me. Understand?" She laughs, loudly. "But I'm doing better. I am. Sometimes I take my medication for five or ten days straight. It's my own choice, after all. My daughter gets me nervous. You know that? She does. *She* has a problem and I'm the one who gets nervous. That you can understand, no doubt. And my mother lives with me, twenty-four hours a day. So. I get upset for a day, but I don't let it linger. I really don't let it linger. Thank God for that. I go to my daughter's place and if she's hos-tile, I accept it. And my son-in-law, the schmuck, I stay away from him and he stays away from me. But I know how he treats my daughter, I know. I don't like hands like his. You know what I mean? He's got ugly hands. His mouth is bad enough, the putz. Excuse me. But you know, tomorrow has to be better, so I accept things. I rely on my medication and when I feel I'm getting uptight, then I can see things realistically. I just don't want to keep on pills the rest of my life. You know, Doctor, I could be my own psychiatrist."

Kirshbaum, wondering if she'd allow any doctor to treat her, suggests she come back in a month for another talk. The opportunity for another monologue should entice her.

The next patient is one Kirshbaum has seen before, often. Peter Parker is 32, a dapper, upper-middle-class man with a psychiatric history dating back to age 18. He's been an inpatient at Bellevue. Now he is out and having trouble with being there.

"My weekend was sheer hell," he tells Kirshbaum. His manner is understated, never shrill. "I stayed in bed all weekend. I felt very weak. It was hard for me to do anything. In bed, I just tossed and turned."

"What were you thinking about?"

"How incapacitated I was. So many years of lost time, like the world has passed me by. Today I felt weak, down and out." He doesn't look down and out. His clothes are well tailored, not cheap. He has a tan he acquired during several months in Mexico, financed by his family.

"I can't stand this feeling. I came to the hospital today for a blood test, to find out what's wrong with me. It's so hard just to think. If I want to start to do something, I can't. I'm conscious of losing a day. It's my life and I don't want to defeat myself. I come and talk to you. I'm not as insanely distraught as I am physically down, perhaps caused by my mind."

He tells Kirshbaum that he had hoped to go on welfare, a move Kirshbaum had endorsed to give him one step toward independence. But he waited more than two hours to see a welfare clerk for three minutes, to discover that he needed a letter he didn't have.

"Okay. So I get the welfare money to live on. Where? In a hotel full of junkies and gutter rats, despicable types. So what? And another weekend will come up soon. God, I don't have any dignity of any kind. Where do I go from here? To welfare? To a vocational workshop? I can't relate to *anything* I'm doing."

"You assume your weakness will continue," Kirshbaum says.

"Sure I do. When I walk, I get pains in my left side. My gall bladder? God, I'm nothing. I *have* nothing. I can't provide for myself. My wife left me because I had no money. I'm deprived of seeing my children. The alternative seems to be death. I can whimper and cry, but I can't sleep and my days are so long. There's no place to hide."

"Can you accept all this, Peter?" Kirshbaum asks.

"Well, I'm still alive."

"Then pursue the welfare matter first. Proceed from the bottom up."

"I see guys my age being productive, having niceties, a decent life."

"Do you think it's hopeless?"

"I'm hanging on, day to day, knowing there are things I'll never attain."

"It isn't easy, but you can't run and hide."

"But what if it is physical?"

"You'll know. You've had tests. But the symptoms can be either physical or emotional. I can't tell yet."

"What do I do with my time? Watch others? Pass time? It's like being on a life raft alone. I'm like a business that keeps losing money. Should you invest strength and courage to prolong the agony or just give up?"

"I don't give up," Kirshbaum says. It is vital, for him, that he make the point.

"Okay. I'm putting myself in your hands."

"I'll outline the plan of action. You follow it. Step one is welfare."

"All right," Parker says. He gets up, wearily, and leaves.

It is almost 6 P.M. Kirshbaum hadn't noticed the passage of time this afternoon. He has to pick up his wife at her parents' apartment, then drive home. He walks out of the building, to his car. As he turns the key in the ignition, he stops. He wonders: if Parker stands too close to the edge of a subway platform as a train approaches, will he jump? Kirshbaum doesn't have the answer.

Lanie Eagleton's day begins with the pooling of diagnostic information, the 9 A.M. staff conference. A new patient has been admitted to the Chest Service during the night. He's a 68-year-old man being held in the Emergency Ward. One of the Chest Service residents, who was on duty when the man arrived, presents the case to the assembled staff.

The man has a long history of chest disease, TB and gastrointestinal bleeding. He was transferred from another hospital in dehydrated condition, with acute bronchitis. An alcoholic, he has not been cooperative, but the resident was able to get him on a Bird respirator, which as he breathes transports carbon dioxide out of the body and supplies oxygen to it. An EKG showed nothing of concern. What does concern the resident is that the man is retaining a large amount of carbon dioxide, creating an imbalance in his blood. Low oxygen content in the blood can be fatal. Eagleton agrees to visit the man later in the morning.

After the conference, Eagleton checks on the state of his bronchoscope. Out for ten days, it is still not repaired. He has several bronchoscopies he must perform so he plans to use a smaller unit, one that cannot perform a biopsy.

He walks through the wards, talking to interns, residents, nurses and patients. His conversations are sprinkled with the names of drugs common to the service: isoniazid (INH), rifampin, ethambutol. A resident asks him about yesterday's pathology conference, wonders how the organs displayed were obtained. Eagleton explains that he phoned the son of the patient who had died and obtained permission for an autopsy. Such approval is mandatory, he instructs the resident.

Similar approval must be obtained for a bronchoscopy. The old, frail woman who awaits Eagleton has given that permission, marking an "X" on the form; the resident treating her witnesses it. Eagleton has assembled his equipment on a cart and, joined by a nurse, brings it to the patient's bedside.

The old woman is in precarious health, so Eagleton has decided not to give her medication prior to the bronchoscopy. He is careful. A bronchoscopy tube clumsily inserted can impair breathing, cause bleeding. Normally, he would give a sedative, an anticough medication, a medication to diminish secretions and a local anesthetic. In this case, local anesthetic and an injection of atropine, to dry up secretions and help prevent fainting, will do.

Eagleton approaches the old woman, who is sitting lifelessly in a wheelchair beside her bed. IV fluid is dripping into her arm. He checks her chart, discovers that she is 86, with a history of stroke, cancer and heart trouble. Miraculously, so far she has survived them all. He listens to her breathing with a stethoscope.

"How are you doing?" he asks her.

She grimaces, but does not speak.

"How are you doing?" he repeats.

She grimaces again and does not speak.

Eagleton realizes that he is stepping on her toes and moves his foot. She stops grimacing. She is wearing a wrinkled white hospital gown and a pair of drooping support stockings bearing the stamp "BELLEVUE."

Eagleton attempts to explain what he's about to do.

"I'm going to use this bronchoscope," he tells her. "I'm going to put a tube down your nose to look for an infection or a mass." From X-rays and other findings he suspects that she has a cancerous mass, but he does not use the term. She listens to him without seeming to hear what he is saying. She stares.

"This will take about a half-hour," he tells her. She doesn't react.

He checks his equipment, assembles the bronchoscope, an electronic and optical device with a tube containing a small light at its tip. The tip is flexible, controlled remotely. As the doctor peers through the lens at one end, he can see through the tube into the patient and by moving a knob can alter what the tip views. A small brush attachment can sweep up cellular matter for analysis later; if this were the larger model, it could remove tissue for a biopsy.

Eagleton is ready. There are several nurses around if he needs their help.

He pours the patient a small paper cup of Xylocaine, the local anesthetic.

"This tastes really bad," he warns her, "so don't swallow it. Just gargle it and spit it out. Don't swallow it."

She swallows it.

"It's a benign drug," Eagleton says to the nurse. "She'll absorb it."

He sprays local anesthetic into her nose, gently pats her on the head. Her hair is white and thin; her scalp is visible through it.

With the help of several nurses, Eagleton lifts the old woman from her chair onto the bed, cranked up to elevate her head. The patient begins to react, for the first time, groaning softly. A nurse pulls curtains around the bed, so the other ward patients, also old women, won't see.

Eagleton sprays the woman's throat. He tries to get her to stick out her tongue, so he can grab it between pieces of gauze and spray a wider area. After several attempts, he succeeds. A nurse injects the atropine into the woman's right arm. Eagleton plugs in an electronic suction unit and turns to the patient.

"This will be a little uncomfortable, but it won't hurt you," he tells her. "You can talk to me all the time." The woman is frightened, but remains silent.

Eagleton lubricates the end of the tube and begins to insert it into the patient's left nostril. She shrieks. He feeds the tube along, slowly. She calms down. He continues feeding it, carefully, peering into the viewing eyepiece as it progresses.

"Relax now, dear, you're doing fine," he says.

He tries to get the patient to cough, so he can get a sputum sample to analyze. She won't, or can't. He studies, through the bronchoscope, all he can see, then slowly removes the tube and pats the woman on her head again.

She is now groaning again, meekly.

Eagleton has not seen much he can use. He has obtained secretions for a TB culture and cancer analysis. The small scope has limited penetration; he could not see any lesions, just inflammation. It will take six weeks for the TB to grow in culture, if it is there. Her cancer history is ominous, so, at her age, treating it may be useless, Eagleton feels. If the TB test is positive, that can be treated. She'll remain on the ward, getting TB care, until all the findings are in.

Eagleton says good-bye to the woman and goes to the Emergency Ward, as he has before, looking for candidates for the Chest Service. If he wants to use a particular respirator, he tries to find a new patient who can benefit from it. He wants to keep his staff busy and challenged and this is one of the ways of doing that. As he enters the EW, he meets an intern who has served a rotation on the Chest Service and has moved on.

"I miss you," the resident says. "It sure was quiet and peaceful up there. I sweat twenty-four hours a day now."

Eagleton smiles. He surveys the EW's assortment of cases; if he wants to admit a patient, he may have to compete with Medicine and Surgery for him. Today, there's just one and the Chest Service resident on duty last night has already claimed him for the service. It is the alcoholic whose case was discussed at the morning conference. Four Chest Service residents meet Eagleton beside the man's bed. This gives Eagleton a chance to do what he likes best, teach.

Eagleton sees the Chest Service as a strong teaching service.

He sees himself as both doctor and teacher. As he moderates the discussion of this case, he tries to get the residents to come to conclusions, correct ones, without leading them. He prods them. He asks questions, some of which he knows the answers to, and provides answers only when the residents seem baffled. His knowledge is comprehensive, his approach firm but benevolent. He can speak to these residents for minutes without using a common English sentence, restricting his speech to the specialized medical language of the service.

Surrounded by doctors, the alcoholic comes to life. What he says does not make sense, but he is, suddenly, animated. Over and over, he repeats, "Land of the living." As he babbles, Eagleton examines him meticulously, talking to the residents as he does. Then the group moves on to view the man's X-rays. Again, Eagleton, without being overbearingly pedantic, lectures. He is able to say to the residents, "When I was a young man . . ." without seeming pompous. He is 33 and they are in their middle twenties, and the difference in experience and knowledge is profound.

In this case, Eagleton cannot make a precise diagnosis and admits it. There is too much wrong with this man to single out one source of trouble. The residents will have to monitor his condition and keep Eagleton informed if developments puzzle them. He goes to lunch.

Today's menu includes an unidentifiable egg dish of Italian ancestry covered with tomato sauce, brown potatoes, canned fruit salad and, for Eagleton, his single conspicuous excess, two glasses of iced tea.

Today he lunches with members of his own staff. For those courageous enough to take him on, it can turn into a debate. One resident wants to talk about sedating asthmatics. He believes it can be done and he defends his position. When he's done, Eagleton looks at him and says, "You try not to sedate a sick asthmatic. It can be lethal." The resident, without realizing it, begins to slide his chair away from the table, as if in retreat.

"The overwhelming number of deaths from asthma, which isn't a killing disease, come when the patients are very ill and are given sedatives," Eagleton adds.

There is mumbled agreement with him on the part of the others at the table. The resident who originated the question timidly picks up his tray and leaves.

At a nearby table in the doctors' cafeteria, a Dermatology

resident and a medical student talk. The student, thinking about his own future, is full of questions.

"What can I expect in Dermatology?"

"Syphilis. Skin cancer. We do the penicillin skin tests for the entire hospital. You know, when a disease must be treated with penicillin and the patient may be allergic to it."

"What kind of facilities do you have?"

"We've got thirty-four beds in two wards, one male, one female."

"Any crazy cases?" the student asks.

"Sure. I remember one, a nineteen-year-old girl from Puerto Rico who was visiting New York. She had hypopigmented lesions on one arm. It wasn't bothering her. It wasn't getting bigger. But her parents, who brought her in, thought someone ought to look at it. One of our residents took a look. The area was anesthetic. She didn't have any feeling in it."

The student has been seduced by the mystery. He puts down his fork and listens.

"They called me and I came down and took a look, too. Leprosy, I thought. There are several tests you can do for it. For pain, feeling. We can scratch the area and put a drop of histamine on it. Normally, that would cause a flare, a redness. If it doesn't, there's damage already done. We admitted the girl and got a Neurology consult, to find out what kind of nerve damage was involved. It turned out that she had tuberculoid leprosy. For that, dapsone is the drug we use. It arrests the development of the disease, but what damage is done, is done. She took it all calmly."

"I didn't realize you saw leprosy at Bellevue," the student says.

"Sure. We had one from India not long ago. The guy felt he was stigmatized and he was right. And another from Thailand. Some from Central America. We don't see the ones who really look like animals. And we don't isolate the patients in our wards, unless the disease gets much worse suddenly. That's possible, by the way. They can get fevers of 106, life-threatening, if they're reacting to dapsone, which can happen. In those cases, the drug of choice, believe it or not, is thalidomide. And it's not easy to get."

"What about being at Bellevue? What about the patients you get here?"

"Well, nothing's worse than being poor and sick. At Bellevue, the quality of the medical care is very good. The waiting, the red tape are not so good. Then there's the language barrier. I speak Spanish. Good for me. But some of our patients, who've been here for five or ten years, don't speak English. Why not? Why must we be blamed for not speaking *their* language in *our* country?"

The student hasn't made up his mind about that. The conversation halts when both men see an attractive Oriental nurse-anesthetist slinking toward their table.

After lunch, Lanie Eagleton keeps in motion. His work is an endorsement of the value of Bellevue's affiliation with the N.Y.U. Medical School. Bellevue is a teaching hospital and Eagleton is a teacher. The affiliation, by definition, supports that. N.Y.U. Medical School faculty members, most of them practicing physicians, are found regularly in the halls of Bellevue, teaching residents and interns the realities of medicine in a setting far removed from the controlled environment of the classroom. Residents taught well in turn teach others. Eagleton, a particularly conscientious chief resident, has many to teach. The process gratifies him.

Today he will spend his afternoon pacing the wards, conferring with nurses, talking to patients, studying charts, advising residents, encouraging interns. His manner remains controlled, disciplined, but those who listen to him attentively have confidence in his skills as a doctor. He is not chummy with them, not interested in the fads and fashions of the outside world; their personal lives, and his, are not relative to what they are doing together. It is the patient who commands their attention.

Late in the afternoon, Eagleton devotes time to preparing a written proposal for a grant he is applying for, to do research next year when his tour as chief resident is over. He will go home to his family tonight; he has a day off tomorrow. He will spend some of that day continuing to work on his proposal.

Diane Rahman moves from bed to bed, making rounds, her two visiting medical students in line behind her, checking on women who have already delivered, on others who will be delivering soon. She explains the taking and processing of blood samples. One medical student has done it before. He seems blasé. The other hasn't. He pays attention. The trio goes from room to room, seeing nine patients. Seven are Puerto Rican, one black, one white. The exchanges are brief, pointed.

"How do you feel? You can go home tomorrow."

"How's the baby doing?"

"Your baby was a breech?" Rahman asks one woman. No answer. "Feet first?"

"*Sí.*"

She shows the students how to fill out forms for blood-test analyses. White, blue, pink. She must remember to sign each form or she'll hear about it and they'll be sent back to her for signature, delaying test results.

There are three women in the abortion room. The young woman who had been given saline solution yesterday has been vomiting. When Rahman moves toward her, she can see that the woman has a pillow over her head, her legs drawn up. Rahman orders medication for the nausea, theorizes aloud to the students, "If the fetus is dead from the saline, the uterus ought to expel it."

The teen-age black girl awaiting another abortion attempt sits propped up in bed, staring numbly out the window. Rahman checks her chart and discovers that a Psychiatry consult was requested. The psychiatrist who interviewed the girl noted that she "was sexually involved with her father, but says the father of this child is her boyfriend."

Rahman goes to the nursing station, to ask one of the nurses to do a urinalysis test on a patient for her.

"I've done eight of those on her already," the nurse snaps.

"She's scheduled to go home today and I'd like the test repeated," Rahman says, calmly.

"I'll try," the nurse replies, stalking off.

A well-dressed young Puerto Rican woman arrives with an application for an abortion. She has one child and has had a previous abortion. Rahman and the senior resident collaborate on the examination.

"This fetus may be too big to abort," the senior resident concludes.

"I'd say she's about twenty weeks," the senior resident adds. By New York law, an abortion can't be performed beyond twenty-four weeks; the state medical association opposes abortions beyond twenty weeks.

In Spanish, the senior resident tells the woman it is too late for an abortion. He asks her if that creates a problem.

Yes, it does. She's supposed to visit her sister in San Juan and she doesn't know she's pregnant. She is upset.

"It's unfortunate," Rahman says.

"Maybe not," the senior resident says. "Let's do an Ultrasound on her. I could be wrong."

At 9:30, Rahman and her medical students head for the clinic. The atmosphere is bustling, with lines of patients, many in their teens, waiting to be seen. Nurses, social workers and administrators dart from room to room.

Rahman can see as many as sixteen patients in two hours. Today there isn't time. She sees four women, then heads for coffee. She is scheduled to be part of a team performing a Caesarean section in a few minutes. At the snack bar, she sits restlessly waiting for her cup of coffee. "You learn to have patience at Bellevue," she says stoically.

What is it like being a first-year resident? one of the students asks her.

"Well, when you start medical school, the hospital seems so far away. You get through school, year by year, and then it's time. I really didn't know I'd be at Bellevue after graduation, but when I visited OB, as you're doing right now, I liked it and I wanted to stay on. As a matter of fact, about a third of the graduates in my class, about 48 out of 130, stayed at Bellevue."

The coffee arrives and is quickly consumed. Rahman stops at the Blood Bank to check on the blood needed on hand for the Caesarean section. It's already been picked up by another resident. Rahman and her escorts head for the delivery room.

The patient is a 34-year-old Puerto Rican woman. She has had a Caesarean in the past, so it was decided to do another. The medical cast assembles. The chief resident, a woman, will do most of the work. An attending physician will stand by, to advise. The senior resident will play a primary role. Rahman will assist. Three nurses, a nurse-anesthetist, an anesthesiologist and two interns from Pediatrics, to claim the baby for their care, are present.

The procedure, which will take two hours, begins at 10:50 A.M. Two nurses are the first to arrive, in gowns, masks, gloves. The delivery table is lit from above by two large movable lights. Equipment is spread on carts, ready for use. Two nurses wheel in the patient and transfer her from bed to table. The nurse-anesthetist and the anesthesiologist check their equipment. The senior resident enters, talks to the patient, who is awake. She is nervous.

The anesthetist gives the woman an epidural anesthetic, near the base of the spine, inserts a catheter to inject more of it when needed. One of the nurses holds the patient's hand, strokes her head.

"You're shaking. Are you scared?" she asks. "Don't be."

The attending, clearly older than all the others, enters; a nurse dries his hands, helps him into his gown and gloves.

All the doctors are now around the table. The anesthetist tests the effect of the epidural with pinpricks; the patient does not respond. A nurse and the senior resident paint her stomach with Betadine, then drape it with a plastic adhesive sterile skin barrier. It adheres to her abdomen, where the incision will be made. Layers of sterile cloth go over it until, finally, only the area of the incision is visible. The end of the cloth is draped so the patient cannot see what will take place. She seems to be in labor, in pain. The anesthetist checks her blood pressure, gives her oxygen.

The chief resident makes the first cut, a horizontal line, with a scalpel across her lower abdomen. The doctor is very careful, tracing the line lightly over and over in the same channel. As she does this, the senior resident ties off blood vessels. With their fingers the two residents separate flesh from muscle. Rahman helps sponge the blood that oozes from the incision.

The senior resident wants more light. He reaches up, moves one of the overhead fixtures. In doing that, he contaminates his right glove. A nurse helps him put a new one over the old one. The attending quietly offers advice, guiding the residents. They split and separate muscle tissue to get to the peritoneum, which they carefully cut through with a scissors, cautiously avoiding the bladder nearby. If they see blood, fine; if they see yellow fluid, it means they've nicked the bladder.

There are now eight people around the patient. A Pediatrics intern stands a few feet away, holding a tray to receive the baby.

The two residents cut into the uterus, delicately, and the entire area of the incision is retracted and held open.

The membranes rupture and amniotic fluid comes splashing out; immediately, it is suctioned away. The chief resident reaches in and the senior resident pushes on the woman's stomach. There is tension, tugging and pushing. The incision does not appear to be wide enough for an easy exit. Air has entered and the baby has begun to cry, although it is not visible yet. Finally, after a struggle, the baby's head emerges, then the rest of its body. Its nose and mouth are suctioned promptly. The placenta follows it out and is preserved for study. What began as a delivery now becomes basic surgery, repairing what has been done to deliver the baby.

A nurse takes the baby's footprints, wraps it up in a blanket and shows it to the mother. "It's a girl," she says. The mother looks at the baby but is not distracted; she is in pain, groaning, pleading, writhing, making it difficult for the doctors to close the incision. She appeals to God, in Spanish. The anesthetist has been monitoring the woman's blood pressure and pulse and announces that both are fine.

"Terrific," the senior resident shouts. "But we need this patient to be unconscious. *Unconscious.*"

The anesthetist notices that the residents have stopped working and are staring at her. She quickly sends more anesthetic into the IV line and, after one spasm, the patient is out. The residents resume their work.

A nurse is talking to the baby. "Come on, child, cry. Get mad." She wants the baby to work up excess fluids; she inserts a suction tube into the baby's mouth and nose. The baby howls.

The attending leaves while the residents stitch. Rahman is working closely with them now.

The Pediatrics intern has examined the baby and carts it off to the nursery. The room is quiet, as the residents work.

"Keep your head up," the senior resident says to Rahman; when she leans over the incision, she obscures his vision.

By 1 P.M., the work is done. Appropriately, the only ones left with the patient are women: Rahman, the chief resident, one nurse and the anesthetist.

Moments later, outside the delivery room, Rahman and the senior resident lean against a wall, exhausted after the intensity of the Caesarean section. It was not as "routine" as originally expected. The unexpected tests obstetricians.

"A vertical incision would have been safer," the senior resident says, "but the last Caesarean she had was done with a smile incision, so we did another."

"What didn't you expect?" Rahman asks.

"There was that difficulty in getting the baby out, in grasping the head. When the air got in, after the fluid came gushing out, I had to stick my finger in the baby's mouth and get a suction tube into it. So the baby wouldn't breathe that fluid. I had to improvise. I used the back of a forceps."

What about the patient moving around on the table?

"She was agitated, not in pain. She did complain of chest pain and I don't know what that is all about. I do know that she needed something and if the anesthetist had been more experienced, she would have anticipated that. You can't work on a patient who's moving around, for God's sake."

What about that chest pain?

"Do an EKG on her right away, then a blood gas and a chest X-ray. It could be nothing. It could be muscle strain. It could be a pulmonary embolism, dangerous. If it is, the blood gas will show that her oxygen level has dropped."

Rahman and the senior resident are exhausted. Neither has had lunch. Neither will. As they separate, he turns to Rahman.

"A secret," he says. "You remember when I pushed on her stomach, just before the membranes ruptured? Keep in mind that I pushed toward the chief resident. When it splashed, it splashed on her."

Another woman may be ready to deliver and Rahman takes a look at her. She is a very short, very fat diabetic Puerto Rican woman, a cheerful and confident mother of six. As Rahman palpates her enormous stomach, a bearded African senior resident walks up. It is time, he feels, to induce labor.

"I'm going to burn my boats," he says.

"Your bridges?" Rahman asks.

"We don't have many bridges in Africa," he answers, a wide smile on his face.

He inserts tubing into the woman's vagina. Fluid drains out. He attaches electrodes to the woman's stomach, measuring the fetal heartbeat and uterine contractions, the latter on graph paper, the former on an audible beep emerging from the monitor at the woman's bedside.

The medical students have returned from lunch and are huddled around, listening. The African resident turns to them and says, "It tells us what the baby is doing during labor."

The patient looks up and says, "I'll be more happy when I see the baby out there."

It is time to wait. The woman has been given medication to induce labor. It may be several hours before she is ready to deliver.

Rahman goes to the ward pantry, smears peanut butter on a slice of white bread and devours it. The students, perpetually loyal, watch her. When she's done, she instructs them in doing an EKG on the woman who just gave birth by Caesarean section. Tired though she is, her explanation of the workings of the machine is precise. They proceed to do the EKG as Rahman sits and watches. They complete it—nothing alarming is revealed by it—and start to leave.

A nurse sees them and sticks out her arm.

"No. No. No. You don't just walk away," she says. "Wipe off each plate with alcohol, because the jelly corrodes the plates."

Sheepishly, they oblige.

It is now late in the afternoon and Rahman is thinking more about the dinner she hopes to eat than the lunch she missed. First, she has to see a new patient, a woman with cardiac complications, and that will require a consultation with the woman's cardiologist at Bellevue. She has to complete forms on the Caesarean delivery. She has a number of discharge examinations to do, so eager mothers can pick up their babies and take them home. The nursery wants her to do a circumcision.

She's on duty tonight, which means she'll be available through the night, to help with deliveries, deal with emergencies, confront any patient complaints. She will be lucky to get any sleep. There's a lecture she wants to attend at 8 A.M., if she's sufficiently alert and interested at 8 A.M. to make it.

Today is Bob Nachtigall's day to schlepp, as he puts it. As a first-year resident, he's responsible for running medical errands delegated to him by the residents to whom he is subordinate. As he arrives in GYN, a third-year resident spots him.

"Dr. Nachtigall, it is a real pleasure to have you with us. I'd like you to meet the nurses and your fellow doctors. It is important on this service to keep your eyes open. No slits allowed."

"I had advance information that today would be a slow day," Nachtigall counters, laughing.

Their confrontation is cut short by the appearance of a woman in her mid-twenties, on the ward to have an abortion today. She is frantic. She wants to see the psychiatrist she's been seeing at Bellevue's clinic, because she's "very nervous." The third-year resident assures her he'll call the psychiatrist, but the patient wants him to "do it now." He does.

When she realizes that her psychiatrist is on his way, she retreats. The resident asks a junior resident what sort of sedative he's given the woman. Five mg. of Valium, the resident tells him.

"Could you spare it? *You* need five. She should get ten," the third-year resident orders.

The woman returns, wanting to know when she's going to the operating room. A time isn't set yet. She shuffles off to her bed, distracted, muttering.

Nachtigall goes to Radiology to arrange for X-rays on a woman who has had plastic surgery on her Fallopian tubes, in an effort to repair a tubal ligation she had in Puerto Rico after having had six children. She is 21 and now has a new husband, who wants a child of his own.

While Nachtigall is reserving the time for her X-rays, a Radiology technician seems unwilling to be cooperative about the appointment. Nachtigall hasn't time to waste, but he tries to remain polite.

"Too many doctors get smart with me," the technician, a tall, thin, twitching man in his thirties, screams.

Nachtigall turns and leaves in mid-shout. "It's a nice day," he says to himself. "I'm in no mood to fight with a skinny creep like that."

He is used to rudeness at Bellevue. "He's going to do his job, for which he gets paid, as a personal favor to me," Nachtigall says.

He goes to the Blood Bank to pick up a unit of blood for a cancer patient who has become anemic and needs it badly. Then he goes up to the operating room area, to confirm today's GYN operating schedule. He makes small talk, attempting to be ingratiating, with one of the nurses. When he leaves, he says, "A ball-buster extraordinaire."

Back on one of the GYN wards, he hooks up the unit of blood to the patient's IV.

"I'll piggyback it with a bottle of saline solution," he tells a nurse on duty, "so if you don't catch it when the blood stops dripping, the line will stay open." It is a procedure he knows is wasteful of the equipment required, but he doesn't trust the nurse to observe the blood running out, despite the fact that only nine of the twenty beds in this ward are filled.

As he gives the patient the blood, he seems depressed. "She has that look, the look of a terminal cancer patient," he tells the nurse. "The tissues seem to melt away, the bones become prominent. And she has lost weight, fifty pounds since she came in here."

The ward itself is quiet. It is a long room, with a row of ten beds facing another row of ten. There are curtains that can be drawn for privacy around each bed. At the far end of the ward there is a small table with chairs and a TV set.

Nachtigall leaves the ward to make a few phone calls. He calls for the result of a Pap test taken six days earlier. He calls Hematology for the results of a bone-marrow analysis on a cancer patient who doesn't know she has cancer. It is a confusing, frustrating matter for Nachtigall to handle. One of the medical students has been lingering near the phone, eavesdropping. Nachtigall addresses him.

"If there's a family, they're told. But the patient knows, too, if he's on cobalt or gets radical surgery. They *know* without anyone telling them. They go through a series of reactions, from denial to anger to either acceptance or rejection. As far as I'm concerned, I don't believe in forcing a patient to confront the diagnosis. Patients rarely ask. We may hedge if they do, but we don't lie. We certainly try to let them know that all is not right, that something serious is wrong, even if we don't use that word. Patients aren't eager to have their worst fears confirmed, to be told about death. We tell them they have a tumor, a mass, but 'cancer' is such an emotionally laden term.

"The family knows, as I said, and they know the prognosis. It's important that the family unit be supportive. The patient's main fear is that of being abandoned and doctors often can't deal with that, because of their own fears and frustrations. The family is what matters. But if I'm asked by a patient, I try to deal with the positive aspects. 'There's no reason to believe you're not cured,' I might say to a patient. Somebody will live for ten years with the disease. I know that. Why not *this* patient? And the patients we get are terribly unsophisticated about what they have. We care for them. Why torment them?"

One of Nachtigall's patients is the 41-year-old Finnish

woman, who has four children. Yesterday Nachtigall performed a D&C on her; Pathology will decide if the specimens he obtained are cancerous or not. The chief resident believes she needs a hysterectomy, to correct her prolapsed bladder. Removing the uterus, the chief feels, will help her long-term health. However, it must all be explained to her, for her approval, and she does not speak English.

Nachtigall calls the page operator, who pages anyone in Bellevue with a knowledge of Finnish. No one responds. A GYN nurse remembers that there is a patient on another service who speaks Finnish. She goes to find him.

The Finnish woman has been joined by members of her family, including her husband; they sit calmly in a waiting room. In a few minutes, the nurse brings the patient from the other service, a man in a wheelchair. Nachtigall, the translator and the Finnish family meet.

Through the man in the wheelchair, Nachtigall explains the operation. The Finnish woman agrees to it.

"We will do it Thursday," Nachtigall says, "and there will be no cutting in the belly. She will feel well and will go home in a week. We can write a letter to her job, saying she should stay home to rest for a few weeks. After the operation, she will have no more periods, but it will not affect her as a woman."

The translator passes along the message. The husband has a question. Can she have more children?

"No," Nachtigall says to the translator, "but tell him she will still have desire for her husband."

The woman and her husband sign the necessary form. Nachtigall goes immediately to type the letter to her employer that he promised. He delivers it to the husband. The translator is wheeled back to his ward. The Finns remain, to talk. The woman, with the face of a peasant, has a placid, beautiful expression. She holds her husband's hand; they smile at each other.

After lunch Nachtigall stops off at GYN to pick up an empty pathology jar and head for University Hospital. Once or twice a month he sells semen (at $25 per contribution) to the artificial-insemination program at UH. "I'd like to do it more often," he says, grinning, to the third-year resident standing nearby. "It's a dinner out. And look how much good I'm doing for the human race."

On the way back from UH, he stops off at the GYN clinic, "the closest thing to private practice," and sees several patients. Then he heads to Radiology to perform a hysterosalpingogram on one of his patients. It's a long word for a simple process: simultaneously X-raying and fluoroscoping the inside of a woman's uterus and Fallopian tubes. As Nachtigall arrives, in the background another resident is battling a Radiology clerk. "At least you could be civil to me," he is shouting. Nachtigall, used to it, doesn't even notice.

The woman in for the test is from West Germany, a childless woman who has had surgery in an effort to correct deformed tubes, possibly damaged by TB while she lived in Europe. Dye is injected and its course followed on a screen. When the test, brief and painless, is done, Nachtigall and a senior resident check the results.

Their conclusion, tentative, is that the surgery was successful. Her tubes seem to be open; dye has flowed smoothly. If she is capable of having a child and the tubes were her problem, she should be able to have a child now. Nachtigall takes her back to the ward himself, rather than wait for a messenger to do it. The woman has not said a word throughout the procedure.

When Nachtigall gets back to the wards, he sees a psychiatrist with the nervous abortion case. The abortion has been done and the woman is desperately anxious to go home. Nachtigall talks to the Psychiatry resident, prescribes Valium for the woman and tells her she can leave whenever she feels ready.

It is now 3 P.M., time for chart rounds in the chief resident's office. The chief announces that he wants to do the hysterectomy on the Finnish woman on Friday. Nachtigall groans; he had told her it would be done on Thursday and now, he says, he'll have to retrieve the translator to change the date. The chief doesn't comment; it is Nachtigall's problem.

A young woman arrives, asks to see one of the residents. Her message is carried into chart rounds by a medical student.

"There's this very cute girl out there with big jugs who says she wants to get undressed just for you," the medical student announces.

The resident in question perks up.

"She looks like one of your girl friends. You know, about fourteen or fifteen."

"If she's one of *my* girl friends, she's a virgin, too," the resident says, going out to see the woman.

A resident brings up the matter of a 23-year-old woman, with three children, who was in for an abortion. The chief resident feels she needs more than an abortion. "She doesn't need more kids," he says. He thinks she ought to have a tubal ligation and he feels, as do several other residents present, that she's a psychiatric case, too.

"She wants to go home," the resident says.

"Tough. Not yet," the chief overrules. "When she's fine, she can go. Let's talk to her about what we think ought to be done."

Finally, the chief wants to talk about one of the ward patients, an 83-year-old woman with cancer. He doesn't want to wait. "That lady has to have a hysterectomy, and she's too ill to give consent," he says, emphatically. "Tonight, you get a relative to approve it. I don't give a shit how you do it. This lady has cancer and she must be operated on this week, without delay."

The OR schedule for the rest of the week is planned and approved. Nachtigall has been taking notes, passing charts back and forth from the rack to the chief's desk. All the charts have now been reviewed. It is 5 P.M. when the rounds end. Nachtigall stuffs his notes into the pocket of his white jacket and heads for home.

At his early morning meeting with the on-call resident, Bruce Mack is interested in one of the cases the resident recites.

Last night at 6:39 P.M., a 56-year-old black woman named Norma Bacon was admitted to the Emergency Ward in a coma. She had been found in her apartment, unconscious. She was unable to provide any medical history and a Neuro consult was requested. The resident tells Mack that when the woman arrived she was breathing, but little else. Her extremities were unresponsive. Her blood pressure was high. Her pupils were pinpoints, unreactive to light. The resident thought she might have some brain-stem dysfunction; he suspected possible bleeding. He wondered if she could be saved.

She was placed on IV fluids, a respirator and a cardiac monitor, the resident reports. Several drugs were tried. Mannitol was used to attack the edema in the brain (if it works, it reduces such pressure) and steroids to stabilize the membranes of the neurons in the brain. Within a half-hour, some improvement was seen. She regained some eye function, but she could move her eyes only to the mid-line, not from corner to corner.

Mack is encouraged by that fact. It suggests that there was not intrinsic bleeding into the brain stem. Had it been intracerebral bleeding, he tells the resident, "No surgeon would have touched it." It could be a lesion in one of the hemispheres of the cerebrum, but Mack discounts that; the evidence doesn't seem to support it. It could be bleeding resulting in the compression of the cerebellum against the brain stem. If he's correct, an angiogram might reveal it. Then surgery might be possible. If the bleeding is superficial, the clot can be suctioned out, along with tissue, relieving the pressure; a small area of the cerebellum might have to be removed as well. That could cause side effects, like an altered gait, but surgery may be essential to save the woman's life, whatever such side effects. There is a risk: if the brain-stem condition cannot be corrected, or if the stem doesn't recover from surgery, the woman could live out her life as a vegetable. Mack thinks aloud; the resident listens.

They visit the woman in the Emergency Ward. Mack tells a nurse that the woman should be moved immediately to Neuroradiology for the angiogram. The nurse resists. She doesn't have the proper authorization, the signed document, to permit that, she says to Mack.

"This woman has no family as far as we know and this is an emergency, a life-saving situation," Mack says, firmly. The nurse backs down and Mack and the resident wheel the woman's bed into the Neuroradiology lab.

Coming out of Neuroradiology, Mack sees another Neurology resident racing toward him. He has a report on Mary Rollins. The EEG is ominously flat, indicating that her brain function is gone. More important, a few more toxicology tests were done and the lab has concluded that the woman consumed a lethal amount of methyl alcohol (wood alcohol), which in its pure state is as tasteless as vodka. It turns to acid quickly and attacks all the systems of the body.

Mack listens intently. When the resident is done, Mack says, "I've never seen one like this recover," and heads for the ICU to see the woman again.

The Medical resident tells him that hemodialysis has been

attempted, the mechanical filtering of the blood system, without any sign of success. It is too late to purify her blood, to eliminate the attacking alcohol. Mary Rollins is pale, without any apparent sign of life.

"Futile," Mack mutters. He is confused by her consumption of methyl alcohol. "It is not a sophisticated way, not quick or unobtrusive, to poison someone or to commit suicide," he says. He stares at the patient, turns to the Medical resident. They agree that she'll be supported mechanically until cardiac arrest makes its inevitable intervention.

There is a macabre terminology, a grim series of jokes, that some Bellevue doctors use to describe terminal patients. An "O" is a patient in bed with mouth wide open. A "Q" is a patient with mouth open and tongue dangling out. A "3-OJ" is a patient with three orange juice stains on the lips and half-empty glasses on the bedside table. There are patients in the "one-fly," "two-fly" and "three-fly" categories, for the number of flies they can tolerate on their bodies; the higher the number, the closer they are to death.

As Mack leaves the ICU, he notices that there are three flies on Mary Rollins' arm. He doesn't make the joke.

He heads back to Neuroradiology, for the angiogram. The patient is in place, ready for the test. Mack trusts that to the skills of the neuroradiologists. He leaves to meet with the residents and the attending who will join them today.

The attending is middle-aged, trim, dignified, with gray hair, glasses and a pipe. It is a typical teaching situation at Bellevue. The attending is there to help the residents solve problems.

The first case is that of Norma Bacon, now undergoing the angiogram. The attending agrees with Mack's diagnosis. One of the residents notes that he phoned Miss Bacon's employer, who said she had no history of complaints at her job, so "we can assume that the attack was sudden."

Mack describes, for the attending's opinion, the case of Mary Rollins. One of the residents interrupts to say that he has talked with her boyfriend. "He thinks he drank the same vodka she did," the resident says, "but he did add that she had been despondent for the past month, after her younger brother died. He insisted that she wasn't suicidal. I asked him to bring in the bottle of vodka, so we could analyze it. He said he would and he seemed straight and serious to me. I just couldn't ask him if he poisoned her."

"Nevertheless," the attending says, "I think a medical detective is called for now." Mack assures him that the police will be notified, if they're not already involved.

The group discusses, briefly, the case of a crusty old woman with a possible aneurysm. She's been causing trouble on the ward.

"What did the physical exam show?" the attending asks.

"A nasty old woman," Mack replies. "The Psych consult who saw her said she was 'a paranoid psychotic' and recommended Thorazine."

After the meeting, Mack thinks of the cafeteria food and decides to skip lunch.

He is on his way to Neuroradiology, to check on Norma Bacon's angiogram, when he meets the chief resident from Neurosurgery. Mack alerts him to the possible need for immediate surgery on the woman. The chief resident says he'll be ready if Mack needs him.

In Neuroradiology, the films have been studied. The neuroradiologist's verdict: a cerebellum hemorrhage is the cause of the trouble; there is a hematoma visible on the X-rays. Mack picks up the phone to check with Neurosurgery about operating on her today. He learns that the chief resident has been called away suddenly, but a senior resident is ready to operate. Mack, talking to the neuroradiologist, says, "The results might not be dramatic, immediately evident. It could take weeks to determine if the surgery is successful. But it's worth the risk." He is glad that his diagnosis stood up and led to positive action, promptly.

Mack realizes that he hasn't had a moment alone all day. Preoccupied with two major cases, one depressingly terminal, the other with some hope, he has grown weary. He is scheduled to attend a neurology conference at the Veterans Administration Hospital. He walks over and discovers that the conference has been canceled. He sits around with a few other residents who hadn't gotten the news either. At 4 P.M., he decides to head for the crosstown bus, to meet his wife at home.

At 8:05, Kalman Post's patient from the VA Hospital, the man due to have the embolization, is wheeled into Neuroradiology. He is sedated but awake. Post has already explained the procedure to him; he has agreed to undergo it.

The patient is strapped to a table. Nurses have arranged all the instruments and equipment needed. Above the table, a fluoroscopic apparatus surveys its field; the embolization will be projected on a TV-like screen.

Embolization is not a common procedure; in two years, not more than a dozen have been done at University Hospital and Bellevue combined. In this case, if the embolization works, it could minimize surgery later.

The neuroradiologists scurry around while Post simply observes. An angiogram will be done first; it will take more than two hours. From the map of the man's brain it will provide, the doctors can define the area that will be the target of the embolization.

"This is a procedure that needs a lot of malpractice insurance," one of the neuroradiologists sighs. In fact, the patient had to be transferred from the VA to Bellevue, officially, and admitted to Bellevue, officially, in order to be certain that Neuroradiology would be fully covered. There are some risks in sending pellets into the brain.

Post has observed angiograms before; he does not have to witness this one. He decides to check a few patients at the VA, but as he is on his way out the door, another Neurosurgery resident stops him with a report. Last night's jumper, brought in by police, died in the operating room. Both sides of his chest were filled with blood and he died before the source of the bleeding could be determined. Neurosurgery never got the chance to study his fractured spine. Post makes a note to check with the Medical Examiner's office to see if he can attend the autopsy.

At 9 A.M., he is at the VA. When he gets there, he discovers that one of his patients, an old man with a possible brain-stem tumor, a perplexing case, is surrounded by white: two residents, two nurses and a nurse's aide. One of the residents explains to Post that at 3 A.M. the old man pulled out a ventricular drain in his head, designed to remove excess fluid, causing pressure on his brain.

Post is mystified. How did the man manage to pull out the drain? He had restraints on, tying his wrists to the side of the bed. It seems impossible.

"He had to do it with his hands," Post says. "There's no other way. It had two stitches in it. And he was zonked out."

He is angry, but tries to keep it under control. The man's intracranial pressure has risen.

"Maybe it was a faulty connection in the drain," one of the residents suggests.

"Impossible," Post says. "Once you get a guy on drainage, you've got to keep him on it. And he's the sickest guy on the floor."

The day head nurse is there. She shares Post's concern.

"The night shift will hear from me," she tells him.

Post waits until the drain has been replaced and the man has been given oxygen. Then, accompanied by a nurse, he visits several patients.

One man, who sits in bed unresponsively, does not acknowledge Post's arrival. He has had a tracheotomy and Post suctions through the opening in his throat. He reminds the nurse that when a doctor does that he must hold his breath, to know how much deprivation the patient can take, with the trach tube blocked.

"If you stand and suction endlessly, blocking the tracheostomy [the opening] with the suction tube, you can forget that the patient needs the opening to breathe. Respiratory arrest can occur," Post instructs. He inserts a new trach tube, delicately. The patient gags. The tube is in.

Post drops in on a middle-aged black man, in traction to correct a fracture of his upper spine. The man is in pain.

"How are you doing?" Post asks him.

"How am I doing? Man, I've been here a month and a week. And, man, I can't cut it. I mean, I can't sleep like this. I'm human, Doctor, and I just can't stay like this," the man bellows.

Post explains why the traction is necessary. "I know it's difficult for you," he tells the patient, "but we wouldn't do it to you unless we thought it would help make you better."

Post and the nurse walk down the long, clean, bright corridor. They pass a room and Post simply looks in, pauses and resumes walking. In the room, a young man in his twenties, with a terminal brain tumor, is staring into space. His young wife sits beside him, staring at him.

"What can you do for him?" the nurse asks.

"Nothing, I'm afraid. It's right smack in the center of his brain and we can't operate on it."

At 10:30, Post returns to Bellevue. The angiogram on the man due to be embolized is in progress. Post walks over to the Medical Examiner's office, on Thirtieth Street.

He peers into the main autopsy room, where seven bodies are being worked on simultaneously. The room smells of foul air and chemicals, and the bodies, like a squad of bombed soldiers, give the place a hideous warlike quality. Post grimaces and backs out of the room. He asks a clerk if the autopsy on the Chinese jumper has been scheduled.

"I don't know, Doctor," the clerk tells him. "But the story is like this. The guy killed another man and when the police got there he jumped out a fifth-floor window to escape. He had to be nutty to do that."

The clerk confirms the resident's report: the man died in the OR, making it a self-solving crime. He shows Post the report filled out by the surgical resident, one of the team that worked on him before he died. It reads: "Jumped from Fifth Floor. Semi-stuperous. No complaints."

Post laughs, looks at the clerk, who is laughing, too.

"No complaints," Post says.

"No complaints," the clerk echoes.

The resident, used to dealing with complaining patients, could not be deterred from seeking another.

Post leaves the ME's office and returns to Neuroradiology. The embolization, he's told, will begin at noon. Post paces. Another resident, wearing a thick bandage around his head, walks in. Post sees him, looks alarmed.

"What happened to you?" Post asks.

"Hair transplants," the resident says.

The two chat. The other resident is from Medicine and he suggests that neurosurgeons often have to settle for less than a cure.

"Sure," Post agrees. "If we can give a patient three more years of better life, we think we've succeeded. You have to be objective about it, not easily depressed by the frustrations involved. Making someone more functional for a time, even for a few months, may be all we can do. It's very important to have that time, to set your life straight. This is something I had to come to terms with early, to the limitations in what I do. And my own emotional response to it all."

The embolization has begun and Post watches. The

neuroradiologist has the tube into the man's groin and is injecting the small pellets into it. They are so small they are almost invisible. As they make their way through the tube to the brain, X-rays are taken.

Blocking off 10 to 30 percent of the troubling blood vessels with pellets would be considered satisfactory, a 40 to 50 percent blockage a success, enabling the neurosurgeons to remove the vessels surgically. On earlier X-rays, they seemed to be superficial vessels, making such surgery easier. However, as the new X-rays are developed, some of the pellets seem to be soaring beyond the area in which they're needed. The crew of neuroradiologists pauses, to evaluate what's been done so far.

Post is not happy with the first results. He expresses his ambivalent feelings to the neuroradiologists, who assure him that they'll continue to work on it. Post, unsettled, walks out.

After lunch, Post confers with the chief resident in Neuroradiology about the embolization.

"We changed nothing," Post suggests.

"It certainly isn't too encouraging," the chief resident says. He decides to get the advice of the chief of his service. He phones him, and within a few minutes the chief is there.

Studying the X-rays, the chief tells Post and the chief resident that a larger-size pellet must be used. The small ones might be passing right through, without adhering to the blood vessels.

Thirty-five larger pellets are introduced through the tube and another series of X-rays, taken and developed immediately, reveal improved results. A cluster of pellets has adhered to the vessels. More large pellets are sent in, to expand the coverage. A chest X-ray is taken, to determine if any of the pellets have made their way into the lungs. None is evident.

The patient remains under general anesthesia, as he has from the beginning, with an anesthesiologist monitoring him. Post pulls up a stool and watches as the neuroradiologists continue their effort. Hours pass. Post gets up, phones the patient's wife and tells her she can be with him very soon. At 5:30, the embolization is over.

The doctors involved in it discuss it. "One patient needed, and got, the bulk of our time today," a resident notes. "More than two hundred X-rays were taken," a technician adds. According to the chief of the service, if all the costs were totaled, the embolization would amount to an expenditure of $10,000.

"At a private hospital, the patient would get a bill for $1,000. They'd absorb the excess. At Bellevue, he'll be billed for one day in the hospital, less than $140, and then only if he can afford to pay it," the chief tells the others.

When Lori Chiarelli gets to the Emergency Ward, before 8 A.M., she finds eight patients in its beds.

Among them are: the man recovering from exposure to the weather. The nurses' notes reveal that at 1:30 A.M. his temperature had returned to normal, his other vital signs were normal and X-rays were negative. He is sitting up in bed when Chiarelli passes by. Another nurse says to Chiarelli, "For *him*, this is the Ritz." The businessman with heart irregularity and lung complications may be a diabetic; tests are being done to find out, and to rule out myocardial infarction. The old woman who fell in her bathroom may not have had a stroke after all; her brain scan was negative. Her condition may be reversible. An old man with a broken leg, compound fracture, open, of the right femur, is in traction. An old woman is suffering from acute anemia and assorted other maladies, the products of decades of neglect. A young Puerto Rican man was admitted at 2 A.M., a methadone overdose victim. He aspirated his own vomit and is being watched for pneumonia and treated with steroids to attack the inflammation doctors spotted. A 56-year-old black woman, brought in last night with a brain hemorrhage, is motionless. An old man, an alcoholic, coughs and spits; it's a respiratory matter and someone from the Chest Service will be down to see him.

"*Cómo esta, amigo?*" the Roman Catholic chaplain asks the Puerto Rican. The OD just nods, inconclusively.

At 8:15, while Chiarelli continues to compile the Board, breakfast for those who can eat is wheeled in on a double-tiered cart. There are six nurses on duty, in addition to Chiarelli, and they're all busy, drawing curtains around beds, cleaning patients, offering bedpans. They are a young and attractive group, making the EW a paradise for male chauvinist doctors.

At 8:25, eight Medical residents arrive to survey the cases in the EW; they find the old woman who has enough symptoms to test them all. At 8:45, an AES resident wheels in a new case, an old black woman. The resident tells Chiarelli, "She's a poor creature from a nursing home. It's an old stroke and a new seizure disorder." Nine more Medical residents file in, to study the woman who fell in her bathroom. The EW is getting crowded. A few minutes later, a group of Trauma Service residents walks in, too.

Chiarelli keeps busy, systematizing everything. She is a meticulous record-keeper, supply-checker. A new staff nurse comes up to her and asks her what she's doing.

"It's important to understand the routine," Chiarelli tells her, "so you don't come to expect constant excitement. You can't wait for that in here. You've got to get everything done the way it ought to be done, with or without excitement."

At 9:30, she joins several other nurses for a coffee break in the snack bar. It's the only place to have coffee, unless you brew it yourself, so the nurses tolerate the high noise level. They exchange tidbits of news and gossip and experiences. One is planning a week at the Club Méditerranée in Martinique. Another, new to Bellevue, recalls her days with the Peace Corps in Colombia.

"It was on the Colombia-Venezuela border and I was the only nurse there," she says. "There were always military skirmishes going on. Our equipment included hundreds of vaginal speculums, don't ask me why, but antiseptic was hard to find. I would have settled for Listerine. We were treating troops hacked by machetes. After that, this place seems calm."

At 10:30, the warmed-up exposure victim is transferred out of the EW to a Medical ward. His bed is made ready for a new patient.

The anemic old lady is causing concern. Her white-cell count is rising rapidly, doubling in a matter of hours to 150,000. Her temperature is 104. A hypothermia machine is wheeled to her bedside; it is used to pump ice water into a blanket beneath her, to cool her down. Her red-cell production, a resident reports, is minimal and the white cells are immature, incapable of fighting infection. As Chiarelli passes the woman's bed, surrounded by residents, one doctor looks at her and says, "Her prognosis is zilch."

An attending and four residents are examining the OD. He is 22 and was found on a street in the East Village. He had taken 150 mg. of methadone, given to him by a friend, he says. He insists that it was the first time he ever took it, or any other drug. True or false, it was enough to put him out.

"This experiment you did," one of the residents tells him, "it almost cost you your life."

As the attending and the residents examine the man, it is clear that the teaching process has been reversed. One of the residents has treated fifty such cases at Bellevue. The attending, in private practice most of his time, rarely sees such patients. The residents tell the attending about drugs used to counteract ODs. In this case, the overdose has been dealt with; pneumonia is now the potential problem.

At 11:15, the businessman with the cardiac problem is shifted to the Coronary Care Unit. Chiarelli chats with the resident on the case; she wants information about heart block. The resident explains patiently and she thanks him, cordially. She's gotten the information she wanted and charmed him at the same time.

Lanie Eagleton shows up again looking for patients and finds the old alcoholic with respiratory problems. Bruce Mack visits the 56-year-old woman with the brain hemorrhage, Norma Bacon. He decides to take her to Neuroradiology for an angiogram.

Chiarelli thrives on this sort of detail, the kind that defines the EW itself. She's been at it longer than most nurses, many of whom would want a transfer to a more leisurely ward after two or three years in the EW. It's something she talks about to another EW veteran nurse.

"I can't say I don't *feel.* I do," she says. "But for my own sanity, I won't allow myself to relate, emotionally, to patients. Once a year, I don't know when it's going to happen, a patient gets through to me. I'll see a face, or blood, in my nightmares. I can't say *why.* Maybe it happens when I'm tired or am questioning what I do.

"I really don't have the time to get involved with patients and their families. I keep busy, because there's a lot to be done. If I were on another sort of ward, I suppose I would get involved.

"Maybe that's why I'm on the EW. You know, sometimes a face appeals to you, God only knows why. I've seen it all by now. Even decapitation. And I know you just can't feel for every patient. At times you feel, at times you don't give a damn. As long as you're honest and do your job, that's what is important. If you just stop and tell yourself that it's a trauma and shut off your emotions, you're better off. I mean, do people really believe all that stuff on *Marcus Welby?*"

A resident passes by, taps her on the shoulder and says, "You're looking good, Chiarelli. Really good. I hear you're two months pregnant."

"I'm not," she answers. "I watch my diet."

When Chiarelli gets back from lunch, half of the sixteen beds in the Emergency Ward are empty. A porter is mopping the floor, very slowly. On a phone, a woman resident is talking to a staff doctor at the nursing home where the old black woman had lived. She wants to get more information on the woman, her medical history, her medication. The staff doctor tells her that the woman is 63, has had seizures and has a lesion on the brain. On another phone, a nurse is trying to locate the brother of the man with the compound leg fracture.

The calls end and the ward is quiet.

"Put your hands in it and think pee," a cheerful nurse is saying to the Puerto Rican OD, who hasn't urinated in thirteen hours. She hands him a urine container and a bowl of warm water.

"It's silly, I know, but it works," she says to him. She goes to a nearby faucet and turns it on. "Listen to that, too, while you're at it."

She brings the man two glasses of fruit juice and puts them beside his bed. "I know, I know," she says, "it's really hard to pee under pressure." He looks oppressed and grateful at the same time.

Chiarelli continues to be in motion, and as she takes care of various chores, the time passes. At 2:30, she meets with a new man in administration, in charge of maintaining and repairing equipment. EW equipment can't fail; if it does, it could mean a life lost. Chiarelli reminds the man of that. He listens, respectfully.

At 3 P.M., a Psychiatry resident, a woman, arrives to talk to the Puerto Rican OD. She has heard part of his story before, but she wants more of it.

"When you left home at fourteen, did you live alone or with your father?" she asks him. She encourages him to talk about his past. He fought with his parents. Then he lived with his father, who drank. His father died not long ago. Then the patient began to drink, too. He couldn't get a job. He's seen a psychiatrist in the past, but not for long. The resident looks at his chart; he's on antibiotics and will be in the hospital for several more days, so she can see him again, to try to direct him toward the Psychiatry clinic.

A male nurse, coming on duty early for the evening shift, stops to ask the clerk if there's much going on.

"It's been quiet today," she says, "but all hell might break loose tonight. Who knows?"

The day nurses gather to talk, before they leave for home. One of them mentions Chiarelli's compulsion to drive strangers out of the EW; people who simply wander in, and don't belong there, bother her. It's a useful compulsion, but it doesn't always work.

"One day I was sitting here when a man came in complaining of lower-back pain. I told him he was in the wrong place, that he should walk over to the AES and see a clinic doctor there," Chiarelli says. "He said that the pain was really bothering him and I just repeated my directions. He shrugged, still mumbling, and walked off.

"As he turned, I looked at him. There was a large butcher knife sticking out of his lower back. I screamed 'Sir' and he turned around. I got him into a bed and then the doctors got him up to the OR as fast as possible. It made me a little less compulsive for a while."

The knife, she points out to the group, was not removed because it defined the area traumatized and it acted as a hemostat, compressing blood vessels. Such a knife should not be touched, she instructs, until the patient is in the OR.

At 3:45, as the evening shift has wandered in and Chiarelli and her staff are almost ready to leave, there's an acute admission, a middle-aged Puerto Rican woman who is semiconscious. She's a Psychiatry patient and one of the Neurology residents had gone over to see her in Psychiatry an hour ago. She's been rushed over to the EW; her brain is herniating, pushing out under pressure into existing space, threatening to compress tissue and cause severe brain dysfunction, or worse. Several Neurology residents run in to work on her. One of them is frustrated and angry.

"I saw her just an hour ago," he shouts, "and she was fine. She'd been complaining of headaches, but when I examined her, the symptoms were mild, not alarming. An hour ago, for

God's sake. She was fine. This is a vascular event as far as I'm concerned, an accident."

Mannitol is administered, IV, to decrease brain pressure. Oxygen is given. The woman is prepared for an angiogram. As the bustle around her bed increases, with nurses from both shifts involved, another bed makes its way into the EW from the AES corridor.

On it is a crusty, 62-year-old Irishman who's sitting up. "It's the pollution," he shrieks hoarsely. "The stagnation. I just collapsed on the street." He smiles at Chiarelli, who smiles back at him, puts on her coat and goes out the door. He's a problem for the evening staff. He may or may not be around when Chiarelli arrives at work tomorrow.

Although George Feldman had only two hours of sleep last night, rounds begin at 8:00 A.M. in the Medical ICU for Feldman and his troupe of interns and medical students. An old Puerto Rican woman Feldman has been worried about is now off the respirator; her chest X-ray is clear and she has no fever. The improvement, since yesterday, cheers Feldman. A smiling old Jewish woman tells Feldman that she has no more chest pain. One of the interns reassures her, by explaining, "You didn't have a heart attack." He tells her that he has spoken with her private physician, who will follow up on her care tomorrow when she is discharged.

An old woman from a nursing home, who was brought in after having a stroke and who had a cardiac arrest on the ward (a defibrillator revived her heart), is unimproved. One of the medical students tells Feldman that he called the nursing home for her medical history, without success. "I talked to a know-nothing secretary who told me she was too busy," he tells Feldman. Feldman tells him to check her X-rays, her sputum and her white count and maintain her on antibiotics. Feldman feels she's almost ready to be shifted from the ICU to a ward, but the intern doesn't want her moved while she has a trach tube in place. "I've had bad experience with patients having trach tubes on the ward," he says. "They can get clogged and go unnoticed."

At 8:35, Feldman leads his crew from the ICU to the ward.

He greets the man with lymphoma, who lies in bed, stoically.

"Move your bowels?" Feldman asks him.

"Yeah," the man says.

"Passing gas?"

"Yeah."

Feldman turns to the intern on the case: "His belly is down. Keep him on clear fluids. You might try some Jello."

A middle-aged alcoholic man is in a nearby bed. One of the medical students has a theory about the case, based on an article he read in a medical journal. He quotes from it exhaustively.

"What happened to the patient in that case?" Feldman asks.

"He died," the student answers.

"I'm against that approach," Feldman says, smiling. He suggests a liver biopsy as a diagnostic tool in this case. One of the interns objects.

"I wouldn't hit my own father with that needle. I know a patient who bled to death from it. This man can be treated clinically, without it," he insists.

"He's your patient," Feldman tells him, trying to be fair. "If we had no history, maybe we would try a liver biopsy. You may be right. The procedure may not be justified here."

Feldman looks at the chain-smoking patient with heart trouble, relaxing comfortably in bed, and turns to an intern and says, "Let's get him out of here by Friday."

A nurse interrupts to tell Feldman that one of the ward patients has a temperature of 95.

"Take it again," he tells her, "and work her up." "Work up" is the conventional medical expression for taking an applicable batch of tests.

After a 9:30 coffee break, Feldman is back on the ward, to see several patients with one of the attendings. As they're moving toward one of the patients, a page announces a cardiac arrest on a ward downstairs. Feldman and several interns race to the ward, running down a flight of stairs, but they're not fast enough to be there first. Three doctors are there when Feldman arrives. He returns to rejoin the attending.

As he walks through the hall, an old woman patient stops him.

"Something has to be done about those people who shout those awful words at night. I mean it. Something has to be done. You know the words. That horrible one that begins with 'F' and the rest of those words. It's bad for my peace of mind," she instructs.

Feldman, looking exhausted, simply listens.

In the ward, the attending examines the old ninety-pound woman with the enlarged abdomen. She looks incongruously pregnant, but appears untroubled, reading her Bible.

Joined by several residents and two medical students, Feldman and the attending encircle a 29-year-old Puerto Rican woman with five children. She's told Feldman that she has high blood pressure; her chart indicates that she had a tubal ligation after the birth of her last child. In examining her, the attending, who conducts a running lecture for the benefit of the others with him, concludes that "They may have done it improperly. The tubal ligation." X-rays have revealed that the woman has one very small kidney (the other is normal); further tests will be necessary on it, although it was not the complaint that brought her to Bellevue. While these tests are ordered, a GYN consult is requested.

The attending finishes his visit and leaves, to return to his private practice. Feldman and an intern stroll over to the bed side of the man with lymphoma. Feldman is fond of the man, who has borne inconvenience, pain, even the threat of death, with grace and tranquillity. Feldman would prefer not to be resigned to the man's inevitable and premature death. It is difficult

"Chemotherapy is the only avenue for us on this case," he says to the intern, as they leave the ward and are out in the corridor, where they can't be heard by the patient. "The condi tion is now generalized, beyond surgery, and it has attacked his liver as well. It's bad. It can obstruct nerves, infiltrate the brain, make him prone to infections that will be difficult to treat. We thought he might have pneumonia, too, but I don't think he does. Just fluid in the chest, between the lungs and the chest wall. But that's obviously not his problem. The treatment for lymphoma is not benign. Radiation can scar and burn. Chemicals can depress the bone marrow, the production of blood. It can cause hair loss, vomiting, diarrhea, loss of power in the extremities. He could go on for two years like this, a very delicate balance. We'll do what we can, then he has to be followed by a hematologist because research *does* produce new drug treatments all the time.

"Too bad. He's such a nice man."

It is noon. The day has gone its ordered way, fortunately for Feldman, without any unexpected developments. He is moving in slow motion now, suffering from sleep deprivation. He walks over to the snack bar, slowly.

At 12:30, having left the snack bar unsatisfied by the tokenism of the bar's hamburger and growing edgy from lack of sleep, Feldman goes back to Medicine, to study recent EKGs on seven patients. He is alone and slumps over the table, shifting the ribbons of graph paper from left hand to right, making notes. An attending cardiologist will double-check his comments, then the EKGs will make their way onto patients' charts. Feldman studies them silently, his brown hair framing his face, falling over his ears. He looks serene; a tentative smile seems to be on his face most of the time.

At 1 P.M., in a room used for meetings and classes on the ward, he reads charts done by the medical students as practice. He corrects them, with comments and questions in the margins. The medical students meander in and out, conversations are started, cut off, started again in new directions. Feldman finishes his reading, looks up and sees a medical student sitting beside him. The student wants to know how Feldman feels about treating terminal patients. The question awakens Feldman, who wasn't expecting it.

"You assess what you think the patient's potential is. You try harder to save a young person. But whatever the age, you usually know when a patient isn't responding to therapy. You can only try a number of things, then you're out of tries. You will try to save an alert patient longer than someone who you know has deteriorated. If someone who seems to be alive but is in a coma, is on a respirator, you can keep him alive on it indefinitely. I know of one case where the respirator simply wasn't adjusted on a terminal patient. And I know of times when entire families are polled by doctors.

"I once kept a woman alive, a woman who had renal failure, diabetes, heart disease, for several weeks. There are times when you can turn off the epinephrine drip without turning off the respirator. Those are the patients you *know* are going, beyond all miracles. Instead of dying in twelve hours, they die in one. It is a tough decision and I don't think it ought to be left to the doctor. But if you had a panel evaluating each case separately, you'd have the danger of *that* power to deal with."

At 2 P.M., Feldman planned to meet with the medical students, to lecture to them on the use of respirators, therapy and blood gases. He is weary but game. One of the medical students tells him that two others won't be there.

"One went to the dentist. The other was up all night, so he went to sleep," the student tells Feldman.

"If he can go home to sleep, I should go home to sleep," Feldman says, with mild anger. "I got to bed this morning at 5:30 A.M. and was up at 7:30."

Two students do show up. They are two in the current batch of medical students who have Ph D s in biochemistry.

Feldman is visibly tired, but he manages a lucid explanation of analyzing blood gases, the body's intake of oxygen and its release of carbon dioxide. One of the students, well grounded academically, says, "I want to pick on you now, before you're awake." But it turns out that Feldman's knowledge, and his awareness of applying it to patients, exceeds that of the students. Finally, one of them mutters disconsolately, "We should know this simple shit. We ought to go home and review the physiology."

Feldman doesn't want the lecture to end, so he encourages the students to remember their medical school training. They come up with several formulas for evaluating blood gases.

"It's good to have you guys around," Feldman tells them, "because you can remember that stuff."

He tells them about respirators, the two basic kinds: pressure (limited by the patient's lung capacity to accept oxygen) and volume (limited to the fixed amount the doctor sets for intake by the patient), their limitations, their dangers.

At 3:30, he stops. His supply of words and his energy have been depleted. The two medical students are tired, too, stifling yawns, but they are scheduled to work on the wards tonight. Feldman will not. He gets up, plucks his coat from a rack, tosses it over his shoulder. He waves at the students as he walks, very slowly, toward the stairway.

Sol Zimmerman had a relatively quiet night in the Pediatrics ICU, studying charts and pacing from infant to infant, until 2 A.M., when he was summoned to OB for a delivery. For two hours he watched and waited, while the obstetricians delivered twins. There was reason for his being there: the mother had previously lost two premature babies. The twins emerged in good health.

By the time the twins were safely tucked away in the nursery, it was almost time for Zimmerman to begin a new day. He managed two hours of sleep in the residents' on-call room, a spartan chamber in the hall between the ICU and the Premature Care Unit.

On morning rounds in the ICU he finds that the burned little girl is lethargic, consuming only milk and Maalox, but showing some signs of improvement. The surgeons have recommended skin grafts, which means more work for the ICU staff, changing dressings. The girl is still septic, although the doctors are beginning to win the battle against infection. The surgeons want to begin grafting on her feet and see how it goes. On rounds, Zimmerman is instructed by the chief resident to tell them to go ahead. He is concerned about her nutrition; her protein loss troubles him and he wants her fed by mouth rather than by tube. He wants to cut her Paregoric intake as well. The chief resident agrees.

The tiny girl with the chest deformity, among other problems, is stable. Zimmerman wants to try her on room air today, trying to wean her off the respirator.

The male twin has overwhelming edema; his lungs are hyperaerated. He looks better, but he isn't. He needs food. His weight is down. The staff is having trouble getting an IV line into him; his veins are clogged and there are few left to hit. The female twin, worse at birth, seems to be fighting back. She has had multiple arrests and has been close to death, but summons the strength to survive.

At 8 A.M., Zimmerman is in the Premature Unit. Most of the babies are asleep. The black baby who worried Zimmerman yesterday had a normal stool last night. Several other cultures are pending, results due today. Zimmerman decides to resume feeding the baby. After he makes rounds with the other doctors in the Premature Unit, he trudges off to OB, to check today's delivery schedule, then to the nursery to visit the new twins he watched delivered last night. One has a black and blue smudge on an upper lip and a swollen cheek from the pressure of the forceps. Both mementos should vanish in a short time.

At 9:30, Zimmerman goes to an X-ray conference with a batch of films of the black boy. The Pediatrics radiologist sees nothing to worry about. Although Zimmerman respects the radiologist, he is more comforted by the normal stool than the radiologist's interpretation of the X-rays. An X-ray might not show signs of trouble until it had arrived, full-blown. Zimmerman has brought along an X-ray of the male twin in the ICU. It shows signs of heart failure and pulmonary complications. "I've never seen a baby survive with that kind of picture," the radiologist says.

Zimmerman returns to the Premature Unit, to do two circumcisions, working with the woman senior resident on a set of twins.

"Here it comes, shmendrick," Zimmerman says to the infant. "Your ding-dong. Don't cry, now. Your whole future is in the hands of a professional."

The baby cries.

Zimmerman puts it in a Circumstraint, a molded plastic tray shaped to hold the baby, who is strapped into it. A small drape is placed over the baby's abdomen. Two clamps hold the foreskin, a probe separates it from the phallus itself. A small scissors cut is made and a large clamp placed over the area, leaving only superfluous foreskin exposed. It is trimmed away. Vaseline gauze is wrapped around the penis, to keep it moist. In fifteen minutes both babies are back in their beds.

At 11:10, there is a "stat" page for Zimmerman. That is the announcement in which the doctor wanted is paged and given a phone number. If he knows the location of the number, he must head for it immediately. In this case, Zimmerman recognizes it, the delivery room, and speeds down several flights of stairs to get there.

The intern awaiting the delivery on behalf of Pediatrics has been having trouble; the newborn infant is not breathing properly. By the time Zimmerman comes crashing through the door and into the room, the intern has managed to suction out secretions and the baby is both breathing and crying. The intern tells Zimmerman that he was worried because the baby was "too quiet."

"You're right. Quiet is bad," Zimmerman tells him. "When I'm coming down that hall and I hear the baby crying, I feel better. If I don't hear a sound, I get worried."

From OB, Zimmerman goes to the nursery, where a group of new mothers are watching a film on caring for their babies.

Zimmerman pauses beside an infant with a conspicuous case of the jitters. He can't explain it and that bothers him. The mother had been on many different medications, but insists that none was a narcotic. It is hard for Zimmerman to tell which one, or which combination, caused the baby to react in a manner similar to that of babies suffering from withdrawal. The baby is the only one crying in the nursery, and it is crying emphatically and without pause. Zimmerman decides to wait; he hopes that the baby will eat properly, will get better and can go home. If it needs treatment, it can get it. If withdrawal is confirmed, the case can be reported to the Bureau of Child Welfare.

After a listless lunch, he picks up some test results in the Hematology lab, spends a few minutes in the Pediatrics library, on his way back to the Premature Unit. When he gets back, one of the interns tells him that chromosome studies have come back on the infant girl in the ICU, the one with the chest deformity.

The studies reveal that the girl is actually a boy; an endocrine problem has led to a phenomenon known as testicular feminization. There is little that can be done about it. The child must be raised as a girl. The testes, which are present, can be removed surgically later, because they might become malignant, if the baby survives that long. Zimmerman is astounded by the news. For three months, the baby has been carried in the ICU as a girl; the parents have been told about their daughter's progress. Now, Zimmerman realizes, he must tell them that the girl is a boy, and hardly a normal boy. The parents are already distressed about their shattered child.

The baby, if it lives, will grow up to look like a woman, but will have only a rudimentary vagina and will be sterile. Several other residents arrive. They begin to chat, first about the odd nature of the boy-girl problem, then about assorted unfortunate events they've known at Bellevue.

Last week, Zimmerman tells them, one of the obstetricians left several sponges in a woman; she had to be taken back to the delivery room. The other residents smirk; it is not an outlandish Bellevue story.

"I remember the medical student who was busy in the EW," one resident recites, "when he got a call from a Medical ward, telling him to hustle up there right away, because one of the patients had a fever of 103. The medical student said he couldn't get up right then, because he had plenty to do in the

EW, but he suggested that the nurse give the patient two aspirin. When the student finished his work in the EW, he called the ward and the nurse told him not to worry, that the patient's temperature had gone down to 101. The student checked again a few minutes later and it had gone down to 99. He felt okay about it and walked up to the ward. He took a look at the patient and the guy was dead. Obviously, he had died when his temperature was 103 and the nurse just kept taking his rectal temperature."

"When I was an intern, we had a patient in traction who just decided to give up," another resident says. "He just hung himself on the traction. A nurse saw him hanging there and drew the curtains around his bed. What she didn't realize was that his purple face hovered above the curtain, so when people passed by his bed, they saw that floating purple head over the curtain. Ghastly."

Today, after rounds and her fifteen-minute breakfast, Mary Williamson is in the operating room by 8 A.M. She is scheduled to excise a lipoma (a benign mass), do skin grafts on a burn patient and a man with a leg ulcer, and do a muscle biopsy. However, when she arrives at the operating room, she is told that there is an emergency case: a 70-year-old Italian man dying of renal failure, with a liver problem, possible bile duct obstruction, pneumonia and congestive heart failure, the latter seemingly under control. Like many Bellevue patients, he is a mass of symptoms and diseases. This operation will be done to explore his gall bladder; if necessary, a tube will be inserted to drain the bile, to prevent it from entering the blood stream.

Williamson is ready to begin by 8:15. The patient is cadaverous and toothless. His skin is jaundiced. The fourth-year resident working with Williamson is trying to find a vein for IV use; he is having trouble. He does a cutdown, entering the skin and through it, to find a vein near the patient's left shoulder. He succeeds. While he is at it, the patient is moaning nonsense syllables, groaning loudly.

"We're going to need some good restraints for his arms and legs," the resident announces. The patient will be given a local, not a general, anesthetic.

"Wait a minute, Doc. Just wait a minute," the patient mumbles.

At 9 A.M., the resident is still working on the cutdown, with an anesthetist looking on. The latter comments, "He looks better than I thought he would look, considering his history." A nurse puts leather-belt restraints on the patient's arms. He is given oxygen. The resident starts a second cutdown on the patient's right arm.

"We've gone into innumerable veins," he says. "They don't go up more than a couple of inches." Then, still working, he says, "I think I've got one here, finally."

"If the operation goes like this, we'll be here all day," Williamson says.

At 9:30, they're ready to begin. Williamson swabs the patient's stomach with Betadine. He is draped, except for his right upper abdomen, where a mass can be felt. Williamson gives him a local anesthetic. An attending has joined the group and watches, as the fourth-year resident begins to cut. The patient groans. More anesthetic is injected. A horizontal incision approximately three inches long is made. Williamson holds a retractor while the resident's fingers poke into the opening, looking at and feeling organs. The gall bladder pops up, blue, smooth and normal-looking. The liver looks abnormal, tender and enlarged. A liver needle biopsy is done and sent on to Pathology. A portable X-ray unit is brought in and fluid is injected into the gall bladder, to visualize it under X-ray. The patient groans again.

"He shouldn't be bothered by this," the attending says.

"He is just uncomfortable," the anesthetist notes.

The X-ray is developed within minutes. It shows a perfectly normal gall bladder, no gallstones, no obstructions. The biopsy puncture in the liver is cauterized.

"I'm sorry we didn't make him any better," the attending tells the others, "but the morbidity of this isn't greater than a cutdown."

Williamson and the resident close the incision. By 10:50 A.M., the incision is sewn.

Williamson had thought the man didn't have gall bladder trouble; it was an educated guess, tested by the investigative surgery.

"I couldn't prove what I thought," she says to the other resident. "And this isn't such a costly procedure."

"You know surgeons," the resident says, "frequently wrong but never in doubt."

"You're a good man," Williamson says to the patient.

"And a lucky one," the resident adds. "Your gall bladder is normal."

The patient stares blankly at him.

Williamson and the fourth-year resident accompany the patient back to the ward. The man's wife is waiting there. She is old and very nervous.

"Everything's okay," the resident tells her. "His gall bladder is fine."

The wife smiles, weakly. "God bless you all," she says.

Williamson and the resident leave the ward. As they do, she turns to him and says, "Another diagnostic non-coup for Surgery. At least we didn't make the patient worse."

At 11:45, the black woman with the lipoma is wheeled into the OR. It is a benign growth on her buttock, where it meets her upper thigh. It looks like a Ping-Pong ball pushing the skin out, perfectly round. It is a quick, simple procedure. With the help of a first-year resident, who does most of the work, the growth is easy for Williamson to remove.

She stretches the skin away from the lipoma with long strips of wide adhesive tape.

"Are you comfortable?" she asks the patient. The woman grunts.

She coats the lipoma and the area around it with Betadine and drapes everything but the small round bulge. The resident reaches over and touches it. The patient jumps.

"Don't worry," Williamson tells her. "We're going to numb it. You'll feel a little stick and a little burning, then some pushing, then nothing." She turns to the resident and says, "This reminds me of Shakespeare. Much ado about nothing."

It is noon. The resident runs his scalpel around the base of the growth, then cuts progressively deeper, in a "V," toward the center below. His cuts meet and the lipoma comes out in his hand.

The patient whines.

"That hurts?" Williamson asks.

"Yes," the woman answers.

"Tell us, because we can give you more anesthetic."

The resident does just that, injecting Xylocaine.

"We're just about finished. The worst is over," Williamson tells the woman.

The resident holds the lipoma in his gloved hand, pokes it with his scalpel. It bursts, spewing gray mush.

"Yech," the scrub nurse blurts out.

"A sebaceous cyst," Williamson says.

"Want it?" the resident asks the nurse, holding it out to her.

"Thanks a lot," she smirks.

The resident begins suturing the gap that remains in the absence of the growth. "It's fine now," Williamson tells the patient. "You can go home today or tomorrow."

By 12:25, the wound is sutured and taped. Williamson has faint feelings of hunger, but there is no time for lunch. The next case is waiting outside the OR.

Her two afternoon cases are a skin graft, one of a long series, on a severely burned 37-year-old Puerto Rican woman, and a skin graft on the ulcerated leg of a partially paralyzed old man. By 2:50, Williamson is done with both.

She leaves the OR and is told that a muscle biopsy, slated to be the last procedure of the day, has been canceled. She changes from surgical green to white skirt and jacket, her silver crucifix dangling from her neck, her white veil replacing her pink surgical hood. She gets to the Surgical ICU by 3:15.

The old GI bleeder's bed, the one that carried him to Radiology and then to the OR last night, is back in place, clean and empty.

Williamson wants to begin rounds, but a number of residents haven't appeared. It is now 3:30, too late to begin and finish rounds today in one tour. She must attend two conferences, didactic moments in an otherwise pragmatic life. At 4 and again at 5 P.M., conferences offer her an academic view of surgery. She abandons rounds, to do them later, for the conferences. In a few months, when her residency comes to an end, she won't be able to attend such conferences, so she tries to fit them in now, when she can, between surgery and rounds.

She gets back to the ICU at 6 P.M., ready for rounds with several other residents who have reported in. She wants to make a point to a couple of them: "You can't know what surgery is all about unless you understand how important rounds are to us. It's our chance to *know* the patients, before we see them in the OR."

She leads the group through the ICU, the point at which rounds begin. Three surgical wards will be covered, in all.

In the ICU, the burned boy she treated in the OR yesterday has a 101 temperature. He is not passing urine, a resident tells Williamson. She tells him to use a Foley catheter if the boy does not pass urine within a few hours.

With Williamson in the lead, the group makes its way from ward to ward. On one ward, an old woman tells Williamson, "I still have pain."

"That's because you had an incision, a cut," Williamson tells her. "If your ulcer gets worse, we'll operate. Anything is better than the pain you've had from it."

"You're right, Doctor, but I gotta prepare myself," the woman says.

An old toothless woman is awakened by the arrival of the residents. "You're feeling much better, aren't you?" one of the residents asks her.

"I'm feelin' better," she says, "but not *much* better." She begins to tremble.

"Stop shaking," the resident says. "You only do that when we're here. Do we make you nervous?"

She looks at him grimly, without answering.

An 85-year-old woman grabs Williamson's arm. "Maybe I'm dying," she murmurs. "I sure feel it."

"Don't say that," Williamson tells her.

As the group moves through ward after ward, Williamson notices that one of the senior residents, who was on duty all night and all day, is still tagging along.

"Go home," she tells him. "I don't want your wife to beat me up."

He smiles, wearily, and leaves.

On one of the wards, an old woman appears to be asleep. When the doctors arrive, she wakes up. Williamson tells her, "You've got to go home soon. You've been here longer than I have."

The woman becomes acutely alert. "Oy, oy, oy," she moans. "The pain. The pain." She points to an IV tube in the back of her hand. The resident on the case walks over and removes it, quickly.

"Oy, oy, oy," she cries. "It hurts to take it out."

"We have to do one more test tonight, with a tube in your nose," Williamson tells her.

"Oy, oy," the woman groans. "Please, no, Doctor, not in the nose, not in mine nose."

Williamson sighs and leads the other doctors out of the ward. The woman returns to sleep.

A patient with a colostomy, a middle-aged man, is recovering; the riddle of his GI bleeding was solved and the colostomy is a price he was willing to pay. He is pleasant and gregarious.

"You should eat," Williamson tells him. "It's good for you."

"Okay, okay," he says, smiling at her. "I'll eat. I don't want you to feel bad." There is intense affection in his words.

Rounds end at 7 P.M. tonight; they can be done expeditiously at times or stretch well into the night, depending upon the nature of the problems encountered.

Williamson starts to leave. One of the residents says, loud enough for her to hear him, "After I promised Mary I'd never practice medicine in Ghana, everything was uphill in my relationship with her."

When Tom Spencer arrives at the AES for his four-to-midnight shift, the place is bustling.

A pregnant Puerto Rican woman, moaning *"Madre de Dios,"* waddles through the AES on her way to OB. Two policemen arrive with a handcuffed prisoner, bleeding from a cut on his forehead. A young black man sits contemplatively soaking a swollen finger; his girl friend bit it, playfully, and it ballooned. A woman with a fractured wrist, confirmed by X-ray, and a small puncture wound on her arm, screams, "Fuck this shit. I'm splitting," and runs out the door. A pursuing doctor stops. "We'll see that bitch when she gets lockjaw," he says. A well-dressed businessman, who sprained his ankle diving for a cab in midtown traffic, has been treated, bandaged, given a cane. "If I hurry," he says to Spencer, "I can make the four-thirty train."

An EKG has been done on a Puerto Rican woman, accompanied by her daughter. It shows an abnormality.

"Has she ever had a cardiac problem before?" Spencer asks the daughter. She stares at him, unresponsively.

"Here," he says, pointing to his chest. "Any trouble there before?"

"Yes, two months ago," the daughter says.

Spencer discovers that the old woman was hospitalized then, in a Brooklyn hospital. The resident on the case tonight would like the records from that hospital summarized on the phone, so Spencer calls. Shuttled from extension to extension at the Brooklyn hospital, Spencer returns a half-hour later, unsuccessful; they've lost the records.

The daughter now remembers the name of the family physician. Spencer phones him. The doctor tells him that the new EKG is not alarming; it is identical to an earlier one. Spencer passes the message along to the Bellevue resident.

"She should be coming to our Cardiac clinic, whatever the EKG shows," he says. Spencer forwards the message to the woman and her daughter.

At 4:30, the police drag in an incoherent OD. He is young, scabrous. "Narcan," Spencer yells to one of the other nurses.

By 4:40, sixteen patients have been registered. A policeman waiting for his prisoner to be treated pats an attractive nurse on the head. A jealous resident, standing nearby, mumbles, "Sick, sick, how sex permeates the air." As the nurse walks away, the resident's eyes follow her.

A woman complaining of a headache tells the triage nurse she must be seen immediately.

"We'll see you, but it will be a long wait, a couple of hours," the triage nurse tells her.

A man is on the public phone near the entrance, shouting into it, "Now, don't get excited, Marilyn. I'm at Bellevue Hospital. Yes, Bellevue. I had a bad nosebleed on the train. Get my Blue Cross card. My Blue Cross card. It's in the closet."

On a bed in the corridor, a drunken old woman sleeps it off. In the next bed, there's a middle-aged woman with a badly fractured right ankle; it is conspicuously distorted and she is in pain. In a third bed a few feet away, a hungry man has lost patience; he slides off the bed and limps toward the snack bar for a hamburger.

The head nurse announces to the staff that Channel 2 News is sending over a crew at 8 P.M. to get background footage for a story they're doing on the high cost of health care.

A short, spindly, intense man reaches up and taps Spencer on the shoulder. Spencer wheels around, looks down.

"I work here," the man says.

"No, you don't," Spencer replies.

"Not *here*," the man says. "At Bellevue. I'm a technician."

"What's wrong?"

"Well, I was working this afternoon and I got thirsty, so I reached over and picked up a glass and drank what I thought was water."

"What was it?"

"Formaldehyde."

"Formaldehyde?" Spencer asks, rhetorically.

"Formaldehyde."

"You better see a doctor."

"Yes, I better see a doctor," the man says. He clutches his stomach, looks pale. "I'm nauseated and very weak."

Spencer escorts him to a resident, who phones Poison Control for the antidote.

"You'll have to drink milk, take some Ipecac to encourage vomiting and stay here for two hours, so we can observe you," the resident tells him.

The man is nervous, twitching. "I don't want to hang around here. It makes me more nervous," he says. "Just give me the stuff and I'll take it home and drink it. I promise."

The resident hands over a bottle of Ipecac. The man grabs it and struts out.

"Formaldehyde?" the resident says, smiling. "I don't believe it."

"Jesus, he could have smelled it," one of the nurses says.

"Next case," Spencer says, resuming his tour of the AES; he is perpetually making rounds.

By 5:55 P.M., thirty-two patients have been registered. It is busy, but so far the complaints have stopped short of panic.

At the front desk, the parade continues. An alcoholic having the DTs, a city bus driver who has had a seizure, an old Bowery bum in bare feet.

A middle-aged woman, her once chic dress hopelessly stained with grease and dirt, comes stumbling through the front door. She gropes for the registration desk, doubles over it.

"God, God," she moans. "We were in an accident, me and my husband. Charlie was hurt, hurt bad. They took him away and I don't know where they took him. Is he here? I hope to God he's here. Please help me find him."

A policeman standing near her comes up. "Are *you* all right?" he asks.

"I guess so. Please, please help me find Charlie."

He goes to a phone, checks accident reports, tracks down the injured man. He's at a hospital on the West Side. He puts his arm around the woman and helps her into his squad car.

The procession resumes.

A parking lot attendant, the name "Waldo" emblazoned on his blue jump suit, weaves in, one hand around the other wrist. His finger got caught in a closing car door.

An ambulance brings a young man who has taken too much LSD. He is violent, bouncing around the walls of the ambulance. An AES doctor has to check him before they can drive him over to Psychiatry for treatment. "I wouldn't get too close to him if I were you, Doc," the ambulance driver tells the resident. The resident leans into the rear of the ambulance, looks at the man, who is screaming and writhing. "Okay, tell Psychiatry I looked at him. He belongs to them," the resident says. The driver locks the rear door and heads for Psychiatry.

A young, handsome, impeccably dressed Indian man walks up to the triage nurse. He smiles at her. She smiles back. "I fainted in the subway," he tells her. She sends him back to see a doctor.

An enormous woman with a long, elaborate platinum wig and a pink pant suit, the garb of a hooker, complains of abdominal pain. She goes into the waiting room to be summoned inside for treatment.

At 8 P.M., the TV crew crashes through the double doors, with mikes, camera, lights, and marches through the corridors. They decide to interview one of the nurses; she is delighted. When they leave, she rushes to a phone and calls her baby-sitter. "Watch the news at eleven on Channel 2," she says. "You don't usually watch the news on Channel 2? Well, tonight watch it. I may be on it."

Spencer talks to an old woman, neat and prim, in an examining room. She is a proper old woman, wears a little straw hat and peers at Spencer through her bifocals. "You know, Doctor," she says to Spencer, "I could go at any minute. At any minute." She laughs. "I have high blood pressure, that's what," she says, "and I just dropped in to have it checked. I was in the neighborhood, you know." Spencer asks her where she lives and she can't remember; he is concerned and persuades her to rest in the Observation Unit until the morning, when a social worker can help her.

There is little time for dinner. Doctors munch hamburgers on the run. Spencer springs free for fifteen minutes at the snack bar. When he returns, it is in time to hear the shout "Doctor, up front" from the triage nurse.

The front doors fly open and ambulance attendants, nurses and doctors surround a young black man; he has been stabbed in the face and chest. He cannot be much older than 18. He wears a single gold stud earring in his left ear. He is transferred from stretcher to high wheeled bed and taken directly into the Emergency Ward, where he is surrounded by the EW crew, with Spencer staying on to assist.

The seven doctors and nurses around the table quickly assess the case. The wounds seem superficial. The man's clothing is removed; his shirt is bloody and fright has led him to defecate. A clerk puts his personal possessions in an envelope: a leaflet from the Revolutionary Youth Movement saying that the CIA is training the police to kill black youths in Brooklyn, a pack of Winstons, a single playing card (the 4 of diamonds) and $2.22.

"We saw him on Avenue C," one of the policemen who found him tells a doctor. "He was being carried along by a friend. That's all we know."

The doctors persuade the patient to sit up, to look for other wounds. They don't find any. An X-ray unit is moved in, for thorough diagnosis. By 8:30, the bleeding has been halted, no apparent danger discerned.

A few minutes later, three friends show up to see the patient. They are his age, his compatriots; they are angry. One of them, in a leather jacket lavishly decorated with silver studs, is carrying a golf club. A hospital policeman asks for it; the youth hands it over. The three are told that they can't see their friend; he must rest.

"We'll see him," one of them says, "now or later. And when he tells us what we want to know, we'll take care of the rest." As a unit, they do an about-face and leave the AES.

In the waiting room, the hooker has crossed her legs, thrust out her chest. There are six men in the room with her. They all stare at her: she is aware of them. "Phew," she sighs and takes a copy of *The Guinness Book of Records* from her purse. She begins to read and all the men, one by one, get up and leave the room.

It is 9 P.M. and fifty-six patients have been logged in.

An aged woman on a stretcher-bed near the front desk is

moaning rhythmically, "Oh God, oh God, oh God," and coughing fiercely. "She is homeless," the triage nurse tells a doctor, "and there's a good chance she may have pneumonia." The doctor, who looks exhausted, doesn't seem pleased by the news.

A black hospital policeman, off duty, walks in and tells Spencer that "some cat scratched me." Spencer looks at his finger, which has begun to swell. "Cat scratch," Spencer writes on the policeman's form. "You need a tetanus shot," he tells him. "Fine with me," the policeman says. Spencer cleans the wound and gives him the tetanus injection. "Bad thing about cats," Spencer says. "Man, this cat had two legs. I was trying to bust him," the policeman says. They both laugh.

By 10 P.M., there are only two patients left on stretcher-beds in the corridors; the others have all been seen and treated. It is almost silent throughout the AES. Again, that tranquillity vanishes when two policemen bring in a skinny black cleaning woman who was shot in the right leg.

"I was just working, Lord knows, just working," she says to Spencer, who has greeted her. "I don't even remember how I got shot. Can you believe that? I don't even remember. I heard a door slam and then I saw some blood on my leg and this here little hole. Goodness gracious. Goodness gracious," she says.

There is a small puncture wound in her right calf. A doctor gives her a tetanus shot, has her leg X-rayed. "Goodness gracious," she keeps repeating. The 22-caliber bullet is there, but there is no immediate need to remove it. She can be seen later in Surgery clinic.

"Don't you worry, Tillie," the doctor says to her. "Did you say your name was Tillie?"

"Millie. Goodness."

"Yes, Millie. Well, don't you worry. We'll take care of you. We'll fix you up so you can go home and take it easy. But I really do have to tell you that the leg will be sore in the morning. So don't plan on going right back to work."

"I really would not want to stay here overnight," she tells him. "I got my own doctor and I can see him. And I don't want to miss no work. My boss is not what you'd call a friendly man."

The AES resident patches up her leg. Spencer extends his arm and she grabs it. Together, they walk through the front door out into the driveway, an unlikely couple in almost every way. Outside, Spencer puts her in a chair and runs out into the street to flag down a cab. He gives her some of his own money to get home.

By 11 P.M., eighty-one patients have gone through the AES. Ambulances come and go. Stretcher-beds are shifted; empty ones are assembled at the front door for sudden use. Relatives sit in the waiting room, chewing candy, drinking Pepsi. The police come in and out. An OD is asleep. Doctors in examining rooms suture small wounds, listen to complaints. Nurses fill out forms for lab tests. An old man in a wheelchair, oddly tattered in appearance with worn suit and vintage derby, clutches a mop he inexplicably brought with him.

It is almost midnight and Spencer is ready to leave when a Puerto Rican family enters. Father, mother, daughter, all neatly dressed, all grim.

"I heard today my other daughter she dead here today," the father says to Spencer. The mother and daughter are crying. Spencer asks for the name and checks the morning's records.

"Yes, I'm afraid that's so. A drug overdose. She was dead when she got here. There was nothing we could do."

The father begins crying, too, and speaks in rapid Spanish, too rapid for Spencer to understand any of it. A Puerto Rican nurse's aide joins them.

"He just wants to claim the body," the nurse's aide tells Spencer.

"Yes. Yes," Spencer says. "It will be at the Medical Examiner's office tomorrow. The morgue." The nurse's aide translates. Father, mother and daughter are all crying now. Spencer lifts his arms in a gesture of futility. The family walks slowly out of the AES. Spencer, his head down, walks slowly, too, to his room upstairs.

WEDNESDAY

Nursing Service Report

G-5—José Martinez, 15 year old, Clorox ingestion—fled while he had visitors.

K-3—Anita Lee admitted for iodine ingestion.

L-4—Tony Marco admitted for thumb reconstruction—severely lacerated thumb—he was fixing his motorcycle. He is a member of Hell's Angels Gang.

Emergency Ward—Mary Johnson—has 50 to 60% 2nd degree burns of upper extremities and buttocks. She was brought in from fire in Brooklyn where four people died—three of them were her children. The patient does not know at this time that her children are dead. Her condition is fair.

F-7—Unknown black infant, possibly 8 months old, was brought in from the street on the evening tour. They are ruling out seizure disorder and his condition is fair. They are attempting to make a positive identification.

Bernard Weinstein gets to Bellevue in time for the 8 A.M. meeting with the medical board, to consider Antioch College's offer to train Physicians' Associates in conjunction with Bellevue. The table is lined with distinguished doctors and teachers, an encyclopedic array of medical knowledge and a wide range of personalities.

Weinstein, who is intrigued by the Antioch proposal, says, "We do have, Bellevue has, a moral commitment to do more than take care of itself. Would the community benefit? That's what is important. If PAs are useful, then we should have them."

The consensus is opposed. N.Y.U. Medical School can train PAs (a group with more medical skills than nurses, less skills than M.D.s), the doctors feel. Such a program with Antioch might conflict with N.Y.U.'s present teaching function at Bellevue; all the directors of services present are faculty members at N.Y.U. as well. One of them notes that nurses can be trained to fill the PA role, if its need is ever confirmed. Weinstein is not convinced, but it is not a battle he chooses to wage at this time.

Weinstein is back behind his desk at 9:45 A.M., in time for a meeting of his own immediate staff. The conversation speeds from point to point: an article in the *Times* predicting new demands from city employees; budget matters; an effort to cut down the preoperation stays of patients; a problem with a surgeon who is holding down two jobs, legitimately, and getting a paycheck for only one; the impending visit of the mayor of Naples, who is also a doctor, a lung specialist and a professor of medicine ("He's a handsome bachelor," Weinstein informs one of his staff, a woman who is Italian, but she's not eager to escort the mayor around Bellevue); an N.Y.U. request for more funds; programming the elevators in the new hospital to include express routes; the new X-ray technician training school which is graduating its first class in a few months.

"Is it helping or hurting?" Weinstein asks.

"I think it may be of minimal use to Bellevue and could be a liability," Doris Lesser tells him.

"So are medical students," he says. "What kind of shit is that? We have an *educational* obligation. Let's go over the evaluation when you have it."

"If we don't continue the school, we'll have a strong union reaction," Lesser tells him.

"Well, that's another matter. If we're running a lousy school, we shouldn't run it," he tells her.

At 11 A.M., the meeting ends and Bellevue's Director of Engineering and Maintenance, Richard Nemeth, shows up to take Weinstein on a tour of his problems. He is young, in his early thirties, and came to Bellevue after experience at another local hospital, less than a year ago.

"This job," he says to Weinstein as they move toward the basement, "is either a nightmare or a challenge."

They make their way through the bowels of the hospital to an area beneath the Psychiatry building. An old pipe is gushing water.

"We've got to take some immediate action," Nemeth tells

Weinstein. "We've got the manpower to do a temporary repair only."

A permanent repair, he says, will cost $40,000. He'll have to turn off the system at night and repair it as well as he can. The two walk through the basement, peering carefully as they go.

There are pools of water on the floor, low-hanging pipes, debris of all sorts, ancient, crumbling equipment, indefinable slush. A community of cats thrives. At times, the East River tide rises and so does the water level in the basement. The smell of rot is everywhere.

Nemeth speaks the language of maintenance: pipes, valves, tanks, connections, pumps. Thick gusts of steam come between the two men as they duck, twist, bend around equipment, some of which appears to be rusting into oblivion.

Nemeth looks discouraged; his smile is a weak one. He seeks guidance from Weinstein.

"If something is usable, let's use it," Weinstein tells him. "If not, get rid of it."

"You wanna see some of the better points?" Nemeth asks.

Weinstein nods, enthusiastically.

Nemeth takes him through the shops: carpentry, glazier, electric, mason, steamfitters. "All I need is money and material," Nemeth says.

"You've got no problems in the new building?" Weinstein asks.

"They're different," Nemeth says.

At 12:30, Weinstein is back in his office, for lunch with Richard Miller, a partner in the architectural firm that has produced a plan for Bellevue's next twenty-five years, for the demolition, reuse, reallocation and construction of its campus. They eat sandwiches and discuss a presentation that Miller will make at a medical board meeting at 2 P.M.

Weinstein explains to Miller, a large shaggy man, the bizarre ways in which the bureaucracy moves and the idiosyncrasies of the members of the medical board. Weinstein favors the master plan and wants Miller to be prepared for the encounter. He mentions the sometimes abrasive nature of the competition for space in the new hospital. While they are talking, Weinstein's phone rings. He listens, says nothing, hangs up.

"The fire alarms have gone off in the new building. They don't know why," Weinstein says. "If it burns down, we can deal with *this* problem later." He goes on with his briefing of Miller. "The more global you get, the less picky the questions will be," he says.

Miller takes his projector, slides and sketches and goes off to set them up in the conference room. Weinstein dashes over to the new hospital, to check on the fire alarm system.

He's greeted in the spacious, almost elegant lobby by a batch of staff members. "The alarms just went off, in no order, for five minutes, then they stopped," one of the men tells Weinstein.

As he speaks, the alarm goes off again, in rings not conforming to the established code. Weinstein, trailed by several others, goes up to the thirteenth-floor control panel, where an intricate, sophisticated computer is supposed to reveal the location of smoke and fire. Richard Nemeth has beaten Weinstein to the board. When Weinstein arrives, Nemeth has found a defective switch and has repaired it, temporarily, with masking tape. Weinstein leaves the solution to Nemeth and heads back to the medical board meeting.

Miller shows his slides, pictures of models of the future Bellevue, an integrated series of buildings, modern and functional, stretched across the area now occupied by Bellevue's antiquated and haphazardly strewn architectural maze. The photos are impressive.

"It won't be a megastructure, at one stroke, but incremental, piece by piece, self-sustaining, as funds become available," Miller tells the doctors. There are a few innocuous questions, then silence. No one has fought over space. Miller leaves and the meeting continues.

Dr. Rudolf L. Baer, chairman of the medical board and Director of Dermatology, presides, gracefully, his Middle European accent never rising above a level of dignified calm. He cites the reports of various committees, already distributed to those present, then turns the floor over to Weinstein.

Weinstein endorses Miller's report. The architectural firm's comprehensive plan for the future of Bellevue has been passed out to the doctors.

Dr. Frank Spencer, the chief of Surgery, hasn't had time to read the report, but states that "pragmatically, you know that everything in this can't be right."

Weinstein, ready, says that it is the basis for future decisions, not an irrevocable course.

Dr. Baer resumes his control over the agenda. The use of the top four floors in the new Bellevue seems inextricably linked to the needs and goals of Psychiatry. However, the HHC seems determined to locate the prison wards, both medical and psychiatric, on the eighteenth floor, consuming two-thirds of the space on that floor. If the decision holds, it will eliminate the creation of a burn center for Bellevue in that space.

"The care of burns here is outrageous," Dr. Spencer says. "I've seen better care by an osteopath. And where's our transplant unit? Are we going to continue to do them in a closet? I have a lot of needs in Surgery that can't be met without the use of the eighteenth floor."

There are outcries, nods, grunts of disapproval. Feelings are expressed around the table. The surgeons are forthright, emphatic. The psychiatrist is calm, contemplative. The chief of Medicine is uncertain. The chief of the Trauma Service is strong, aggressive. The Director of Radiology is in search of verification, documentation. The head of Pediatrics is firm and fatherly. The ranking dermatologist, Dr. Baer, remains gentle, open to persuasion.

The consensus is that the HHC is responding to political pressure to place the prison wards on the eighteenth floor.

"The press has criticized us before for not protesting political decisions that affect medical care," one of the doctors says. "This is such a case. A prison ward or a burn unit?"

One of the chiefs suggests going directly to the mayor with the problem. Another concurs.

Dr. Baer says he will appoint a committee to review the situation and choose a course of action for the others to consider.

Dr. A. Keegan of Radiology presents some samples of how X-ray films can be miniaturized, to store them for years and protect against the loss of full-sized plates. He shows old, conventional X-rays and smaller versions of the same subjects. There is little difference in quality. He proposes converting to the new process.

"We can get eighty to a hundred thousand of these in an electric retriever," Keegan says.

The meeting has gone on for almost two hours and the members are restless, although only two have left. Keegan is popular, likable, witty. The board supports him, as last-minute chaos invades the room. No formal vote is taken on Keegan's proposal, no talk of funding the plan, although Dr. Baer's mild voice is heard asking the question about funds as the meeting seems to end itself, spontaneously, and the doctors rush out of the room.

Weinstein goes back to his office, makes a few phone calls, awaits a visit from a member of the community board, a woman who wants to discuss Bellevue finances for the next year, as budgeted by the HHC. She has seen the HHC's allocations for Bellevue and Bellevue's request for funds for projects beyond the conventional budget. She hopes to inspire the community board to support some of those projects.

The woman arrives, after 4 P.M. A middle-aged patrician, she wears a beige shirt-dress in cotton-suede. She has horn-rimmed glasses and her hair is teased and sprayed. Her mouth is permanently pursed, to denote seriousness. She talks incessantly, politely, and shuffles papers constantly, referring to one, then another. Her brow remains furrowed throughout. Her manner is upper class, a departure from the earthy quality most community board members display.

After a few minutes, Weinstein's eyelids are at half-mast. He chews his Dentyne, unsmiling, and stares at the woman almost catatonically. She wants to help somehow, but she is confused by all the figures on the sheets she keeps moving around in front of her.

Finally, she looks at Weinstein and asks, "What have we resolved?"

"Nothing," he says, shrugging.

They are not antagonists, although the community board can and does attempt to exercise its power as an advisory body.

Weinstein is tired and the woman is tireless, a combination difficult to reconcile. She leaves at 5:15. Weinstein sighs, heavily. He has dictation to do, aides to talk with, mail to read, the engineer's grievances to assess, his article to work on. He shuts the door to his office and, one by one, gets everything done. He gets to his car by 8:15 for the drive to New Jersey. An aide who worked late, too, meets him in the parking garage.

"You know," Weinstein says to the aide, "when my head is working right, I can take good advantage of it and work late. My wife is used to it. She just goes ahead and eats dinner."

At 8:30 A.M. on Ward NO–6, Dirk Berger and his staff (twenty-one of them are present this morning) gather for rounds. The young head nurse, her blond hair in a ponytail, cradles the communication book, in which staff members make notes about patients around the clock. She reads the newest entries.

The little, emaciated old woman from the Aberdeen inspires a line. "Her color is ghastly," the head nurse says.

"That's her normal color," Berger comments, smiling.

Howard Walker, the man who says he is a biology professor, spent much of the night in a wheelchair, disorganized. Berger and the resident on the case decide to meet with him later in the day.

Another patient, an introspective, brooding black woman, went to a group therapy session, but sat there silently, wringing her hands. Berger is not put off by her behavior; he thinks she is almost ready to be discharged.

"About two or three days before her discharge, call the Aberdeen for a room for her. But don't discharge her on Friday, because weekends are chaotic at the Aberdeen," he says.

A young Vietnam veteran spent time on the ward with his wife, who visited him last night. She, in turn, met with a resident and threatened to commit suicide.

"It's her husband I'm worried about," the resident says, "but we can't let her get away either."

"She's sick of the attention her husband is getting and she wants some for herself," Berger says.

"How about getting them both into family therapy?" the head nurse suggests.

The conversation flows to the husband's plight. Unemployed and tormented ever since he got back from the Army, he walks to the nearest police station once a month ("When the moon is full," one of the residents notes) and picks a fight with a policeman. He has threatened to kill himself several times. Essentially a nonviolent person, he turns his anger against himself. A few weeks ago, he went out, got drunk, returned home to cut the "bad thoughts" out of his head with a razor. He was on NO–6 a few hours later.

The resident offers to treat both husband and wife. Berger thinks it's a good idea.

The fat woman who writes poems reported that someone tried to rape her during the night and someone else stole money and cigarettes from her. The toothless old woman still roams the ward, drooling, incoherent.

As the rounds end, the social worker adds, "Another successful evening without an incident."

As Berger sees a clinic patient privately, the drooling hag lingers outside his office, taunting his secretary. She corners a resident, tells him a few dirty jokes, kisses him, drinks coffee, smokes incessantly. When the resident attempts to escape, she rushes over to him and tells him, "I owe you something." He stares at her and answers, "What?"

"This," she shouts and punches him in the jaw. He recoils. Behind them, a line of patients has assembled for their morning medication, served in paper cups, with grapefruit juice chasers.

Berger emerges, as his patient leaves, and announces that he is going to have his breakfast. He opens a can of Tab. "Ever see Tab withdrawal?" he asks his secretary.

He phones a resident in the clinic to find out if Johnny Rogers, whom he saw yesterday at the Aberdeen, has shown up for an appointment. He hasn't. Berger explains Rogers' suicidal behavior to the resident in case Rogers shows up.

A patient interrupts to ask for a Winchester from the ward pack, kept in Berger's secretary's desk.

Berger's frail friend from the Aberdeen comes rushing in, to ask him to phone the hotel for her to find out if she left some money in her room. Berger obliges her, and as he talks to a friend at the hotel, the woman puts her head next to Berger's and screams into the phone, "I'm a hundred percent okay. If you come over here, I'll give you the one-two." Berger finishes his conversation, then turns to her.

"Look, we're going to find out how much money you've got. Don't worry about it. Just start eating, will you? You've got to have more than coffee."

The woman, who looks like a babbling crone, is treated gently, courteously, by Berger. She smiles and parades off to her bed.

As she leaves, an argument can be heard in the corridor outside Berger's office.

A young black man is telling an older, agitated black woman, "I am Superman."

"You ain't nothin' but Super Sick," she yells. "You can kiss my black ass." A nurse separates them.

The resident who has been treating Howard Walker enters Berger's office to talk about Walker. He's done some checking,

on the phone. Bellevue records show that the man did indeed
have a lobotomy several years ago. He is a biology professor,
confirmed by the chairman of the department at the school
listed in the patient's chart. From various sources, the resident
has compiled a portrait of Walker similar to the one Walker has
given. He has had a number of breakdowns, hospitalizations,
shock treatments. For years, he spent much of his time each day
washing his hands. He got to Bellevue after his wife died, when
he was found lurching down the street.

"I want to see him today," Berger tells the resident.

A second resident, the one treating Sarah Morgan, enters. He
has gotten a report from the Chest Service. Test results, now
thoroughly analyzed, show lung cancer. The surgeon involved
doesn't feel that the "old woman" can survive surgery. The
resident tells Berger that he feels surgery must be done and he
will go to the chief of Psychiatry to lean on the surgeon if he has
to do so. Berger agrees. He feels it is possible that the tumor
may have caused her psychiatric condition. "It is possible," he
says, "and she *looks* old. She's forty-five."

At that moment, Howard Walker limps into Berger's office.

As the resident leaves, to do battle with the surgeon, Walker
sits down, between Berger and the resident on the case.

"I'm feeling a great deal better today," he says. "Yesterday I
cried a bit, but a friend visited me and I felt better immediately."

"You were found unconscious? Or just reeling around the
street?" Berger asks.

"I don't remember. I was feeling bad. I had taken some tranquilizers and a pint of gin."

"What was going on?"

"I guess I must have felt that I had no reason to live since my
wife died a few weeks ago."

"Why?"

"Well, I lived with my wife for twelve years. She died in just
four days. Like that. She had a headache and a pain in her chest
and I thought she had the flu, so I gave her some pills I had. The
medicine I gave her really killed her. She was right. She thought
it was a heart attack. I was wrong."

"It is tough to try to treat your own family. Beside losing her,
you missed the diagnosis."

"Unconsciously I knew she was having a heart attack. I

thought it was flu. But then her priest came over. She was a Catholic, I'm not. And he seemed to help her. She seemed to feel better. She was devout. I never really understood it."

"You've never attempted suicide before?"

"No. Just previous depressions."

"How do you feel now?"

"On the road to recovery."

Walker is pale and worn, like a man who has not slept in days. He is a husky man, a once strong man who has gone chunky from self-abuse, neglect. He is wearing a suit, clinging to a standard he was taught years ago, but his tie is gone and his shirt tails dangle out beneath his jacket. He is wearing shoes, but no socks. His language is not that of the streets, but closer to that of the classroom. He is an educated man, rare in the wards at Bellevue.

"What are you thinking about?" Berger asks.

"That you can't be responsible for your unconscious if you're not aware of it."

"What were you like before the lobotomy?"

"Well, I had a hip accident more than a dozen years ago. I had started teaching before that and was doing well, but the hip trouble affected my work. I couldn't sit or stand or walk. I was in pain, slowed down. I began to take Dexedrine, more and more and more. Then I learned how to inject it. I developed a paranoid psychosis. I went into a hospital, stopped the Dexedrine, but then I got out and resumed taking it. And I began to drink. A fifth of gin a day. But I knew then that eating just a few scrambled eggs each day, and doing the rest of it, would put me away."

"Then?"

"I got treatment and got a job doing biological research. But I'd come home at night and take Librium, some gin and go to bed."

"How did you feel?"

"I had a kind of chronic mild depression. Alcohol. Drugs. Depression. One ball of wax."

"How did you get to a lobotomy?"

"I wasn't satisfied in my work. I wanted help. I had read everything I could find about lobotomy. I called an experienced doctor, who recommended a surgeon. That was five years ago and I've had no trouble since, until a few weeks ago. I don't drink much now, really. Actually, I was depressed after the lobotomy and—"

"A lobotomy doesn't cure depression."

"I had trouble getting work. I had some shock therapy then. I was obsessive-compulsive and depressive. I would look at doorknobs for hours, retracing a line from the knob to the ceiling over and over."

"Do you see a psychiatrist now?"

"Once every six months."

"Medication?"

"Yes. And I found a job, too, because with my history it was hard to get a job in a university. I went to work every day. Last week I worked on Friday, made an attempt on my life on Saturday."

"Do you remember how?"

"I drank a couple of ounces of gin and a half of a bottle of Carbona. But I knew it no longer contained carbon tet, so it wasn't really an all-out attempt."

"It sounds like a pretty seriously planned attempt to me."

"Yes. I did think about it for several days and even wrote a note giving my money away and asking the lady who cares for my cats to find a home for them."

"You have children?"

"Yes. One runs a restaurant. The other is in medical school. I write to both of them."

"Okay."

"I don't know how I got here, do you?"

"No."

"A lady I know says I was heard screaming that night. I don't know, I just want to go back to work. It's hard to overcome a lag in work."

"Fine. Let's work on it. We're aware of your job. We want you out, too, so you won't get seven-eighths of the way, or all the way, next time."

"I appreciate that. I appreciate you seeing me."

Walker gets up, clutching his hip, and limps out. Berger turns to the resident. "Maybe the way to deal with him is intellectual rather than purely psychological. He's bright. Talk to him. Listen to him. Watch him."

"I am. I will," the resident says. "I saw his wheelchair in front of the shower room last night and I rushed in to check. He was just taking a shower, that's all."

"Well, tell the head nurse to check on him at night, too. And put him on Thorazine to get some antipsychotic effect, to help him back to reality."

They're cut off by the arrival, unannounced, of one of Berger's clinic patients. She wants to see him privately, so he searches for an empty office; there's too much traffic in his. He puts a key into a locked door down the hall. It doesn't open. "I put the wrong key in," he tells his secretary. "Maybe my unconscious is telling me not to see her."

But he does. A young and attractive blonde, well dressed and well constructed, she is in despair. Her boyfriend, as she calls him, has moved out. In the past, she would have slashed herself or gotten drunk or both; now she feels she can depend upon Berger to get her through it. She wants him to know about this problem. She'll talk about it later in the day, when she has a regular appointment with him. Meanwhile, Berger arranges for her to see a social worker, one he likes and trusts, to see if there's anything she can do for her. It is now 12:15 and Berger must preside at a meeting of all the Psychiatry residents. He tells the patient he'll see her later and picks up his lunch, a bottle of diet Dr Pepper, before dashing to the residents' meeting.

Bellevue Psychiatry, on the hospital's northern boundary, has dark corridors; its rooms are musty. Cheer is not to be found in its decor, only in the manner of those who work there. There is some joy in the manner of the twenty-five residents who have shown up to meet with Berger in an unused library. Talking to one another is slightly easier than deciphering the riddles of their patients.

Berger is the ranking resident in Psychiatry, but he is not one to flash his rank. He moderates, almost invisibly, as the residents confront their problems. Issues are raised, debated, discarded, noted.

There is a grievance about salary. The average first-year resident earns $14,000, but no two residents seem to receive identical paychecks; they have compared amounts. Deductions seem impossible to define. One of the residents will turn detective and try to find out.

There's a rumor that hospital parking will be leased to a company that will charge high prices. One resident wants a bicycle rack installed.

Overcrowded offices have a negative effect on therapy; even patients who aren't claustrophobic feel cramped. Bureaucrats, responsible for most administrative matters in New York hospitals, plague the lives of doctors. "Psychiatrists. Shit on them," Berger says, mockingly.

There is trouble on the wards. The nursing staff is inadequate. Attendings resist the complaints of residents.

"On my ward," Berger says, "we are getting screwed. We have just lost another practical nurse because she failed her math exam. I saw the exam. It brought beads of perspiration to my forehead. One of those things with bushels and pecks. Of Thorazine. The Nursing department is unmovable, a totally feudal hierarchy almost impossible to touch. And the aides are rigidly controlled by Nursing, too, and protected by their union."

A resident adds his wrath. "On one ward, the aides were pulled off and the patients ganged up on the nurses."

Another resident: "Well, get an elephant gun. If the patients get violent and you haven't got help, knock them down with it."

"You know, if we wrote a letter to the *Times* about these conditions, if we wrote to a flock of politicians . . ." Berger says.

"Okay. If we get together to talk about our problems and act on them, I'm ready. If we try that, we might get some action."

The residents file out of the room. As they do, one of them sighs and says, "Very depressing."

At 1:30, Berger is back in his office on NO–6.

He talks to a social worker, the young woman not long out of school, about the talk she had with his distraught woman patient while he was at the residents' meeting. It was not the emergency it seemed to be, the social worker tells him. The woman is in a work program at the hospital and that has helped to distract her, to keep her busy. She's there now, on the seventh floor.

That floor in Psychiatry has rooms for crafts, music rooms, a gym, a library and a branch of the public school system. Patients who are in the hospital get to use these facilities and, if the work has been therapeutic, can continue to use them once they're released. Skills are taught. Further training is available through the office of vocational rehabilitation, as a transition to an outside job. Berger works closely with the therapists on the seventh floor. He also runs a weekly group therapy session for former ward patients; he visits troubled patients at home as well.

When the social worker leaves, she's replaced by a medical student Berger knows, a young man who is surveying hospitals, getting ready to apply. He wants to know something about Bellevue Psychiatry, about which he has heard both good and bad.

"The building sucks," he says, cynically, "I know that, I've looked at it. But the case load is heavy and good and maybe that's the best thing. Everybody works hard and learns. That's what they say. When I'm here, just looking around, I see patients who are zonked out and I wonder what that *means*. Is that treatment? Or is it like freezing some cat until you think you *can* treat him? I guess I could go elsewhere for my training, but there is something about Bellevue."

"Look, it's like this," Berger says. "The director of resident training here is a Freudian analyst, but the methods we use are eclectic. Sure, the new residents read Freud. Then they go into Horney, Sullivan and others. Later, there's strong emphasis on psychopharmacology. We're strong here on drug education, on treating schizophrenia, on the whole idea of continuing education. Other hospitals can be rigid. We're not. I can do a lot of things on my own if I feel they're intelligent to do."

The student listens, without comment.

"Treating schizophrenia is not slick and easy. It can't simply be treated with drugs. You're right about that, if that's what you meant by zonking people. You've got to have follow-up psychotherapy. To get the patient into the outside world, to get him to function responsibly without pain and without departing from reality. That's the goal. You don't hear us use the word 'cure' very often. You just take them one at a time because to philosophize or generalize is very, very risky."

The student leaves, to make up his own mind. It is 2:30 and Berger has an appointment with one of his head nurses, a gray-haired black man, who arrives on time. Before they can begin their conversation, a resident bursts in.

A patient has deliberately held a cigarette to her finger and burned it badly. Is there any ointment around? Yes, Berger tells him.

"You know what's weird? I tested her yesterday and she couldn't differentiate between feelings of hot and cold," the resident says to Berger.

"Could be a by-product of her psychosis," Berger suggests.

The resident shakes his head in disbelief, but has no time to debate it. He leaves to find the ointment and Berger turns back to his head nurse.

They are together to talk about one of the best staff nurses on the ward. She wants to get her master's in psychology and wants to continue to work on the ward, part-time. The Nursing department, down through channels, has returned a negative decision. The nurse is angry and is threatening to quit. Berger knows her value to the ward. If she is allowed to get away, he would have just two R.N.s on duty during the day, not enough. The head nurse understands, but he has accepted the verdict from above. Berger does not. He phones the chief of Psychiatry, tells him about his need for nurses, that he's lost four R.N.s in four months. The chief tells him he didn't realize the problem existed; he'll check and call him back.

"At a rich voluntary hospital, there'd be five R.N.s on duty during the day," Berger says to the head nurse as he leaves. It is as close as Berger gets to a shout.

The resident treating the biology professor comes in. He's phoned Walker's private psychiatrist, who confesses that he can't make much sense out of the patient's life history. After all, he doesn't see Walker very often. Berger is suspicious, but unable to do anything about it. Obviously, they can't rely on that doctor for help. He tells the resident to get back to Walker.

He signs a form for the discharge of the man found drunk in Penn Station. He's now sober and certainly not psychotic.

At 3:15, Berger sees the young woman whose man has fled. He shuts the door to his office, defending their privacy against the intrusions of residents in need, for an hour. She emerges smiling, happier, and Berger escorts her to the door to the ward. He unlocks it and lets her out. By the time he gets back, a resident has taken over a chair in Berger's office, seizing a moment's relaxation and a cigarette.

The resident, a few months out of medical school, is happy to be on the ward, he tells Berger. It is a good one, he says, as if he knew others as well. He has developed a loyalty to Berger and to the other staff members and this is his way of expressing it.

"It's true that the doctors are less experienced than those on other wards here. Sure. But there are fewer patients per doctor. And the entire staff is enthusiastic about what we do," Berger tells him. "We're not overcrowded. We respect our capacity. And there's a sense of community here. We serve our community, with the help of the Aberdeen. And we try to get some continuity in our work with patients. You've seen that. Not in and out and forgotten."

Just as Berger finishes, eight staff members come in. One is carrying a birthday cake. It's a party for one of the activity therapists on the ward. They all like her. She is young, attractive, dedicated to her work, intense about the work the ward does. The candles are lit; she is summoned. "Happy Birthday" is sung. She blushes, pleased. The cake is devoured rapidly, amid exchanges about patients. There is no small talk. One by one, the staff members go back to their jobs. Finally, Berger is alone.

He sits on top of his desk, almost hypnotically wiping streaks of frosting from the top of his desk, staring into space. It is after 6 now. Whatever he is thinking is his secret. People pass his door, but do not intrude. Tonight, he must go to a methadone clinic where he moonlights, picking up extra money for a few hours' work each week. He'll be there for three hours tonight, before he can drive home, get some sleep and resume his life at Bellevue in the morning.

At 9 A.M., Ken Kirshbaum attends another teaching conference, a two-session exploration of a young girl's psyche supervised by a psychiatrist who specializes in adolescents.

The psychiatrist, an elegant man in his forties, is well known to the residents, and well liked by them; more than twenty residents and social workers are present. The patient, who is being seen in the clinic, is brought in and seated next to the resident who interviews her.

She is a teen-age black, born in Haiti. The resident asks her questions; she answers directly. She lived in Port au Prince, in various American cities, a nomadic life. Her father was a difficult man, unpredictable, erratic. She calls him "crazy." When two other children left home, the father began persecuting her. He would become angry if he found out that she was seeing boys. She "snuck out once or twice a week," when she was 14, to do just that. "I wanted to get out of there," she tells the resident, a woman with an ingratiating manner. Her father and mother, the patient says, fought constantly and didn't sleep together. "He may have cared for her, but he didn't know how to express it," she says.

A year ago, she left their house in Haiti and came to New York with her mother. Her father had told her he wanted to have sex with her. "It was the first time he ever said anything like that," she says. "It scared me. He had a crazy look in his eyes." One day while the father was at work, mother and daughter left.

What about her mother?

"My mother is sane. She does everything that people think is normal. She's not exciting. I am. I'm daring. I take my chances. I have sex with my boyfriend without using birth control. My mother would get mad, but I figure she knows and doesn't approve. I have sex with other boys, too. I enjoy it. I feel it's all right." If she got pregnant, she'd have an abortion, she says.

The future baffles her. "I have to decide what I want to do after school. Mother says I put value on material things. I know that material things don't make you happy, but she's right. And I go out with poor boys, uneducated ones. She thinks I have an inferiority complex. I do like people who are raw, not polished. I guess I feel mixed up about men."

She is tall, slim, buxom. She goes to modeling school. Most of her friends work, don't go to college. "Sometimes I'm sick of school, but then I want to be different, too. I want to be well-off. Not an apartment for me. A house."

She confesses that there are moments of stress that immobilize her. "I go crazy. I can't stand much noise. I can't stand it when little kids make noise. I get angry and want to throw them out the window. But I don't really hurt anyone."

She would like to control her anger, but it builds and builds. Later, she feels sorry. But her rage persists.

"I used to plan to kill my father. With poison. I didn't do it because I was afraid I'd get caught."

She is calm throughout the exchanges with the resident, despite the fact that she is surrounded by a semicircle of residents and social workers, staring at her. She seems controlled, oblivious of them, aware only of the resident who is talking with her, a woman she considers her friend.

"If I sit around and think about it, I can get sad, so I try to go out with my friends. Sometimes I feel I can't get out of it and think of getting rid of myself. I cry a lot, have trouble sleeping. I think about taking sleeping pills, but we don't have any sleeping pills. Whenever I'm upset, I eat. Anything I can find."

She has tried to talk to her mother about her frustrations, but "if I can't understand them, how can she?"

She has trouble concentrating. She's able to listen in classes and she enjoys school, but "if I'm reading a book I can read the same sentence twenty times."

What was her past like? What does she remember about it?

She remembers that when she was very small, she was hit by a car and spent time in a hospital. It was a comforting place. Her earliest memories, between the ages of two and five, are pleasant; she lived with her grandmother, a good woman. Between six and ten, she lived with her mother in a house in a New York suburb. Otherwise, life has been a shuffle, with her father appearing and disappearing, living in Cleveland, in Haiti, in Brooklyn.

The resident thanks her and the girl leaves.

"She's like many adolescents coming to the clinic today," the resident says. "They come in on their own, having heard about it from their school guidance counselors or from friends. They tell us they want to get their heads together and came to Bellevue to do it."

"I'm encouraged," the presiding psychiatrist says. "The reputation of Bellevue must be improving. It's no longer thought of as a place where crazies are locked up."

The group agrees to discuss her case at tomorrow's session. It's time for all those present to get back to work.

Kirshbaum attends his clinic unit meeting, then takes a sandwich and a can of 7-Up to a meeting of Psychiatry residents. He finds the meeting is in progress when he gets there. He eats his sandwich and listens. Dirk Berger presides, but his manner is so understated that anyone can speak when he or she feels the urge. Although Kirshbaum doesn't see much of Berger—Berger runs Ward NO-6 and Kirshbaum is in the clinic—he likes him. Berger is casual but smart, and Kirshbaum respects that. Also, Kirshbaum would like that job, chief resident, next year when he's eligible for it. There's little he can do to get it, except do the best job he can and hope that it's noticed.

There is a discussion of the resident's right to see, and debate, the evaluation of his work filed by supervisors and attendings, to learn from them and to protest if necessary to the Director of Residency Training. An ill-founded criticism, gone unchallenged, can affect a doctor's career. Kirshbaum casts an affirmative vote for the right to defend himself against buried threats to his future.

When the meeting ends, it is almost 2 P.M. and Kirshbaum must see a procession of clinic patients. Every few minutes a new one appears. Kirshbaum follows a path from his office to the registration desk, picking up charts, leading patients to his office.

A 14-year-old Puerto Rican boy who has threatened his family with a knife. A 6-year-old boy who, according to his mother, sits at home, beside a window, leaning outward, talking to a brother who died in a fire a year ago. He was with his mother, out of the apartment, when it happened, and he heard his mother threaten to kill herself when she heard about her son's death. He has become a severe problem for his teachers. Kirshbaum talks to him simply, affectionately. The boy has little to say; this therapeutic process could take many months, years. Kirshbaum gives the boy a bag of lollipops he's brought especially for him, and hopes the mother will continue to bring him in.

A young woman, frenzied, arrives next, convinced that her own therapist, on vacation, is dead. She is followed by a young black woman, 22, without any history of hospitalization, confused and troubled about sex; a white man in his twenties, retarded, illiterate, worried about his 55-year-old mother's strange behavior; a 33-year-old Latin woman, who looks 60, who has been admitted to Bellevue more than twenty-five times since 1968 for chronic drug abuse.

Kirshbaum, who has seen the Latin woman before, can see immediately that she is in better shape. They chat, briefly, and he gives her a one-week batch of Valium. When she leaves, he hopes that she'll show up in a week and will be improved then, too.

She is out of his office at 5 P.M., giving Kirshbaum a chance to go home. For a change, the waiting room is empty. Tomorrow will be a long day, ending with an eight-to-midnight shift in the Psychiatric Admitting Office. Remembering what that can be like, Kirshbaum hopes to get some rest tonight.

Diane Rahman's day begins at 8 A.M. at the N.Y.U. Medical School, with two hours of conferences. For the first hour, an attending who is on the medical school faculty lectures on urinary-stress incontinence, followed by a film starring the attending, doing a vaginal hysterectomy. The second hour is an OB-GYN conference devoted to unusual cases. There are thirty doctors present.

The first case, presented by a senior resident, is that of a 33-year-old Puerto Rican woman who appeared at Bellevue asking for an abortion. She told the resident that she had had a radical mastectomy, for cancer. The resident, concerned that the pregnancy might stimulate the cancer, consulted the surgeons. The decision was made to do a hysterectomy, on the assumption that cancer cells would be dependent on the estrogen produced by the ovaries during pregnancy. The operation was done, removing fetus, uterus, and ovaries.

"Debatable," one of the older attendings comments, sternly, "but at this point, let's keep an eye on the woman, to watch her remaining breast for any signs of cancer. The surgeons removed the other one, I know, but long-term follow-up is not their strong point."

The next case is presented by Diane Rahman: the Puerto Rican woman who has two problems, obesity and diabetes. When she arrived in OB, Rahman says, she was due to deliver in three weeks. She was extremely heavy. She was on a diet, but hadn't followed it. As she reached her delivery date, she developed an infection of the abdominal wall, which OB treated with antibiotics, successfully. On the ward, she was put on a 1,500-calorie, salt-restricted diet. Her diabetes was controlled with insulin, but because of it the medical staff decided on an early delivery. When her blood-estrogen level dropped drastically, the chief resident decided to induce labor. The African resident did just that. The patient's membranes were ruptured deliberately, risking a Caesarean—extremely difficult in an obese woman—if the technique didn't work. Fortunately, it did work. She went into spontaneous labor and last night gave birth to a normal, healthy daughter.

"Delivery ought to be guided by test data, not necessarily by the fact that the woman is a diabetic," an attending comments. "And you ought to know that with a patient this heavy it is important, in a Caesarean, to ventilate, and because it takes longer to get to the baby, general anesthesia is mandatory."

On her way back to Bellevue, Rahman trudges wearily along First Avenue. Although she managed to seem alert during her presentation of the case, she is tired from a long and busy night on duty. As she walks along, she tells another resident what she encountered during the night.

"Must have been the full moon," she says. "I had a woman whose membranes had ruptured at twenty-eight weeks. A likely miscarriage to deal with. She may have to be delivered, whether the fetus is alive or dead, within twenty-four hours if she shows signs of infection.

"The obese Puerto Rican woman had her girl at 8 P.M. Another woman aborted, twice, at 3 A.M. and 4 A.M. Twins. She lost both. Another one went into labor at home at 4 A.M. When I saw her, it was time, so I admitted her. Her membranes ruptured this morning, so she should be ready to deliver at any minute."

The woman is ready, and as Rahman gets back to OB, two nurses are rushing the woman into the delivery room. It is 10:10. Rahman races off to scrub.

The patient is a young Puerto Rican having her first child. She is small; her stomach seems smaller than most. The nurses spread her legs and strap them into stirrups. Rahman enters, takes a look at her, then walks out. The nurses follow her, leaving the patient alone.

"Please, miss, don't leave. Don't leave," she shrieks. Rahman hears her and returns. The woman is terrified.

"Just relax," Rahman says to her. "There's nothing to worry about. The pain comes and goes. Don't be afraid."

The woman continues to groan. The nurses return to prep her and drape her.

"Be still and breathe. *Breathe,*" one of the nurses tells her. *"Push."*

The senior resident walks in, to watch. The anesthetist has set up blood pressure and pulse monitors and is giving oxygen to the woman; earlier, she had been given Demerol, for pain.

The senior resident walks up to the patient, smiles at her and says, "The baby is almost here and everything is going very well. Just push."

The anesthetist translates into Spanish.

The senior resident, Rahman, the nurses and the anesthetist are all scrubbed, gowned and ready, caps and masks in place, gloves on. This delivery belongs to Rahman.

She can see the top of the baby's head, then it retracts. Thinking aloud, Rahman decides not to use forceps; she wants to avoid the cervical lacerations and damage to the child that are possible with forceps. She wants the woman to push out the baby on her own.

Suddenly, the room is absolutely quiet. The senior resident tells Rahman to watch out for a sudden birth, to be ready, then he leaves.

"*Muy bien,*" the anesthetist says to the patient.

Rahman inserts her fingers, probes. The baby's head emerges, in her hands, easily. The rest of the sleek body follows, slowly, smoothly. At 10:35, the baby is in the outside world, screaming properly. Rahman severs the umbilicus. A nurse suctions the baby's mouth and nose, then holds the baby up for the mother to see.

"*Niña,*" she says.

An intern from Pediatrics has arrived, to claim the baby and take it to the nursery. Rahman does not speak to him; she is pulling on the end of the umbilicus and it slides out, pulling the placenta with it. She cleans the patient, checks for lacerations, finds one and sutures it. She is done by 10:45.

Unassisted, she has delivered a child. She leaves the delivery room to fill out the required forms and give post-partum orders for the nurses. On one form she writes "Pregnancy Unremarkable." As she continues to write, there is a smile on her face. She no longer seems exhausted.

Filling out the forms takes so long there is no time for lunch. A fresh medical student arrives at 2 P.M. They talk about cutting corners at Bellevue.

"You go with your patient to Radiology, so you know you'll get the best X-rays," she tells the student. "If you want something done at Bellevue, you do it yourself."

The student trails along as Rahman checks a woman who has

been in labor since 7 P.M. last night. She's in a labor room, one of four that adjoin the delivery rooms, but she isn't progressing quickly enough. Rahman decides she needs help and orders Pitocin.

She talks to the senior resident about the Puerto Rican woman who seemed to be too far along for the abortion she wanted. Having sent for an Ultrasound test yesterday, she's received a mixed blessing. The pregnancy is not more than twenty weeks, permitting the abortion. However, there's a fibroid tumor next to the fetus—the total mass is what misled the senior resident.

"All right. Let's do the abortion. That tumor may shrink after the pregnancy is over and then it can be handled surgically," the senior resident says.

Rahman keeps in motion, conducting discharge exams for women who want to get out of Bellevue and go home. She checks her ward patients. She remembers that she has a saline abortion to set up, a clinic patient to see. Her stomach tells her that she didn't have lunch. She gets a peanut butter sandwich on white bread and a pear from the OB pantry. While she munches it, she can hear two nurses talking a few feet away.

"The babies born here are so small," one says. "Not like those in private hospitals where I used to work."

"It's a matter of good nutrition," the other answers. "Our mothers have to be told and told what to eat during pregnancy. The ones we get drink Pepsi instead of milk."

The clinic patient arrives to see Rahman. She is a black teenager named Jenny James, who decided to take the day off from school because she wasn't feeling well. She showed up at the clinic, where she became OB's problem; examination revealed that she was eight months pregnant. When Rahman questions her, she discovers that the girl's membranes ruptured this morning, but the girl didn't understand what that meant. Rahman takes a blood sample, checks the girl's blood pressure and pulse and has her admitted to the ward.

In one of the labor rooms, the woman with the fetus and the tumor awaits her abortion. Rahman can go home once the saline drip is finished.

The woman is solemn, silent. Rahman works quickly. Soon the saline has flowed out. The woman begins to cry, softly. Rahman looks at her from the doorway. She is sad, too, and very tired. She removes her white gown, hangs it up and very slowly walks to the elevator.

Bob Nachtigall's day begins in a classroom at the N.Y.U. Medical School, with an 8 A.M. lecture on vulvar lesions, followed by a conference of OB-GYN residents. He gets to Bellevue at 10:15.

When he arrives in the GYN examining room, the center of activity, he sits down at a desk to collect his notes for the day. A buxom, stocky laboratory technician comes up behind him. She massages his neck and tells him she's going home. He tells her he'll be over in a half-hour, but he knows he's kidding and she grudgingly knows it, too.

A resident sticks his head out of one of the examining booths and yells at Nachtigall, "Are we really going to do a tubal ligation on a twenty-three-year-old girl?"

"She has three kids now," Nachtigall tells him, "and doesn't want any more."

Nachtigall goes back to his notes. "I don't see how we can do four tubal ligations, with everything else we have to do today," he tells one of the nurses. She doesn't seem interested in his dilemma. He manages to compile an operating schedule and delivers it to the nursing station on the OR floor. The head nurse quibbles with him about the way GYN schedules its operations. She is looking for trouble, asserting whatever power she thinks she has, but she doesn't want to escalate the debate.

As he walks away, Nachtigall mutters, "There's the right way and the wrong way and the Bellevue way. The Bellevue way is just a paranoid-schizophrenic's view of the Army way."

He gets back to GYN in time to answer the phone. It is a patient describing her pain to Nachtigall.

"The pain you're having is just menstrual cramps. That's good. Okay? It will decrease, don't worry. Take the Darvon and I'll see you next week," he says. He is concerned about her. She is in her twenties and wants a hysterectomy because she's had irregular menstrual bleeding, due to what Nachtigall feels is a hormone deficiency. She hasn't had a period in two months, but the progesterone he's giving her may be working.

"I'm sure it doesn't require surgery," Nachtigall says to another resident who is perched on the edge of the desk. "I'd rather treat her with hormones. I'm trying progesterone now, to get her a normal period. It is really a matter of GYN endocrinology and it takes time, but this problem can be solved. She *can* be regulated. Once you can make the diagnosis, you can always figure out the treatment. Right?"

The other resident nods in agreement. He is distracted, however. A tall blond good-looking nurse is ambling his way; she leans over and kisses him, then slinks away. "Come back later, when I'm not busy," the resident calls to her.

"You get the feeling that it is not pure coincidence that certain guys go into GYN," Nachtigall says to the resident, who has a look of latent satisfaction on his face.

Nachtigall makes a phone call, to get the address of a patient who had an abortion on Monday. The attending performing the abortion discovered a fibroid tumor and Nachtigall wants to follow up on the case. He calls the chief resident about the operating schedule for the rest of the week. He is busy with small matters. "These running-around things have a way of eating up the time," he says.

There are screams from an examining booth.

"Ay, ay, ay!"

A few feet from Nachtigall a Puerto Rican woman is signing the permission form for a tubal ligation. The resident with her asks, "Do you want a hysterectomy?"

"Forget it, man," she says, "not me."

A nurse is playing with a patient's three-month-old daughter. A medical student is taking a blood specimen. The phone rings again. It is a resident at the AES. A woman has walked in with a blood pressure of 80/50 and has just expelled a fetus. The GYN resident taking the call says, "Bring her up here. I can't help her down there." The AES resident tells him he believes she's in shock and shouldn't be moved.

"Okay, okay," the GYN resident says, "I'm on my way." He runs out the door. Ten minutes later, he's back. "It wasn't that urgent," he tells Nachtigall. "She wasn't in shock." He is carrying a small plastic bag with the fetus in it. Nachtigall grimaces.

"Reminds me of the first abortion I was in on," Nachtigall tells him. "A vacuum aspirator. It wasn't working properly, and we went in with a curette to see what we could find. I came out with a small leg. It was gross and horrible, even if I do believe in abortion."

He picks up the phone, as if to wipe out that thought, and calls a patient's husband to get his endorsement of an operation to be done on her.

"I'm calling from Bellevue," Nachtigall says. "No, nothing happened to your wife." There is a rapid flow of Spanish from the other end of the line. Nachtigall waves at a nurse who speaks Spanish. She picks up the phone and explains. The husband can't come in to sign anything. He works. The patient has given her written consent; that will suffice.

More phone calls. The Pap test result Nachtigall has been waiting to get for a week is negative. "Man, I'd make a dynamite secretary," Nachtigall tells a passing resident. "I'm a little overtrained for it, but . . ."

The resident turns to him, not quite hearing what Nachtigall has said, and proclaims, "I follow up on two kinds of cases on my own: fascinating gynecological problems and extraordinarily beautiful women."

Nachtigall gets up, smiling, and walks over to one of the wards. He takes two blood specimens and hand-carries them to the lab on his way to lunch.

Lunch today is a hamburger at the hospital snack bar, minimal relief from the diet at the doctors' cafeteria. Nachtigall sits down beside a nurse he knows and they talk about OB-GYN. The nurse drops an aside about "neurotic doctors."

"Sure, being a doctor, whatever the specialty, is an ego trip, but doctors are a rigid, compulsive lot. They don't get into introspection enough. They believe their press releases. And that's why so many patients feel they aren't really talking to their doctors.

"Doctors rob themselves of their own effectiveness by trying to keep that bullshit fantasy of their invulnerability alive. Doctors are so afraid of making a mistake they'll do anything to avoid admitting one. You can get sucked into it. Maybe it's because people don't want to see doctors behave as human beings. Maybe they really want them to be supermen. If you tell a patient you don't know what's going on, she'll find another doctor.

"Sure, we're well trained, but we make mistakes. We shouldn't have to live up to the myth. But if we don't, there's a big stink."

At 1:30 P.M., Nachtigall is in the GYN clinic. He spends two hours there, seeing one patient after another, without respite.

It is 3:30 when he gets back to GYN. The examining room seems quiet.

"Macy's is having a whale of a sale," a nurse's aide is saying.

"I'm awfully hungry," another adds.

A nurse's daughter, 6, sits primly in a spotless dress and does her homework. Another nurse studies the *Times*. A resident instructs two medical students in a simple pregnancy test.

Behind a closed curtain, one of the residents is examining a woman. She has a nasal, Bronx voice.

"I have mental illness," she tells the resident. "I have no control over my will power."

The resident does not comment.

She tells him that she believes she was raped several days ago, while she was a patient at a state mental hospital. The resident continues to examine her. Outside the curtained booth, residents have begun to assemble, quietly, for chart rounds. The room is silent.

"Tell me, Doctor," the woman says, cutting through the silence. "What is it in a woman that they call the cherry? Is that a medical term?"

The resident's voice tightens. "No. The medical term for it is 'hymen,'" he answers.

"Is that what bleeds?" she asks.

"Not if you've had intercourse before," he answers.

"Is intercourse when they put it in your hole?" she asks.

"Yes," he says, his voice starting to crack.

"Well, that didn't happen to me," she concludes.

The resident excuses himself, emerges from behind the curtain, runs to a corner and doubles up. A few minutes pass; he returns to tell the woman her examination is over. She emerges.

She is middle-aged, with gray hair. She wears blue sneakers and a pink flowered dress. She is clutching her purse and a clear plastic raincoat.

"I'm going to give you some pills," the resident tells her.

"To put in my mouth," she says, calmly.

"No," he says, "to put in your vagina."

"I can't find it," she insists. "Is it a small hole?"

"Use a mirror," he tells her, "or put the pills where I put my fingers."

She is very happy and skips out with the prescription form in her hand. The resident races into the chief resident's office, joining the others.

The chief has been in the OR most of the day. He is exhausted. Nachtigall mans the chart rack, handing them in batches to the chief.

Nachtigall wants to release a woman at 10 A.M. tomorrow rather than holding her until 6 P.M. to await test results he feels are irrelevant. It will save her money on the hospital bill. The chief agrees.

A patient given blood transfusions hasn't shown any progress. "Maybe it's because Bellevue blood self-destructs," the chief says.

The old woman with cancer must be operated upon, the chief insists. "She's going to have a vaginal hysterectomy and we're not going to tell her why," he says.

Nachtigall outlines a case. One of the ward patients has been in for days with a postdelivery infection. Her husband, who's been taking care of the newborn baby, may lose his job. The patient wants to go home to relieve him. Her infection seems cleared up, the chief admits, but the best medicine ought to prevail; he thinks she still needs antibiotics and bed rest. At Nachtigall's request, he'll check her tonight.

The chief says he doesn't want to do a laparoscopic tubal ligation on the 23-year-old woman. He wants to use a technique that will permit possible repair later if she wants more children.

A resident stumbles in during rounds, looking as if he is about to faint. "Man, man, man. The paperwork is getting to me," he says, collapsing into a chair.

The chief describes an episode in the OR today, during an abortion in which the patient refused general anesthesia. "You ain't puttin' that mask on me, baby," she said, sitting upright on the operating table. The chief wants the residents to know that such a problem can arise. "We gave her a little Xylocaine, some Valium, and we talked her through the procedure," he says.

The resident caring for the old woman with cancer wants to revive the discussion of her case. He doesn't want to be the one to tell her she's going to have a hysterectomy. The chief wants him to tell her, but he doesn't want her to know about the cancer, just about the operation itself. The resident resists. The chief orders him to tell the woman.

"You can't beat the fox," Nachtigall says, pointing to the chief. "He'll get 'em, one way or another."

The operating room schedule is revised, some cases shifted from tomorrow to the following day. It is a schedule in revision until the morning. Nachtigall is on call tonight; tomorrow he'll make rounds on the wards early in the morning, check new admissions and see patients with GYN problems referred from other services, in addition to the phone calls, walks to labs, confirming the OR schedule and the unexpected, a constant.

It is 6:30 P.M. Anticipating tomorrow makes Nachtigall feel tired.

At his morning meeting with Dr. Randt, Bruce Mack is reminded that when he discussed Mary Rollins' case with Randt yesterday morning, the chief had suggested that she might be the victim of methyl alcohol poisoning. Mack informs Randt that toxicology tests finally came to that conclusion, too. Randt is pleased to have his judgment confirmed, but not pleased about the plight of the patient. The two men discuss the case of the middle-aged woman, Norma Bacon, in a coma, and before Mack can complete his summary of the case, Randt has made the diagnosis. Mack smiles. It is difficult to trap Randt or find him in error, and Mack's respect for that, and for the man himself, make these morning meetings memorable for Mack.

He leaves Randt's office to return to the ward, to get together with the Neurology nursing supervisor, three head nurses and a staff nurse for a gripe session that Mack encourages. There's no agenda; Mack simply wants the nurses to tell him what's wrong on the wards. While one of the nurses eats her breakfast, a hard-boiled egg in a urine-specimen collection cup, the others tell their problems to Mack.

Neurology residents are not making ward rounds often enough. They pop in to see their patients at times, one nurse says, but often days go by without formal rounds, patient by patient.

"When we want a particular resident, we can't seem to find him, even by paging him. That makes it hard for us to plan our days," a head nurse tells Mack, who makes notes in a small black notebook.

"What can we do about patients who stay on the ward for six months?" a nurse asks.

"Well, you can bronchoscope them every day until they

agree to leave or we can get some social workers up here to place them," Mack says. He knows the problem at Bellevue of dealing with homeless patients who stay in the hospital after being treated.

"The attendings come in and out so fast, they seem afraid to come to the ward unless there's an exciting case on it," another nurse says. "We feel like orphans." She talks to Mack pleasantly; he isn't the object of her wrath, but he's the doctor who can do something about her troubles.

"When there aren't residents around, we have trouble moving the patients, especially the heavy ones, back into bed after they've been sitting in chairs," a nurse says.

"The last time I helped with that, the patient defecated all over me," Mack says.

"It's good to get your hands dirty," the nursing supervisor tells him.

When the meeting ends, Mack sees the neurosurgeon who operated on Norma Bacon last night. Mack wants a report. The neurosurgeon confirms the cerebellum hemorrhage, says he removed a large clot, 20 cc. in size, from the cerebellum. The patient stopped breathing spontaneously, needed a respirator, and her eye movement and reflexes deteriorated rapidly. The prognosis, he tells Mack, is poor. Mack listens attentively, concealing any disappointment he may feel.

At 10:25, Mack joins another attending, not either of the ones who appeared earlier in the week, for rounds. Neurology residents have shown up, too, and the small group makes its way to the male ward. Actually, it is not rounds as the complaining nurse would define it. As if corroborating her complaint, they are visiting one interesting case: a man who suffered from head trauma, is leaking spinal fluid from one ear and has partial paralysis of the face. The attending examines the man, speaks about the case, then moves on to look at another patient. When he does, Mack gathers the residents around him and says, "We'll *all* go on rounds today, so the nurses and the patients know we exist."

The attending rejoins the group as it walks down the long hall toward the female ward and the Neuro ICU. One of the residents tells Mack that he wants to do a pneumoencephalogram on a patient.

"I'm not convinced it's necessary," Mack tells him, "and it

will cause the patient considerable pain."

"You can't treat patients like your relatives," the resident responds.

"And you shouldn't treat patients as academic problems either, doing tests just to get findings which you may not even need, simply to further your own education," Mack tells him.

In the female ward, under Mack's leadership, the attending and residents go from bed to bed. An old woman in one bed stares at them. "I've never seen her before," one of the residents says to Mack. "Did she just arrive?"

"She got here last month," Mack barks.

The ward is filled with immobile old women. When the tour ends, one of the nurses turns to Mack and says, "It's just like a little nursing home here."

At that moment, the Emergency Ward pages a Neuro consult, and Mack decides to take the assignment himself. He waves at the attending and the residents, and heads for the EW.

When he gets there, he finds a prisoner from a city jail. The man, a Puerto Rican with tattoos all over his arms, legs and chest, had attempted suicide in jail. He had scaled the side of his cell, bar by bar, until he was six or seven feet from the concrete floor. Then, he dove headfirst. Mack finds him guarded by two policemen. Although the man has been tied down to his bed, he is shaking violently. One of the residents on duty in the EW suspects that the man is having a seizure. Mack examines the man carefully, discounts a seizure. "This guy," he says, "is simply very frightened."

"Actually, we called you down here to evaluate his tattoos," the EW resident laughs.

The patient is splattered with blood from face to feet, from a deep wound in his head. He is shaking frenetically and mumbling, "I'm jumpin'. I'm jumpin'."

A technician wheels up a portable X-ray unit. "You just want to be sure, first, that he hasn't broken his neck," Mack tells the resident. The X-rays are developed within minutes: no broken neck. "Treat that gash on his head," Mack tells the resident, "and keep an eye on him."

Mack is ready to return to the Neurology wards, but as he is about to leave the EW, a resident from the AES comes charging in pushing a bed bearing a middle-aged woman.

"It's a good thing you're here," he says to Mack. "An ambulance brought her in after she had a seizure at work. She was lucid and was talking to me just fine, but then she deteriorated rapidly, went into respiratory distress, had blurred vision and started to vomit. On the left side of her face I thought I saw the signs of a stroke. If you hadn't been here, I would have called you."

Mack bends over the woman's bed and looks at her. She is still awake, but her face is distorted. When Mack pricks both sides of her face simultaneously with safety pins, she turns toward her left. "They turn toward the side they don't feel," Mack tells another Neurology resident, who has shown up to help out. Two others arrive in minutes.

The woman's wig and clothes are in a heap under the bed. She is an attractive middle-aged woman, perhaps 50. Mack knows nothing about her; he hasn't had time to investigate. He prescribes mannitol, steroids and phenobarbital, and a nurse quickly administers them.

"It might be a deep bleed that will progress," Mack tells the other residents. "But then she is not in a coma. She has some movement and she can speak." As Mack is talking, the woman moans and has another seizure; she twists in bed, quivers for several minutes.

When it is over, a spinal tap is done; it is "grossly bloody" and high intracranial pressure is evident, a sign of a hemorrhage. The woman is getting worse rapidly.

"In a deep intercerebral bleed, when the patient is failing rapidly, ninety-five percent die," Mack tells another resident. But he doesn't want to give up. Surgery might be worth trying, if there's time. An angiogram would be the best move, to outline the nature of the bleeding so the neurosurgeons can decide what to do, whether to cut or not, what the odds might be. If the bleeding turns out to be shallow, there may be hope.

"At best, if the bleed is a deep one, there's a one percent chance. But I can't give up on her and let her die in front of me," Mack says.

An anesthesiologist is called and arrives a few seconds later. She intubates the woman, and as she does it, the woman vomits, spraying a resident who is assisting. Disregarding his own condition, he puts a suction unit into use, so the woman won't aspirate her own fluid.

There is activity on all sides of the bed now. The patient has stiffened and is turning the backs of her arms against her sides, a sign of dysfunction in the mid-brain area. Mack steps back when she does that, and just stares at her. He sighs. "She's surgically unapproachable now," he says. He suspects now that she would die in the middle of an angiogram; there's no point in trying that test now. Unless the drugs produce some improvement, there's nothing left. So far, the mannitol has stimulated urination, no more than that. "Not enough," Mack says. He walks over to the snack bar with the Neurology resident.

It is well beyond the normal lunchtime. Mack orders two fried eggs, but when they come, he sits staring at them. He is disturbed by the rapidity of the disintegration of the woman with the stroke.

"You know, I'm still aghast that I can speak to a patient and a half-hour later know I'll never speak to her again," he says to the Neurology resident. "But what can you do about that? After a while, you become submissive to fate, contemplative about this sort of thing, because you know that the frenzy it once inspired in you is useless."

He finishes his eggs quickly, without pleasure, and gets back to the Emergency Ward, to stand beside the woman's bed. IV lines are in, providing medication; they were inserted as soon as she arrived in the EW, because when blood pressure drops it can be difficult getting a line into a patient. But the IV medication, Mack knows, won't solve the woman's massive problem. She is breathing heavily now. The cardiac monitor beeps irregularly. Mack continues to stare, as if intense concentration will provide him with an answer. Another resident passes by, looks at Mack and at the woman and says, "What can I tell you?"

A nurse walks up to tell Mack that two of the woman's relatives have arrived. Mack whirls and sees them, the woman's son and daughter, in their twenties. They are tense, shaking, on the verge of tears.

"She's never been sick before," the daughter says, suppressing a sob. "She did have high blood pressure and she took pills for it."

"We didn't know that she got sick at work," the son adds. "We didn't know she was here until someone called us." Mack leads them to her bedside. They look at her, look at Mack.

"How is she?" the daughter asks.

"Not good," Mack answers, barely above a whisper.

"Her chances?"

"Very slim."

"But she *could* recover?"

"Not likely. Not likely in cases like this."

"Surgery won't help?"

"We don't think so."

The daughter and the son walk slowly to a nearby waiting room. As they leave, one of the neurosurgeons comes up to Mack. He's discussed the case with the chief resident in Neurosurgery, who wants to do the angiogram, just in case the bleeding is superficial and the signs are misleading. Mack is skeptical, but agrees; the two doctors carefully push the woman's bed toward Neuroradiology. When they get her there, Mack leaves. He will check on her later if she lives. The angiogram should take an hour or more.

Mack goes back to his office on the ward. He has to write a presentation of a case he has researched; when he is done, Dr. Randt will present it at a conference. His loyalty to Randt makes Mack feel guilty about not having gotten the paper done by now. He had assumed it would be a quiet, uneventful week. It has not been. It is now late in the afternoon and there is no point in working on the paper in his office. He collects his notes, to finish it at home tonight.

At 8 A.M., Kalmon Post is in the Neuro ICU, to take a look at the man who had undergone the embolization yesterday to block troubling blood vessels in the brain. The man is sedated, relatively reactive, but conspicuously weak. Post is puzzled. The man could be weak from the nine hours of general anesthesia and the demands of the embolization itself. But there are signs of paralysis, however mild, and that disturbs Post. The man is being given oxygen, and Post makes certain that the ICU nurses watch him carefully.

"If the corner of his mouth twitches, that's a fit. Let me know immediately. I'm not sending him back to the VA until he's better," Post tells the head nurse.

In the next bed, the woman in her thirties who had been studied by the Head Trauma Unit is back in the ICU. The tests were not favorable; there is possible brain-stem damage. She is still on the edge of a coma.

Post leaves the ICU to check the women's ward. As he enters, he can hear the babbling sound of an old woman in a chair near the entrance. She screams monosyllables, meaningless sounds, and claps her hands. Her disorder can't be treated neurologically. She is being sent to a state mental hospital today. As Post watches, a nurse walks up to the woman; the woman leans her head against the nurse's stomach. The nurse pats her head, strokes it, and the woman quiets down. She is clearly regressive. When the nurse walks away, the woman resumes her discordant chanting.

"You hush!" an old black woman trying to sleep yells at her.

Post finishes rounds quickly. There aren't any new patients and the old ones seem stable. He goes back to the Pediatrics ICU to see the 8-year-old boy.

"Say your name for me," Post says.

The boy looks at him and whimpers.

"Don't be afraid," Post says.

There is a trace of muscle movement in the boy's right leg, but his right arm doesn't move and his eyes don't cross mid-line when Post asks him to follow his finger.

"It's still early," Post says to the Pediatrics resident on duty. "But I'm not optimistic. The trouble is that children hesitate to try to speak at all when they have trouble doing it, so I can't tell how he's going to do. It's that first word that counts. But he does seem to understand what I say to him. Nevertheless, he'll be somewhat paralyzed at best. That was a large clot we removed."

It is 9 A.M. and Post goes to Neuroradiology to pick up the X-rays he'll need to discuss the embolization case at the conference later today. They're not ready. He stops at the Hematology lab, to check a blood-gas test on the embolization patient. The blood is low in oxygen. Post phones the nurse in the ICU to tell her to continue the oxygen and take another blood-gas sample in ten minutes. Then he walks over to the VA.

At the VA, Post checks into Radiology, to ascertain the details for a ventriculogram on a VA patient of his. Once there, Post is unsuccessful in getting a room, a technician, a nurse, for the procedure, which involves the injection of oil into the brain and recording its movement on X-rays. Post is angry.

He is rankled by delays, sloppiness, neglect.

"At Bellevue we'd be finished with this study by now," he says to a Neurosurgery resident who tags along. "At University Hospital we'd be finished and the films would be ready."

Post tells the resident to set up the ventriculogram for later and he makes rounds. When he's done, he looks weary. In a few weeks, he'll be out of the VA duty, off to his rotation at University Hospital before returning to Bellevue as Neurosurgery's chief resident for his final year.

At 11 A.M., he is back at Bellevue, to pick up the X-rays. As he waits for them to be collated, he listens to two residents who are discussing a case.

"I've got this patient who is in bad shape," one resident tells the other. "I wanted to talk to his wife about his condition and she comes in to see me. She's an old Jewish woman, and when I tell her that her husband is going downhill, she looks at me with a kind of resigned expression on her face and says, 'Poor Mendel, he's always been a loser. You know something? He was in the Army years ago and he was supposed to get out on December 8, 1941. Believe me, it's true. Always a loser. He's been terribly sick. So now he's got pneumonia and I should say, 'I'm not surprised.'"

It is noon and Post meets Dr. Ransohoff for rounds. As he nears Ransohoff's office, he asks another resident, "Is he in a good mood?"

"He said 'good morning' to me," the resident replies.

Ransohoff and an elderly attending join the residents, led by Post, and make rounds. So far this week, in Post's life, Ransohoff's criticism has not been focused on Post. Rounds go smoothly, ending at 12:35, time for Post to have lunch. He can't. There's a Neuropathology conference he wants to attend and that's more important to him than food.

Post attends the conference in a classroom setting, a room full of doctors, more than forty, and a lecturing pathologist, using samples on trays and slides projected on a large screen.

In one case, the pathologist concludes that a 65-year-old man who died could have been operated upon; according to the pathologist, the man lived for six weeks with a condition that he felt was operable. However, he states, the family opposed surgery; he knows that. The neurosurgeon who treated the man speaks up: the patient was too sick, in and out of consciousness, for an operation. He is defensive.

The pathologist, adhering to a literal academic approach, shows some illustrative brain tissue. There is an obvious aneurysm and a blood clot near the surface.

"I didn't intend to criticize the management of the patient," the pathologist says. While the aura of challenge hovers over the room, several doctors squirm uncomfortably. Another reads the current issue of *Penthouse*. Another sleeps.

The conference ends in time for the Neurosurgery conference to begin, at 2 P.M. There are twenty doctors present, including the chief, Ransohoff, and a number of well-known attendings. Post begins by presenting the case of the 8-year-old boy in the Pediatrics ICU.

"We missed it on this child," he says, indicating that the boy was released from the hospital prematurely and then readmitted too late. What bothers Post is that the clot was enormous, yet the boy did not react to it, apparently, when it occurred, but instead reacted days later. Ransohoff is baffled, too, and suggests an angiogram now, if the boy can endure it, to check the status of his brain after surgery.

Post listens to Ransohoff carefully, notes his suggestion, then begins his presentation of the embolized man. He starts with the case history, from headaches to seizures. Then he outlines the embolization itself. It is hard to evaluate the success of it, he tells the doctors. Some of the pellets can't be accounted for. The patient, who was weak prior to embolization, is now monoplegic, Post tells the group, and the general anesthesia may have something to do with his weakened condition.

The reference to general anesthesia provokes Ransohoff, who seems astonished that it was used. The neuroradiologists, Post testifies, specified general anesthesia. It was *their* procedure.

Ransohoff argues, vigorously, against the use of general anesthesia in an embolization. He insists that the patient's condition should have been monitored throughout the procedure.

"That's impossible to do when the man is unconscious," he shouts. "Wrong and disgraceful, that's what it was."

Post's face reddens and he attempts to explain.

Ransohoff interrupts. "Has anybody from Neuroradiology been up to see the patient? No. So we're the ones who are left to talk to the man's family. The balls went astray without anyone knowing what was happening to the patient. The guy may get better, sure, but Neurosurgery and Neuroradiology have to prevent this kind of thing from happening. We must tighten it up before we do any more embolizations."

Post assures him that he'll check the patient frequently, then sits down as quickly as possible.

Other residents present other cases, from Bellevue, the VA, University Hospital and St. Vincent's, an N.Y.U. affiliate in Neurosurgery. This week there have been several cases in which brain tumors have been removed, cleanly and properly, with subsequent dramatic deterioration of the patients. It is a massive mystery. "A vascular accident" a doctor terms one of the cases.

Ransohoff admits that in one case he had planned to do a subtotal removal of a tumor, but it came out so easily he removed all of it. Then something went wrong. Infarction of the brain stem, perhaps. He simply doesn't know. The brain, at times, is an insoluble riddle, even to the best of surgeons.

As the conference ends, Ransohoff and one of the attendings leave the room together. Ransohoff turns to the attending and says, "We all make mistakes. We all learn."

It is 3:30, time for the final conference of the teaching afternoon, cosponsored by Neurology and Neurosurgery. It is held in a large room; almost a hundred doctors, including chiefs of services, attendings and residents, and a few nurses are present.

Today's conference belongs to the staff of the N.Y.U.-Bellevue Rehabilitation Medicine department. It's their show, and they are eager to keep it lively, not pedantic, in showing how their work relates to what neurologists and neurosurgeons are doing.

There is some suspense, some sense of production, of planning, in the presentation.

A Rehab Medicine doctor narrates.

The first case is that of an older man who had lived with his neck mysteriously locked in a fixed position, turned to his left, making everything he had to do a matter of embarrassment and stress. The patient is invited in and sits in a chair in front of the audience. At the presiding doctor's suggestion, he moves his neck from side to side, easily.

"His problem was corrected with eight weeks of therapy. That was a year ago. Today, he's still untroubled."

The second patient described had a similar problem. "He was in therapy for three months and has been free of his symptoms for a year," the narrator says.

The conference is beginning to take on the quality of a revival meeting. Conversation hums throughout the room.

The third patient is a teen-age girl, a victim of cerebral palsy. For years she wore a brace on one leg. She could not cut her own food; her bent right arm, with its perpetually clenched fist, prevented that. Then Rehab Medicine went to work, teaching her how her muscles functioned. She enters the room, without a brace, and sits down gracefully in the chair. She gets up and walks, almost runs, without any difficulty. Her right hand is still awkward, but she demonstrates that she can now open and close it. She suffers from fewer spasms, she says, and she can use the hand to help cut her food. She's had five one-half hours of therapy sessions on the hand.

When the girl leaves the room, a film is shown, explaining the technique. It involves the electrical stimulation and conditioning of the muscles, moving in reaction to sound waves, to teach the patient to instruct the muscles to behave properly. Eventually, when the muscles have been taught new patterns, stimulation is removed. It is myoelectric feedback therapy, a kind of mind-over-mind, Pavlovian discipline. It amounts to having the patient consciously instruct himself, retraining the brain to rule the body with the encouragement and guidance of a skilled doctor.

In the film, a woman patient describes her suffering from long-standing depression, related to a persistent, involuntary head tremor. Electrodes are attached to her neck and a sound apparatus hooked to them. As she moves her head, a sound can be heard and measured on a dial. When she stops trembling, the sound ceases. At the end of one session, captured on film, she is sitting still, without a tremor. Her history runs a gamut: various doctors treated her with drugs, including Valium and Haldol. She was in group therapy. She spent six years in psychotherapy. The tremor persisted.

"The earlier doctors were treating the mind, not the muscles. We attempt to re-educate the muscles, the manner in which messages are relayed from brain to muscles," the presiding doctor narrates.

When the film is over, the room is filled with the sounds of doctors talking about it. There are questions from skeptics.

Yes, it is experimental and too untested to evaluate firmly, the Rehab Medicine specialist tells the group.

Post wonders if this technique can be considered a "cure,"

but before he can ask the question, the Rehab Medicine doctor anticipates it.

"We don't claim that we are curing anything," he says. "Whatever the disease process is, the technique is something that may help the patients function. It's a treatment that doesn't require surgery or medicine. The concept is one of increased input, increased visual and auditory perception, the disturbing of an old pattern and establishing a new one. After all, we learn how to eat. And, remember, our approach is experimental and, importantly, benign."

He provides some findings, too meager for generalizing. In nine cases studied, three have shown clear improvement sustained for months. Three have been altered for days using feedback techniques. Three others can be helped for periods of up to an hour and can't be classified as successes or failures yet. Some may need a portable electronic device to provide the needed stimulation, so they can "educate" themselves at home.

"That's better than most psychotherapy can provide on such patients," a doctor in the audience says.

"We're not competing," says the Rehab Medicine doctor, minimizing his own elation with a sense of medical propriety. "Call it learning, if you need a label for it. It can be called operational learning or bio-feedback, except that there are so many loonies in that field, under that heading, that I'd rather avoid it. We call it sensory feedback. And it's not brand-new. NIH was into it in the sixties, and we got into it at Bellevue in '68, in Neurology's EEG lab. In the beginning, it seemed to work on psychiatric disturbances. Anxiety. Phobias. Certain kinds of headaches. Tension. We found that seventy-five percent of the patients would learn new patterns of behavior quickly. We taught some to express anger when they didn't seem to be able to, and others to relax. And, most important, to control both. In a technical way, you might say we were using voluntary components to modify involuntary aspects of the central nervous system. Yogas and Zens do the same thing. We do it with electronics."

He explains that feedback was introduced to Rehab Medicine in 1970, to treat certain central nervous system diseases or problems. So far, he says, it's been effective.

"The patient lies down, puts on earphones and listens to clicks or tones or watches a dial, all of which are related to the function of a particular muscle, and thus he learns how to modify and control his movement. The patients have the ability. They just never learned to handle it. And once they incorporate the learning experience, the feedback mechanism can even be abandoned in some cases."

"Is the most important thing making the patient aware of his problem?" a resident asks.

"It's more than that. It is learning specifically, relating it to a single muscle and giving the patient the control, the self-regulation, of it. Without drugs. Without surgery. Without their complications. The worst thing that can happen to us is that the technique simply doesn't work."

He cites an additional case history. A middle-aged painter is unable to work after a stroke. He recovers to a degree, but his right hand won't open. In feedback therapy, he's shown that the good hand, the left one, functions and he can relate its function to readings on a dial and clicks on a sound box. Transferring that learning to the right hand, while the patient monitors his own actions again, is vividly effective. He can pick up a pen and draw again.

"In that case," the doctor points out, "the good hand taught the bad hand."

He leaves the room and the doctors disperse. Post stands at the window of the room, staring out at the East River. He is cautious, thorough, interested, all at once. Tomorrow he'll take the train to Boston for his visit to Massachusetts General. He makes a note to follow up on the myoelectric feedback research when he gets back to Bellevue next week.

After a day off, Eugene Fazzini returns to Surgical Pathology with renewed vigor. His morning begins as it usually does, with the staff conference to consider new tissue specimens. Interns, residents and attendings slowly come in, gradually filling the seats around the long table. The coffee is ready, to assist the rejuvenation process for those who suffer from sleep deprivation, a common Bellevue malady. Fazzini has his collection of slides ready to distribute. He's at his table, beside the others, and has scrawled on a blackboard some of today's cases.

Among them: a rash on the back, a pruritic rash on a leg, a

lacerated spleen, chronic tonsillitis, a cyst of the right knee, a subphrenic abscess, adenoids and a ureter. The slides are passed around. Fazzini peers into his microscope and comments.

A young Puerto Rican man has a rash on his face, a visible lesion. "Is it seborrhea? Lupus? Psoriasis?" Fazzini questions the group. The teaching function becomes an early-morning game show. The doctors present make their guesses. Fazzini renders the official verdict: the rash is confined to the superficial epidermis. That, along with other factors evident on the slides, means it is one of the eczema group. Correct diagnosis: seborrhea.

Fazzini announces that French Hospital has sent over two slides, specimens from a patient with a mass in his liver and a nodule nearby. What is it? Fazzini's conclusion is that it is cancer.

Fazzini has passed out all the slides now; each doctor is kept busy. Fazzini turns to working on the duty schedule for next month. When that's done, he heads for the Pathology library.

An attending takes Fazzini's place at the small table. In the library, Fazzini does research for a paper he's writing. He's looking for a report on a leprosy case; Bellevue still sees a few.

After more than an hour spent reading in the library, Fazzini joins another attending at an autopsy conference. The autopsy room in Pathology is less bleak, less harrowing, than the one in the Medical Examiner's office a block away. It is a spare environment, with large metal tables and stools.

As Fazzini enters the room, several doctors are already there. A young resident rushes in and says, "How do I find that brain from yesterday? Where would it be?" The attending points a finger; the resident, without comment, follows the direction.

The doctors gather around one of the large metal tables. A Pathology resident describes the first case, represented by a tray of organs. The man who once contained those organs was a 48-year-old Puerto Rican who came to Bellevue three times within a period of several months. He suffered from acute abdominal pain, later had seizures and suffered from mental deterioration, becoming psychotic. He was difficult to retain; after each visit, he would "elope." Finally, he came to the AES a few days ago, in pain and having difficulty breathing. He had a seizure at that very moment, suffered cardiac arrest and died. The Pathology resident outlining the history suggests that those who treated the man at Bellevue "probably didn't know what was going on."

The autopsy is an attempt to discover just what did go on. The resident turns things over to the attending, who does an organ-by-organ assessment.

He picks up the heart, which he finds to be enlarged, and points out a needle track from the last, futile attempt to resuscitate the man.

"The coronary arteries are beautiful," he says. "There's no evidence of fibrosis. It's a hypertensive heart, but there's nothing terribly severe there."

He displays the lungs. Nothing there, no congestion or clots or evidence of chronic bronchitis. No pneumonia. There's nothing of use to be seen in the small intestine either. The kidneys, however, have a mottled look.

"They're fairly large and meaty in appearance," the attending says. "Some scarring does indicate a degree of vascular disease. Further analysis needed."

The liver is next. "There's some degree of fatty change in the liver, an insignificant increase in fibrous tissue. It really should look like what you see in a standard butcher shop."

The spleen is firm. The adrenals "don't look bad." The bone marrow is a little soft, with some degree of uremia present.

The patient suffered from hypertension, the attending notes, and that, along with the changes in his kidneys, can lead to a diagnosis of membranous glomerulonephritis, a kidney disease that can kill by causing complications. Kidney sections may tell more, but for now, the attending says, "We can't see much more, grossly."

The autopsy that produced the organs under study was one of approximately three hundred done at Bellevue each year. Family consent is required if there is a family to consent; if there isn't, the director of the hospital can approve a request for an autopsy forty-eight hours after death, but final approval rests with the Medical Examiner. In today's first case, consent was obtained from the man's wife. In the second case, it wasn't necessary. No family was found.

A new tray of organs is put on display. They come from the 26-year-old Chinese who killed a man and leaped out a five-story window to escape police. It is a case that interests several doctors at the hospital, apparently.

"Who ever heard of such a mishegoss in Chinatown?" one of the residents says.

The organs are all a deep reddish-brown; the Medical Examiner preserved them in fluid containing formaldehyde, which makes them more difficult to evaluate. There are sutures in the liver, a sign that the surgeons were busy. The aorta is lacerated. It is a typical traumatic heart, with clots and blood in the cardiac muscle. The lungs show bleeding, too. There is visible bleeding in the kidneys. There is a section of the man's spine, fractured, with visible blood clots; his fractured ribs and pelvis were not removed in the autopsy. His brain, oddly, shows little damage; it is almost intact. He was conscious when he was admitted to Bellevue. He had fallen on his feet. As it turned out, it didn't matter; the impact destroyed him without having to crush his brain.

There are few conclusions to be drawn. The man died violently.

"We don't usually see this kind in Pathology," the attending says.

On that note, the group ends its deliberations. Fazzini returns to his office. He has not spoken during the conference, preferring to defer to the attending.

He adheres to his diet during lunch at his desk, reads the *Times* and is ready to confront the afternoon. Another pathologist comes into his office to tell Fazzini that the sputum sample received earlier in the week, from a patient on the Chest Service, showed nothing alarming. At that moment, the Chest Service resident who delivered that sample shows up with another, a half-inch piece of lung tissue from the same patient.

Fazzini does a frozen section immediately. He cuts a small piece of tissue, freezes it by machine, slices the hardened block, fixes it, washes it, puts it through an alcohol bath, then stains it.

Within five minutes from the time the resident brought it over, Fazzini is peering at it under a microscope. As the resident stands by, Fazzini concentrates on it for several minutes. He suggests that it might be a mysterious microorganism, difficult to treat and usually fatal, Pneumocystis carinii. The resident runs off to transmit the tentative verdict. Stains will be done in an effort to confirm Fazzini's impression.

Fazzini remains at the table. On it there is a small box that bears the label "Interesting Lymph Nodes." Above his head, on a wall blackboard, someone has written, "This could be the day."

It is time for Fazzini to walk over to the VA, for an afternoon Pathology conference there with colleagues from that hospital and University Hospital. The three Pathology departments convene regularly at such conferences, to share insights into odd and pertinent cases.

The conference takes place in a hot, stuffy room and the pathologists are crammed into it. Fazzini, despite his diet, is a very large man. Only the nature of the material—Fazzini is a man fascinated by what he does—keeps his mind off the oppressive air. His insights into the cases discussed, the unequivocating way he offers his analyses, inspires respect among the other pathologists. They know him, of course, as do many of the doctors in the general hospital.

As Fazzini leaves the meeting, at 4 P.M., one of his colleagues walking out behind him turns to another doctor and says, pointing to Fazzini, "The man is brilliant."

It is a pleasant day, and when Fazzini emerges from the VA, he joins another Bellevue attending and a friend from the UH Pathology department for a slow stroll along First Avenue. It is one of the rare moments he can spend outdoors on any day.

At 8 A.M., when Lori Chiarelli goes on duty in the Emergency Ward, there are five men and five women in beds to greet her, some new faces and some old. The seriously anemic old woman is there and so is the old woman from the nursing home. The old Irishman who arrived as Chiarelli was leaving yesterday was found to be in respiratory or cardiac distress; more tests are needed.

The night head nurse, looking sleepy, gives Chiarelli a rundown on the new admissions. While Chiarelli absorbs the information, the OD is sitting up in bed, alert and surly, demanding to be released. A resident walks up to him and says, "You may feel all right, my friend, but you have pneumonia. You can't go home."

"I want this shit off me," the man replies, pointing to his IV tube and blood-pressure cuff.

"Now, be smart," a staff nurse tells him. "You can't go home like this. You're not a doctor."

"I know I'm not a doctor, but I feel okay. I'm twenty-three years old and I can do what I want," the OD screams.

"You do what the doctor wants. He decides," the nurse snaps.

At 8:30, Chiarelli continues her early-morning chores, wending her way through a batch of medical residents making rounds, looking for odd cases. Among the new patients are a 49-year-old construction worker who fell, hitting his chest on a pipe, a 45-year-old Oriental man suffering from hypertension, a 35-year-old black man with kidney stones, a young black woman with a stab wound in the shoulder and a 19-year-old Puerto Rican woman, mother of a 4-year-old child, suffering from abdominal pain and vaginal bleeding. By 9:15, the construction worker, the black woman with the stab wound and the old woman from the nursing home are all transferred out of the EW to other hospital wards.

One of the new admissions, Chiarelli discovers, is an old woman who had tried to commit suicide in a nursing home; as she tried to jump from a window, she had a stroke. She has a history of seizures and is partially paralyzed. Her symptoms are familiar to Chiarelli. Studying her chart, Chiarelli can predict the woman's fate at Bellevue, from the EW to a Medical ward and then, possibly, on to Psychiatry, where many attempted-suicide cases wind up.

At 9:30, a collection of residents join an attending at the OD's bedside. As they arrive, the OD proclaims, "I wanna go home, man."

"Wait a minute. You're not being much of a man. Don't you want to get better?" a resident asks.

The patient's sense of machismo is challenged. "I don't give a damn," he bellows.

"Well, we give a damn. What happens if your family finds you on the floor not breathing? What happens then? You're under our care now. Realize how sick you are."

"I'm not sick, man."

The resident sighs and turns to a compatriot: "One thing you have to realize about dealing with patients like this is that you can't deal with patients like this."

Two of the doctors struggle with the patient, who has been trying to crawl over the side of his bed. They attempt to tie him down, but he resists and they're not successful.

"Why you do this shit to me?" he yells. "Go everybody away."

One of the doctors has whispered instructions to Chiarelli, who's been watching it all, and when the man turns to confront the group of doctors, Chiarelli slips up beside him and injects Valium into his arm. The resident looks at the man and tells him to "relax, lie down and be calm." The man slowly does relax, falls back on his pillow. The doctors leave and Chiarelli goes on to other duties.

Within an hour, the OD is sitting up in bed, peacefully. Then he nods off. The attending returns to wake him up, to tell him that he must remain in the hospital. The patient looks at the attending incredulously, widens his eyes, curses in Spanish and returns to sleep.

An attending and a resident survey the old Irishman, two beds away. He has a history of falling down and fracturing bones. This time he has a lacerated leg, but that is not his main problem. He is weak and has moderate congestive heart failure. The attending summons a cardiologist and a technician does an echocardiogram, a sonar-like device that uses sound waves to study the configuration and movement of the heart, its findings recorded on Polaroid photos.

At 10:40, there is another admission, a 39-year-old black man who complains of having trouble breathing. He looks almost terminally weary. He tells the resident examining him that he is on welfare and lives alone in a decayed hotel. He says he is feeling very weak; his voice is barely audible and the resident leans over the bed to hear him. "Doctor, I spend my days just walking around," he says. Under questioning, he reveals that he is an epileptic; the resident notes that, so the man's medication can be maintained while his respiratory problem can be deciphered. He notes, too, that the man seems to have a heart murmur.

Outside, a police car pulls up. A policeman gets out of the front seat, opens the back door. A man falls out, on his head, becoming a potential head-trauma case, whatever he might have been before.

In the EW, an X-ray technician wheels her portable unit to the OD's bedside, to take a chest X-ray. The patient is standing on the bed, only his head showing above the drawn curtains around his bed. He is trying to urinate.

One of the nurses is making an entry on his chart: "Threatening staff with bedside equipment."

A second nurse, looking over her shoulder, asks, "What does that mean?"

"It means he said he'd shove the respirator up my ass."

The hypertensive Oriental is shifted to a Medical ward upstairs.

At 11:35, Chiarelli and a nursing supervisor meet with most of the EW nurses, privately, "to hash out a staff problem before it gets out of hand." No one else is admitted to the meeting, which takes only a few minutes. When Chiarelli returns, she sees the female Psychiatry resident revisiting the OD. The man tells the psychiatrist that he will stay in the hospital and behave himself if someone will call his mother and sister, so they know where he is and can visit him. He rambles, informatively. His stepmother murdered his father, he says, and he has been drinking two pints of liquor a day since he was 16. He tells her, too, that he is an epileptic, had his last seizure three months ago and takes Dilantin for it. The psychiatrist notes that on his chart, so the residents can give him Dilantin. He had not told them about being epileptic; he is as cordial to the psychiatrist as he is hostile to the Medical residents. She tells him that she will contact his mother and sister and that he should allow himself to be transferred to a ward, where he can recover. He agrees, meekly. Within a few minutes, that transfer takes place.

Chiarelli has stationed herself at the desk in the middle of the ward. A resident walks up and says, "See that patient over there?" pointing down the ward. "Well, the diagnosis is halitosis, severe. Can we please get this guy some mouth wash, so I can examine him?" Chiarelli finds the mouth wash.

A Neurology resident strolls in; like other doctors at Bellevue, when he has a few moments, which isn't often, he visits the EW, where the action is. He finds little he can do and settles for a talk with a fellow resident he hasn't seen in weeks. They talk about the way doctors behave and the Neurology resident issues a proclamation aloud:

"It's a matter of the contemplative versus the aggressive personality. One wants to think. The other wants to act, often egotistically. It's definitely reflected in the way they behave. Surgeons are more temperamental. Pathologists are contemplative. The medical man may be imbedded in the literature.

The surgeon doesn't give a shit about it. Surgeons have a frightening amount of confidence. Some of it is false confidence, but
it enables them to act. A medical man might feel there would
be alternatives to be thought out. Not the surgeon. He decides
and starts cutting."

The monologue ends abruptly when the resident sees
Neurology's chief resident, Bruce Mack, come into the EW. The
resident saunters off and Mack moves quickly to the bedside of
a new admission. The man is the Puerto Rican prisoner who
tried to commit suicide in his jail cell and gashed his head. He
is handcuffed to his bed. Mack takes a look at him; the man is
covered with tattoos. There's little to be done; the man is resisting treatment. Mack discusses the case with another resident,
then starts toward the door. At that moment, an AES resident
wheels in a woman who had had a stroke while being examined
in the AES. Mack rushes over to her.

One of the nurses has been on the phone talking to one of the
neurosurgeons; she reports her conversation to Chiarelli. The
Puerto Rican woman whose brain had herniated yesterday was
taken to the operating room, where a clot was removed successfully. There is little follow-up in the EW; patients move on and
are not heard about. Chiarelli is pleased to get the news in this
case. Better to go to lunch with good news in your head, she
says, than obsessed by some disaster.

When Chiarelli returns from lunch, the Emergency Ward
shows signs of action. The black man having trouble breathing
is surrounded by residents. Chiarelli hurries over. She's told by
one of the residents that the man has been tested thoroughly
and a diagnosis has been made: acute bacterial endocarditis, a
serious matter. It is an infection of a myocardial valve, an infection which eats away the valve. The infection complicates surgery, but open-heart surgery may be done. The doctors can't
treat this case leisurely with antibiotics; there isn't time. The
valve must be replaced. The heart murmur detected when the
man was admitted is now thought to be "not innocent," in other
words a reflection of the condition, an indication of valve failure. A senior attending, a cardiac specialist, is called to help
decide what to do.

As the residents work on the man, feverishly taking blood
samples and giving him morphine to ease his pain, which is
escalating, two emergency cases arrive minutes apart and Chia-

relli rushes to the far end of the ward to meet them.

The first is a middle-aged cab driver; he got out of his cab in midtown traffic and collapsed. The police brought him in and residents rush over to revive him. His face is blue. His pupils are dilated. It is cardiac arrest. The residents work on the man vigorously. He is dead.

A young black woman has been brought in, simultaneously, bleeding from stab wounds in her abdomen—her intestines are protruding from a wound—arms and legs. There is no pulse felt in one arm. An IV line is installed immediately; she's given plasmanate. Blood samples are taken. Trauma doctors arrive. Chiarelli moves in to help. Another nurse joins her. The doctors and the nurses work on the woman with practiced precision, rarely speaking to each other, never showing any sign of alarm. The Trauma doctor turns to see if the cab driver is still on the nearby bed. He isn't.

"What did they do with that guy?" he asks Chiarelli.

"He's gone."

The Trauma surgeon nods.

The stab victim is moaning "please" and her teeth are chattering.

"You're doing fine, just fine," Chiarelli tells her.

"I got stabbed in the house where I live," she says to Chiarelli.

A female resident inserts a Foley catheter into her, to withdraw urine.

"Oh, Lord. Oh please, God, don't do this to me," the woman shouts.

"It's important to know how much urine you've got," the Trauma doctor tells her, softly. "We wouldn't do it to you if it wasn't important." An X-ray technician arrives to take an abdominal film.

At the other end of the EW, eighteen residents, medical students and attendings have lined all sides of the bed of the man with acute bacterial endocarditis. The attending called to rule on the cases has concluded that a cardiac catheterization is essential: injecting dye into the heart to determine the degree of breakdown in the valve. It can be followed, immediately, by the open-heart surgery. A physical exam has revealed little that is specific; in fact, the heart murmur is less evident now, so the attending says he wants to be certain before surgery is initiated. The damage must be located, he says. The patient must be taken to a lab especially equipped for the procedure, and he must consent to it, and the subsequent operation, in writing.

In the background, the stab victim is sent up to the operating room. An attendant from the Mortuary Service paces, waiting to transport the cab driver, whose body has been taken to a holding area for dead bodies in the AES, to the Medical Examiner's office. The old Irishman is transferred to a Medical ward. A nurse lectures a medical student, "Don't walk away from a bed when the side rail is down." He looks repentantly at her and slinks away.

All the doctors leave the bedside of the man with endocarditis, except the resident who first saw him when he arrived in the EW. The resident attempts to explain to the man what is wrong and what must be done. A nurse tries to help.

The patient is deteriorating rapidly, getting weaker and weaker. What was a difficulty breathing now has become a vicious pain in his chest.

The nurse points to his chest and says, "There's something really bad there, so you'll have to go to the operating room, so the doctors can repair it."

The resident explains that they need his written permission, a "Consent for Operation," for both the catheterization and the heart surgery.

"You have to sign here, because there's no tomorrow on this. Understand?" the resident says. The man stares numbly into space, does not reply. Several other doctors file back, beside the bed.

The patient, who is drugged and weak, picks up a pen the nurse is holding and makes an illegible scrawl on a blank piece of paper, a rehearsal. But when he is handed the actual form, he won't sign it, or can't.

"He won't sign," the resident tells the attending, who has joined the increasing group around the bed. Once again, the patient's bed is fenced by doctors.

"Well, that certainly will solve a lot of problems," the attending comments.

A nurse remembers that the patient has no family but does have a friend waiting outside; perhaps he can help, she suggests. She goes to the EW waiting room and returns with him. He is a tall, dignified black man. He came to Bellevue to hold his friend's money for him while he was in the hospital, and he stayed to see how his friend's condition progressed.

He stands beside the bed; the doctors have parted to make room for him. He stands there for minutes, silent, staring at his friend. His head, topped by a glistening gray Afro, shakes almost imperceptibly.

The resident again asks the patient to sign the form. The man's eyes open wide, in fright, and his body, drugged by morphine, is motionless. He seems unable to perceive what is happening. One of the residents says that it may be wise to call a psychiatrist to declare the man incompetent in order to perform the surgery and save his life.

Amid all this, a middle-aged man is wheeled in, complaining of a heart attack. A resident examines him and concludes that it is indigestion, not acute. An EKG and a chest X-ray, done rapidly, are negative. He's sent back to the AES, on his way home.

At 4 P.M., the new nursing staff is on duty, but Chiarelli has lingered, joining the group around the black man's bed.

One resident turns to another and says, "Between you and me, he's dead already. His blood gases get more and more terrible every twenty minutes. He'll die on the table, if not before."

Another resident urges the man to sign the form, again. The man shakes his head from side to side; he cannot speak.

"Tomorrow won't come unless you sign the permission," a resident hollers.

"Don't threaten him," a nurse says.

"I'm not. It's a fact."

The patient's friend edges closer to the bed. He leans over, glaring at his friend, and screams, "You gonna *die*, man. You in bad shape. Sign it, man. Sign it." He begins to cry. A nurse beside the bed hands the patient the pen and the form. Very slowly and almost illegibly, he makes a scrawl that barely resembles his signature, in the wrong space on the form. A delegate from the Bellevue administrative staff, called to affirm the protocol, sees him do it and terms it acceptable. There are now eleven other witnesses, doctors, nurses and the man's friend. Quickly, the patient is shaved, from the neck down, and a catheter is inserted into his penis.

"We need that guy on the house staff," a resident says, pointing to the patient's friend. "He's the only one who said it, really said it."

Three doctors push the man's bed toward an elevator that has been reserved. It is 4:15 and there are just four patients left in the EW. The new shift is on duty. Chiarelli goes home.

The 8 A.M. X-ray conference in Medicine is presided over by an attending radiologist. It begins with abdominal films of one of George Feldman's patients, the man with lymphoma. There is an enlarged mass in his spleen, "encroaching on medial structures," according to the radiologist. There is an unexplained mass in his chest, "expanding bronchopulmonary nodes." The radiologist, who knows the case from earlier X-rays, asks, "Is this a sign of some infiltration process?"

Feldman nods, grimly.

Chest X-rays of a 73-year-old Puerto Rican woman admitted last night show "signs of pneumonia or developing MI [myocardial infarction]." An intern volunteers that her sputum test indicates pneumonia. The radiologist points out that her heart is enlarged and may be "giving out somewhere." He adds, "I won't argue with you that pneumonia is there, but the total picture seems to indicate more than that."

After a fast cup of coffee in the ward kitchen, Feldman makes rounds with two interns and seven medical students. There are three very old women to see in the ICU. On the ward, there are nine more old women, including the new admission and two women ready to be discharged. The array of diseases and symptoms goes with age: diabetes, uremia, pneumonia, congestive heart disease, impaired kidney function. The diagnostic and treatment tools are evident: blood tests, urinalysis, X-rays, oxygen, drugs.

On the male side, there are four patients, including the stoic with lymphoma, who will stay, and three others due to be discharged within a day or two.

By 9:45, the rounds are over. An attending arrives, to accompany the doctors and students on a tour of the new patients. They visit the 73-year-old Puerto Rican woman. "If she's got pneumonia, she should be a lot sicker than she looks," the attending tells Feldman, adding that he suspects she has some sort of congestive heart failure.

"My general approach to elderly women is to treat them gently," the attending announces. He is younger than most, a doctor who spent his residency at Bellevue not long ago and continues to spend all of his time at the hospital, forgoing private practice.

In a room down the hall, there are two more patients to see. The old underweight Puerto Rican woman continues to look quite pregnant; she has a diseased liver. Across the room from her is the young Puerto Rican woman with hypertension and a small kidney, possible renal artery stenosis (narrowing of the artery). She becomes the subject of a debate that goes on for several hours.

According to Feldman, she came into the hospital for an angiogram, to assess kidney function. She is in bed, but does not look or act sick. She smiles, is relaxed. Her toenails are painted in five different colors. She has consented to the angiogram, because she's been told by a clinic resident that her high blood pressure may be due to trouble in her kidney. In the hospital, her blood pressure has dropped. The third-year resident who has seen her in the clinic, a Renal Fellow, is taking the position that people with high blood pressure often get better, their pressure drops, in the hospital. This does not, he feels, eliminate the need for the angiogram and possible kidney surgery afterward.

A second attending, an older man, the prototype of the kindly middle-aged, soft-spoken doctor, opposes both the angiogram and the possible surgery. He joins the group to state his position.

He believes that the high blood pressure can be managed with medication. He does not believe that the angiogram should be done unless it leads directly to necessary surgery determined clinically. He sees it as gratuitous. The Renal Fellow takes the position that the woman would not take her medication regularly; her history would seem to support his claim that only surgery can help her, because she can't be relied upon to help herself. Having explained his position, he rests his case, temporarily. The older attending leaves.

Feldman is sympathetic to the older attending's viewpoint. In cases involving 50 percent renal artery stenosis, the mortality rate in surgery is 5 percent. The mortality rate on angiograms is less than 1 percent, but it is a factor, he feels.

"Why risk it?" Feldman asks. "If her blood pressure gets worse in three years, then you can consider surgery."

The Renal Fellow is provoked. "If you're not going to do it, then just discharge her," he says, petulantly.

The young attending joins in. He feels that it is difficult to predict that the woman's hypertension can be controlled by medication, that her kidney problem could get worse despite such medication.

The Renal Fellow, shuffling his feet nervously, turns to Feldman and says, "Look, she was admitted by your chief resident for a purpose." He is trying to pressure Feldman.

The young attending says, "She is young and could tolerate surgery. It's better now than years from now. But I guess I'm butting into your argument. I tend to err on the side of being surgically aggressive."

"George is being hyper about the angio and the complications that might ensue," the Renal Fellow says.

"It's difficult to control blood pressure in the clinic," the young attending says to Feldman. "You see them once every two or three months. A bold stroke now may be better than expecting the patient's cooperation for forty years. If you wait ten years, it could spread. She might end up with heart disease and you might then be very worried about helping her. Her cooperation is very important in reaching a decision."

"Okay, I'll talk to her," Feldman says.

"She cringed at our mention of surgery, but she didn't rule it out," the Renal Fellow tells him.

"Look at it this way: there are two people who must decide, the patient and the resident in charge of the ward," the young attending says. "But the doctor who sees her regularly later, his opinion is important, too, because it will be his case." He gestures toward the Renal Fellow, who will be the likely doctor to see the woman in the clinic later. "I know," he continues, "that the other attending, a very competent internist, disagrees with me. It depends on how strongly *you* feel," he tells Feldman.

"I'm not deciding now," Feldman says. "I'll talk to her first."

"Fine. Talk to her and see what you think." The young attending goes on to say, "We all disagree. I know I come from a school that says if you can spare a patient from having to take medication the rest of her life, you ought to seriously consider it."

"I asked for your opinion, hoping it would go the other way, to tell the truth," Feldman says to the attending. "I'll leave her on the schedule. You following her in clinic," he says, pointing to the Renal Fellow, "is the best argument for doing it."

"We have to decide what we think is best for the patient," the attending says.

"I agree and I think she must understand these things," Feldman says.

Feldman walks away from the debate, goes to the woman's bed, pulls up a chair and sits down. She smiles at him.

"You know you've got a dangerous disease, high blood pressure," he tells her. "It can cause heart trouble, stroke, make your kidney worse. You went to the clinic and got pills to take and you didn't take them."

"No."

"If we give them to you, would you take them every day?"

"Yes."

"Why would it be different now?"

"I wouldn't need an operation."

"We don't know if you do need one. Would you rather take pills for forty years?"

"Yes."

"If we do the test, it might show a need to operate on you, to operate on what is causing your high blood pressure, and fix it with the operation, so you wouldn't have to take pills."

At this moment, the woman's boyfriend arrives. He is husky, Latin, with a mustache. He kisses her and sits down on the opposite side of the bed from Feldman.

"There are different ways to treat high blood pressure," Feldman tells him. "It is dangerous, but it can be controlled by medication or possibly an operation. If it works, the patient is as well as someone without high blood pressure. It's not a disease we take lightly. The right treatment is important. If you take pills, the blood pressure will be controlled and you can lead a normal life. But in our tests, one kidney is small. That can cause high blood pressure. We don't know for sure. It is possible. The test you came in for will help us tell."

Feldman pauses while the two consider what he's said.

"We can do the test if you will consider the possibility of an operation," he resumes.

"You do the test tomorrow?" the boyfriend asks.

"Yes."

"I'm sure she understands the need for taking the pills now," the boyfriend says.

"The test will show us what to fix in an operation. That's the reason for doing the test. You'd have to take medicine forever otherwise."

"Look, Doctor, she's uptight about an operation. She doesn't like operations."

"Why?"

"She's talked to her family and her friends, who told her not to let them take out a kidney. She's worried about what it will be like after the operation."

"I can understand that."

"I told her to get the test, and if an operation is needed, she can talk to another doctor, to get another opinion."

The boyfriend talks to the woman in Spanish.

"She wants to know if she has the operation, will she have problems later?"

"I'm not sure," Feldman answers. "There is no guarantee. It's the medication or the operation. You have to be good about taking medicine, and it's true, too, that the operation may not work. How well you take your medicine is a factor. If we operate, there's a good chance you won't have to take medicine."

The patient studies Feldman as he speaks. She understands much of what he is saying, but she speaks little English. Her boyfriend discusses it all with her in Spanish.

"She'd prefer pills to the operation," he tells Feldman. "She has a thing about having an operation."

"If the test shows that she needs an operation, you can explain it to her," Feldman says. He gets up and walks out of the room.

He talks to the intern on the case. "This lady may need surgery," Feldman says. "I'm not convinced that she'd take the pills. And she does seem willing to go ahead with the angiogram." The surgery, if it follows, Feldman explains, could range from a bypass to correct the renal artery stenosis, to removal of the kidney itself. As Feldman ponders that, the older attending returns.

"If the renal disease was causing her high blood pressure, it wouldn't result in normal blood pressure while she's in the hospital," the attending says. "This is an honest difference of opinion," he adds, suggesting that the chief of the service might arbitrate. His feeling is based on dealing with reliable middle-class patients in his own practice. Feldman reminds him that Bellevue patients aren't always so reliable.

Feldman returns to see the patient, to take her blood pressure. It is high. "She's hypertensive now," he tells the intern. "She'll get the angiogram." After that, the debate will resume, he tells the Renal Fellow, who has accompanied him to see the woman, because Feldman remains unconvinced about the need for surgery.

After lunch, Feldman's afternoon on Medicine is taken up by meetings.

Five medical students show up to listen to Feldman talk about hypothermia, the opposite of fever, a lowering of the body's temperature. The most common cause, Feldman tells them, is obvious: exposure to cold. In hospitalized patients, it can be due, too, to septicemia, an infectious process. He warns against treating anyone with hypothermia, in or out of the hospital, by allowing them to drink whiskey, the old wives' remedy. "It's not wise," he says, "because it opens the peripheral vessels and doesn't help at all. It's better to give someone a blanket instead."

In cases of acute exposure, which Bellevue doctors see regularly in Bowery types in winter, it's best to cover them with blankets and let the warming process proceed slowly. Trying to warm them up too quickly can create cardiac arrhythmia, extremely dangerous. He admits that there is a debate within medicine about the treatment of exposure cases. The students ask questions; he answers them directly, without ever compromising his basically gentle manner.

After the teaching session, Feldman meets with the ward nurses and the ward social worker, to discuss problems that have arisen in the care of patients, the relationship between the medical staff and the nurses, particular needs for the social worker's services. He deals with all the nurses judiciously; he knows that at some point in weeks ahead he will need them.

It is now late in the afternoon and the ward is quiet. Feldman goes to the nursing station, sits down and makes entries on patients' charts. When he's done, it is time to go home. He wants to read several medical papers, to be ready for a conference tomorrow. He got some sleep last night, but not enough. He fell asleep before dinner, the phone rang and he awoke to cook dinner, then had trouble getting back to sleep. Tonight, he may have better luck.

When Sol Zimmerman gets to the Pediatrics ICU at 7:30 A.M., all the patients are stable. The resident who worked last night sleepily reports to Zimmerman that a new admission was in and out within a few hours. The baby, the newborn child of a drug addict with syphilis, was given an exchange transfusion for neonatal jaundice, new blood for old, in the ICU, where the procedure could be properly monitored, then was transferred to a ward.

Zimmerman strolls back to the Premature Unit, where he patrols his infants until 10 A.M., when he joins other residents and interns at a conference with several attendings, to talk about the jittery baby in the nursery, the baby whose mother had been on multiple medication.

An intern presents the case to the twelve doctors present. The baby is suffering from the jitters, he says, but no other visible symptoms. The single symptom might be disregarded except for the fact that the mother had taken so many different medications during her pregnancy. She had taken Dilantin and Mysoline for a seizure disorder, digoxin, Pronestyl, Esidrix, iron, Bicillin and guanethidine, all for problems not related to the pregnancy itself. One attending, given all the evidence, discounts anything serious. Given the lab results, he says, "This is probably a hyperreactive child, not much more than that. Often jitters are worrisome, but don't develop into anything serious." His verdict: "Worth following up in the Pediatrics clinic."

At 11 A.M., when the conference ends, Zimmerman, the attending and several interns make rounds in the Premature Unit. The baby Zimmerman feared might have bowel complications is improving on antibiotics. A new admission is a newborn baby with a temperature of 102 and persistent diarrhea.

In the ICU, Zimmerman tells the attending that the surgeons have postponed plans to begin grafting skin on the burned child. She urinates and defecates on her thighs, and the surgeons have passed along the message that the risk of infection is too great. She's being given codeine for her pain, Zimmerman notes.

"Let's not make her an addict, please," the attending says.

The little pale baby with the chest deformity, who was thought to be a girl and has turned out to be a boy, looks like it might survive its many problems. The major issue is how to tell the parents.

"It will be a blow for them," the attending says. "A sexual ambiguity. *We* can't quite handle it, so how can we expect the parents to? I wouldn't tell them yet, particularly since the father may have a sense of the inevitable. And as far as I can see, it's like a zero prognosis for this kid, even if it does survive the acute period. The mother, too, keeps saying that she can't understand how her baby has survived."

The twins remain troublesome, but they continue to struggle.

All the babies in the ICU represent some variation on the life-and-death issue. The attending feels it is an issue that must be dealt with in doctors' training. He raises it now.

"What are the ethics of what is going on here?" he asks. "How far do you go with children like this? Do you add a drug? Do you resuscitate? Do you give oxygen? There's every reason to believe that a child has sustained brain damage. What then? You can look at a baby and know in your heart that the baby hasn't got a chance in hell.

"What do you do if the baby stops breathing? There is no policy. It's up to each of you to decide. The situation changes from minute to minute. You don't know when to pull the plug. A lot of people can't bear to watch a baby stop breathing, whatever is wrong with it. In some cases, I can. In others, I can't. You must give a baby every chance, of course, but then what? You have no choice but to try very hard, that's my belief.

"Sometimes there's nothing about a baby that will kill it. We can keep it alive. The question is, should we? In a terminal disease, you know the patient is dying. A baby may not be destined to die at any minute. It won't be a good baby, maybe, but it may not be terribly bad either. You can wrestle with this as a group, but each one of you has to decide for himself. And I didn't bring up the question because I want you to do away with any of these babies. I brought it up because you may face it in a matter of hours."

Zimmerman knows how important it is to remain alert to

sudden changes in the infants he cares for, just as he must recognize the signs of danger in all newborns. Among them: anything irregular in the family history (e.g., diabetes), complications of gestation and delivery, abnormal position of the baby in the uterus, congenital malformations, rapid or difficult respiration, abnormal crying, coughing, irregular pulse, absence of a suck reflex, sweating, vomiting, diarrhea, no stool for forty-eight hours or no urine for twenty-four.

Others: abdominal distention, bleeding of any sort, cord odor, a small head, convulsions or irritability, lethargy, fever, paralysis, pallor or jaundice, and anything that can be categorized by the familiar nurses' expression "not looking right."

After lunch, Sol Zimmerman keeps busy in the Premature Unit. He takes blood samples to the lab. He injects an anticoagulant into one of the infants with a clotting proclivity. He goes from isolette to isolette, checking the charts and bodies of each baby. Most of them have not been named yet, so he talks to them by calling them "Baby Diaz" or "Baby Rodriguez." He strokes them, talks affectionately to them. As he circulates, one of the nurses dresses a set of twins, while their mother and grandmother sit by, smiling.

When he's made his own rounds of the Premature Unit, Zimmerman walks around the ICU, peering, checking, making notes, then goes to the nursery, to sign some forms, finally on to OB. He enters in the middle of a debate about a delivery last week. It shows signs of escalating into an argument between a male first-year resident and an attending. The baby involved was delivered dead. The first-year resident wanted it delivered by Caesarean section when the fetal monitor showed signs of fetal distress. The attending wanted to wait for a normal delivery. Overruled, the first-year resident waited, irritably. The delivery took place. Now the two are reviving the issue. Zimmerman listens, but abstains.

He has spent most of the afternoon in motion. At 3:30, having double-checked that no deliveries are scheduled for this afternoon, he joins sign-off rounds with the chief resident and the senior resident.

The burned girl shows signs of improvement, modest but encouraging. The boy-girl cries soundlessly, mouth open, private pain evident, as the doctors pass it. One of the twins, the boy, has contracted pneumonia and, less dangerous, conjunctivitis, inflammation of the eye linings. New medication will be tried, new tests done. His sister continues her struggle.

The rounds move on to the Premature Unit, where various infants and their needs are discussed. Then the chief resident and the senior resident leave to tour the wards, while Zimmerman settles down to cover his flock. Tonight he is on duty, to watch both the Premature Unit and the ICU and, if needed, any Pediatric emergency that arises in the hospital.

Today's operating room schedule indicates that Mary Williamson will be working in Room 6 and will have four cases: a subtotal gastrectomy and a breast biopsy on a 60-year-old woman; a revision of an amputation below the right knee on a 75-year-old woman; two muscle biopsies, on men 55 and 33.

As Williamson arrives dressed in her green surgical outfit and pink cap, with mask dangling from around her neck, one of the male anesthetists is having an intense conversation with the head nurse.

"I've got a guy I'm supposed to put to sleep," he says. "The guy I'm supposed to put to sleep is named Williams. Okay? The guy in the bed outside the OR has 'Morgan' written on his IV bottle and he says his name isn't Williams. I would like to be sure. *Please.*"

The head nurse says she'll check with the ward where the patient originated and will let him know.

At 9:15, Williamson goes into the OR to check it out. She talks to the scrub nurse about instruments she'll need. The patient, who looks older than 60, is on the table, while the anesthetists are busy around her. The woman sees Williamson and tells her, "This room looks like Patty's Day, with all the green around here. All you need is some shamrocks."

Williamson smiles at her.

"This will take all day, I suppose," the patient says.

"It depends on how long we break for lunch," Williamson tells her, laughing.

The woman is distracted by some inner thought and stares at the ceiling. Then she begins to babble: "He died too soon," she says. "He died too soon. Lung cancer. It was terrible."

No one answers her. Is she speaking about her husband? A

friend? A relative? The nurses and anesthetists go about their work, checking oxygen, injecting anesthetic into the IV line already in place.

The patient goes to sleep. One of the anesthetists intubates her and attaches the oxygen supply to the tube into her lungs. Williamson inserts a Foley catheter for urinary drainage and scrubs the patient. A first-year resident, who will assist, goes over the same area with Betadine. He drapes the patient, covers all of her except the left breast.

"We'll be doing two biopsies," Williamson tells one of the nurses. "We want a piece of each frozen and a piece of each permanent." She wants the nurse to send the samples to Pathology as soon as they're removed. A frozen section can be done, quickly, on part of the tissue and a fast definition returned while the patient is still in the OR. A permanent section, a more comprehensive analysis, can be sent back when ready.

"We need this information quickly," Williamson says. "It will help us decide what to do inside. This woman has a lesion in her stomach and bilateral breast lesions. Probably carcinoma."

The resident feels the mass in the left breast and makes a small incision above it, scarcely more than an inch. He extracts a piece of tissue with his scalpel, then a second. Williamson shouts, "Where's the circulating nurse? This is very important." The nurse ambles in; she does not seem to share Williamson's sense of urgency.

"There are two pieces of tissue, one for frozen and one for permanent," Williamson tells her.

"Which is which?" the nurse asks.

"It doesn't matter," Williamson replies. The nurse walks out, slowly.

"This could turn out to be a bad, bad day," Williamson says to the resident.

Williamson and the resident do the biopsy on the right breast.

"Both mammograms were positive, so we're doing these incisionals to find out," Williamson tells the resident.

"Close it, take the drapes off and take the frozens over to Pathology," Williamson tells the resident. "Call us right away." He grabs two sets of tissue samples, in bottles; the nurse has bottled the first specimens. He heads for Pathology.

An attending surgeon arrives, scrubs in to share the larger procedure—the subtotal gastrectomy (partial removal of the stomach)—with Williamson. He is young and cool.

As Williamson paints the patient's stomach with Betadine, he asks, "Who is she?"

"She told me she worked on Fifth Avenue, and it turned out that she cleaned offices there," Williamson says.

"She looks older than sixty."

"Hard life. When I first saw her, she was rundown and vomiting and bleeding."

Williamson and the attending are joined by another young resident and two nurses, the scrub nurse who will man the instrument tray at the foot of the table and a circulating nurse, to get what is needed.

As the attending moves up to the edge of the table, Williamson looks at him and says, "What plays or musicals have you seen recently, so I'll know what tunes to expect?"

He doesn't answer. He is studying the patient.

"Her blood looks a little dark," Williamson says to the anesthetist, without pausing. The operation begins. Williamson cuts a long vertical incision down the woman's abdomen, approximately seven inches in length. Together, the attending and Williamson work on it, with the attending commenting and instructing. As they deepen the incision, they clamp off and tie blood vessels. Finally, they are through, into the area of the digestive organs. Williamson sticks her hand in and probes.

"I don't feel any lesion in this area," she says, trying to find a lesion that is evident on an X-ray illuminated on a wall across the room.

The cutting resumes. The attending holds tissue and points out areas to be cut. Williamson follows his directions. Their foreheads meet directly above the gaping slash in the woman's abdomen. The cutting goes slowly, bit by bit. It is 11:15.

The dialogue is literal. "And here's the head of the pancreas," the attending says, giving a guided tour of the patient's innards. "Just cut right across there," he points. Williamson cuts. "You have to come down here and cut across there," he tells her. She does.

A nurse pokes her head through the door to the OR. Pathology reports that the frozen sections showed invasive carcinoma of both breasts.

"This was an obviously neglected case," Williamson says to the attending. "With her symptoms, anyone else would have gotten attention."

"You've got to move early on cancer of the stomach, because it destroys quickly," the attending comments.

"We're going to act on the breast cancer very soon, too," Williamson tells him.

"Today?" the scrub nurse asks.

"No. Relax," Williamson replies.

The OR looks like the setting for a group portrait in green. Green tile walls on all sides. Green gowns. The resident is holding a retractor; his neck is beginning to strain. The attending is suctioning. Williamson is cutting. All in silence.

"Keep going. Just be careful," the attending says. "There's a large penetrating gastric ulcer that looks benign. And another one that looks malignant."

It is noon. The young resident changes sides of the operating table. His hand and arm are numb from gripping the retractor, and as he circles around the table, he flexes the hand, waves the arm in the air.

"We need a big right-angle clamp," the attending says to the circulating nurse. "How long will it take to get it?"

"About ten minutes," she says.

"Forget it."

The anesthetist begins to hang a unit of blood on the IV pole, ready to transfuse the patient.

"Wait a minute," the attending bellows at Williamson.

The anesthetist, unnerved, reacts by grabbing for the tubing on the IV pole, tearing the section he's grabbed away from the blood itself. The blood splatters on the floor, on his green pants, on the respirator. He jumps up, puts it all back together. Eyes move toward him, but no one speaks.

The cutting, clamping, tying go on, methodically. By 1:15, after three and a half hours, a crucial step has been reached; most of the stomach, with its threatening ulcers, has been freed and is lifted out by the attending. It, too, will be sent to Pathology. What remains is connected to the upper part of the small intestine.

A second unit of blood is on the IV pole. At 1:30, the original scrub nurse leaves and is replaced. At 2 P.M., the attending leaves. Williamson thanks him. She continues on her own, assisted by the young resident. As the attending guided her, she instructs the resident.

A third-year resident arrives, scrubbed to help if needed, and Williamson tells him to "open the specimen and look at it." The inner work has been done; the gastrectomy has been completed. Now the incision must be closed. It is 2:30. Williamson never took that lunch break she jokingly mentioned hours earlier to the patient. She is still on her feet.

The third-year resident examines the specimen on a nearby tray. He slices it—the stomach and an adjoining accumulation of fatty tissue—and sees two ulcerations, one benign; the other, firm and irregular, seems malignant to him. But he is not certain. Neither is Williamson, who takes a fast peek at it. The tissue looks like a red, slippery, small and apparently uncomplicated organ. There is a line of hard nodules, lymph nodes, that appear cancerous, the resident notes.

"If it's cancer," he says, "the prognosis is very poor and probably means we'll find it elsewhere in her body eventually." Pathology will have its last word on the subject soon.

Williamson and the young resident continue to work. Large sutures now bridge the gap over the incision. Williamson pulls them taut, closing the wound.

The entire operation has consumed six hours. There are three more to do before Williamson's day in the OR is ended. Then she must make rounds. And tonight she is on call.

The anesthesia classroom is on the ninth floor, adjoining the operating rooms. A male nurse-anesthetist is conducting an informal class for one medical student.

The nurse-anesthetist is a stocky man, young, who manages to transmit confidence without appearing pompous. He knows his field and is happy to explain it.

He tells the student that anesthesia is in the hands of anesthesiologists, doctors who have their M.D. degrees, and nurse-anesthetists, registered nurses who have completed an additional two-year course in anesthesia.

Normally, he tells the student, the former outnumber the latter at Bellevue, but when the Anesthesia department lost its accreditation for not having a chairman, most of the staff residents left for work at other hospitals, leaving the anesthetists in command until the department could regain its status (by finding and keeping a chairman). The residents are gone, but a new chairman has been found.

"One of the basics of knowing what you're doing in anesthesia is the classification of the physical status of the patient," he tells the student, referring to a category listing prepared by the American Society of Anesthesiologists:

1. A normal healthy patient
2. A patient with a mild systemic disease
3. A patient with a severe systemic disease that limits activity, but is not incapacitating
4. A patient with an incapacitating systemic disease that is a constant threat to life
5. A moribund patient not expected to survive 24 hours with or without operation

"The anesthetist puts the patient to sleep, with Sodium Pentothal, before the basic anesthesia is employed. He sets up his monitoring devices. Then he gets down to the hard work.

"In the OR, we may use an inhalation agent, a gas. Ether isn't common any more. It's less safe and more explosive than the other anesthetics we can use. And it can cause vomiting. At Bellevue, we use halothane and cyclopropene. The latter causes bronchial constriction, so we precede it with a muscle relaxant and it's not used on patients with asthma or high blood pressure. Halothane does relax muscles, making it easier for us to insert an endotracheal tube. All these gases are carried in nitrous oxide and are given along with a constant flow of oxygen.

"Then, there's a second class of anesthetics, narcotics like morphine, Demerol, fentanyl. Each one has a side effect to be guarded against.

"A third group are all locals. The patient remains awake, but the area to be dealt with is numbed. Xylocaine is common at Bellevue. We usually give it by injection, with epinephrine to slow down the absorption rate. We use spinals, too. Pontocaine by a one-shot injection. Xylocaine can be given in an epidural injection, through a catheter that stays in place so more of it can be given if we have to.

"Finally, patients can always be tranquilized prior to surgery, with drugs like Valium."

The student, who didn't expect all these facts when he inquired about anesthesia, is fascinated. He makes notes in a small black notebook. The room is lined with drawings, photos, dummies, plastic heads to practice intubation.

"You know what it's like to be in anesthesia? It's like becoming a Mason," the anesthetist tells the student. "A closed shop, anesthetists and anesthesiologists. A very ego-inflating experience. A trip. You're it and you know it. Like a cardiac surgeon. The one important thing lacking is communicating with patients.

"But, believe me, there is something special about Bellevue. I think of it as a kind of spiritual experience. Really. I like it here. I stay here for $12,500, when I know I could make $22,000 at some other hospital. I stay. I'm sentimental about the place, if you can appreciate that, about all those ghosts that inhabit the place. There's two centuries' worth of them in these halls. I know that some of the doctors here think it's the asshole of the world, but I don't, and I don't kid myself about what's wrong with Bellevue either.

"Then, of course, there's my job. There are risks. But what's important to know is that you can't be scared of what you're doing, because the patient may be scared out of his wits and that's what you've got to deal with.

"You've got to be careful about what you do and what you say, when the patient is waiting to be operated on. Hearing is the last sense to go, so you've got to be careful. And when a patient is scared, all kinds of things can happen. His blood pressure shoots up. Tachycardia. Lungs constrict. Complications. Arrest. Fear has a lot to do with that, so it's the patient you've got to deal with, in what you say to him and in what you give him.

"Except for some of the horrendos we get at Bellevue—and they'd be tough to treat anywhere—an anesthetist can deal with the problems that come up. He can monitor everything, efficiently. The biggest trick is not putting the patient to sleep. That's easy. The biggest trick is getting him up after the operation is over. If a patient is gorked, you can call it fate, sure. But it usually means that somebody goofed. The day you're not afraid is the day you get out of that indecision that leads to errors.

"If I have a question, I don't want to panic. I ask it, even of the doctors on the case while they're at work. I hang loose and make sure I'm right. I know the drugs I use. I know what they can do, what they can't do, what to do if they produce side effects. You have to know where you are, always. You can't be vague or unsure. It's a technical job and you have to make those decisions you've been trained to make. It's no great big thing. You stop and think and you find out that there aren't any secrets about it."

The session is over. The student walks out, to scrub in on an operation. The anesthetist ties on his mask and moves toward an OR, too, to return to work.

After dinner, Sol Zimmerman goes to OB, where a Caesarean section is in progress. The attending, a large, bearded man looking like an overweight Transylvanian count, is in the gallery supplying directions to the doctors below. Two residents perform the section, which goes smoothly until the baby emerges, a deep shade of blue. While Zimmerman watches, a Pediatrics intern and a subintern take the baby, beating its feet and rubbing its back, suctioning secretions rapidly. Suddenly, the baby girl comes to life, cries and begins turning pink. Then she grunts.

Zimmerman knows the sound. It can mean possible RDS, respiratory distress syndrome. The baby is quickly transported to the Premature Unit by the intern, with Zimmerman racing along.

Minutes later, the baby is still grunting. Her temperature is 95. She is acidotic. Her chest X-ray, taken quickly, shows some haziness, probably due to secretions in the lungs, but not alarmingly like RDS. She will be warmed up in an isolette, Zimmerman decides. But he wants other opinions.

He calls a junior attending, who thinks Zimmerman should act more rapidly, moving the baby to the ICU, getting a line in for medication later and giving bicarb to correct the acidosis, which must be done before further treatment can be initiated. Zimmerman listens, then calls a senior resident, who favors a stay-put approach, waiting for the temperature to rise.

"If she gets better, we lucked out," Zimmerman says to the intern. "If she gets worse, we weren't aggressive enough."

At 7 P.M., he is in the ICU, at 7:15 back in the Premature Unit. The newborn baby's temperature is up to 97. "She's warmer," he says, "but not necessarily better."

He trusts the intern to keep an eye on her. He has to do a spinal tap on a beautiful infant girl who has been running a fever and suffering from diarrhea. She is now on the strongest antibiotic available to her, gentamicin, after three other antibiotics tried didn't bring prompt improvement. As Zimmerman permits a second intern to help him, the intern attempts to get the spinal needle into the baby, to extract spinal fluid for analysis. He has trouble and goes through four needles unsuccessfully. A nurse is watching critically; she tells the intern that her head nurse limits the attempts to four on any single patient at one time.

Zimmerman looks at her and says, "When *she* goes to medical school, she can make rules like that." He asks for another needle, which he inserts, correctly, sparing the intern further nervousness. Test tubes are rushed off to the lab; the intern carries them himself. As he leaves, Zimmerman tells him, "I'm worried about this baby. It's another case of a prematurely ruptured membrane in the mother, and the spinal fluid doesn't look right to me. It could be sepsis with meningitis. But we'll know for sure, I hope, in an hour." The intern dashes out.

Zimmerman sits back wearily to await the results. He can't sit for long. At 8:15, he goes back to the ICU, to check the condition of the infants there. All is calm. At 9, the results of the spinal tap are phoned to the intern, who informs Zimmerman. All the findings are favorable; there is no meningitis. Further cultures may provide new leads. Zimmerman is both relieved and frustrated. "If it isn't meningitis, what is it?"

At 10 P.M., Zimmerman, an intern and a senior resident sit in the nurses' room of the Premature Unit and go over the babies, chart by chart. They talk about the baby with the fever and diarrhea, trying to make educated guesses about what's wrong with her. The tentative consensus: gastroenteritis. They'll know more tomorrow, when more test results are in.

The other resident leaves. Zimmerman and the intern spend the rest of the night in the Premature Unit. It is an uneventful tour for them. Zimmerman gets four hours' sleep.

This afternoon, Tom Spencer worked out at the YMCA. He spends much of his free time there, running, jogging, lifting weights, playing basketball. When he arrives at the AES at 3:30, there is an alcoholic spread out on the sidewalk; a policeman is trying to awaken him. Inside the AES, Spencer finds out from one of the residents that the knifed merchant seaman brought in earlier in the week went through surgery with apparent success, despite the fact that one of the slashes cut through his trachea back to the vertebrae muscles.

While they're talking, the policeman brings in the alcoholic and delivers him to Spencer. The man, shabby and weak, is having trouble breathing. His face is purple. Spencer reaches into his pocket, extracts a pint of vodka and dumps it into a sink. The man is in no condition to be treated at the AES and released, so Spencer helps him into the Emergency Ward.

Within minutes, the man is stripped, put into a bed, given oxygen and IV nourishment. Spencer returns to the AES, where he is accosted by an old man who claims he injured his foot and has been waiting for attention since 8 A.M. Spencer checks. The man arrived at 3 P.M., had X-rays taken. Spencer looks at the X-rays. There is a fracture.

"I was a longshoreman and a trolley motorman in my time," the man blusters to Spencer. "I've done a lot of things. Once I killed a Jew," he laughs. Spencer glares at him, but says nothing. "You know damned well that if I were a black man, I'd have been taken care of here right away," he hollers. "I deserve better treatment. I'm from the First War."

"Which side?" Spencer asks, expressionless. The man does not hear him. Spencer wheels him into the Plastic Surgery room, to have a cast put on the leg. The resident on duty there is an African black. Spencer leaves them together.

A resident comes charging out of an examining room, almost crashing into Spencer. He points to the room and says, "Get that guy out of here. He just wants a sleeping pill and a bed."

On a bed in the corridor, a drunk is mumbling, "I'm cuckoo." A passing resident comments, "Thanks. We never would have known."

At 5:15, there are five patients on beds in the corridors. Among them is an old man suffering from an overdose of mineral oil; after hours in his own private track meet, he is beginning to feel better.

Up front, a small, skinny 70-year-old man weaves his way to the registration desk. "I would like you to know that I am a social drinker, purely a social drinker, a very sociable drinker," he announces to one of the clerks. "Baby, that's all we get here is sociable drinkers," she says to him. The man ambles around the front area for a few minutes, shakes hands with doctors and nurses, then moves rapidly out the front door. No one wants to stop him.

The old bigot now has a cast on his leg; Spencer is instructing him in the use of crutches. He hails a cab for the man, helps him into it. "Whatever he is, I'll feel better if he gets home safely," Spencer says to another nurse.

In the back of the AES, a young black man has been sitting clutching a dislocated thumb. A resident stops in front of him and shouts, "For God's sake, this guy's been here for two hours. Can't we find someone from Plastic to take care of him?"

At 6 P.M., Spencer takes a dinner break. As he returns, a black man, middle-aged, is having a seizure in the waiting room. He had been seen earlier by a resident who didn't see any need to hospitalize him. The man's chart notes that he is epileptic and an alcoholic. Spencer lifts the man onto a bed and wheels him to the resuscitation room. He may be in alcoholic withdrawal; he murmurs that he had a quart of whiskey yesterday. Another patient in the room, reclining on a bed watching it all, asks Spencer, "Mind if I puke up?"

"Yes, I do," Spencer tells him.

In an examining room, a doctor and a nurse are undressing a fashionably dressed woman complaining of abdominal pain. The nurse slips off the woman's underpants. The doctor gapes. "Jesus God," he says, *"balls."*

Spencer keeps moving. He checks a woman, grimy and old, who ODed on five Tuinals. He slaps her face, to keep her awake. A large black man on the bed beside hers tells Spencer, "Man, I got beat up. I really got it." Spencer gives him a tetanus shot. The man's face is puffy, lacerated. A punch in the head can do more than that, Spencer knows; he summons a Neurology consult.

By 7:30, forty patients have been registered.

Spencer has walked to the front desk, to see what action is going on up there. His timing is perfect.

Two hookers have strutted up to the desk. One is in her early twenties, black, bulging, buxom, with a large teased black wig. The other is tiny, young, with straight long blond hair, a red dress with a plunging neckline. "Baby, I do believe I got the clap," the black hooker tells a clerk. She laughs. "Like it's in the

line of duty, you might say." She is sent in to see a doctor, while
her friend waits for her.

The police surround an ugly, fat, pimply woman and her
nervous, emaciated husband.

"That's right. That's what I did," she screams. "I threw the
son of a bitch through a plate-glass window."

"It wasn't *your* plate-glass window," one of the policemen
says. "It belonged to a restaurant."

"Fuck it," she says.

"Then she slashed her wrists," the timid husband wheezes.
His jacket is shredded. Her wrists are bleeding, slightly. She is
wearing dirty, ragged sneakers, baggy pants, a sweat shirt.

"You a psychiatrist?" she asks Spencer. She doesn't wait for
an answer. "Well, if you are, you ought to know that I cut myself
intentionally. I've seen plenty of head doctors in my time and
they don't understand a thing."

"You really should talk to one of ours," Spencer says.

"Why not? What difference is one more gonna make?" she
says.

Spencer gets a messenger to take her to Psychiatry, known
at the AES as "The Banana Factory."

With that taken care of, he goes back to check the Tuinal OD.
He slaps her in the face and she wakes up.

"You *must* stay awake," he tells her. "It's bad to sleep." He
checks her blood pressure, then asks her, "How much is Tuinal
on the street?"

She looks at him, dazed, and says, "A buck and a half."

At 8:15, the black alcoholic-epileptic, on a bed in the corridor,
has another seizure. His breathing is heavy, horselike. Four
nurses and two doctors accompany him back to the resuscitation room, where he's calmed down, given medication.

In the corridor a nurse and an old drunk are debating. "You
must be examined by a doctor before you can leave and you
must have a bath before the doctor examines you," she says,
staying several feet away from him.

"Like hell I do," he says. "I want to go home. I don't want no
bath."

Spencer walks over to help, but at that moment a siren breaks
into the routine. An ambulance screeches into the driveway, its
siren on, and Spencer runs forward.

The rear door flies open and Spencer, with the help of several residents, pulls out the stretcher. A middle-aged man is on it; he is a mess below the waist. One leg is almost completely ripped off above the knee. A policeman accompanying the man tells Spencer, breathlessly, "The guy works for the railroad and the poor bastard must have been run over by a train."

The man is rushed into the Emergency Ward.

On the table in the EW, his clothes are stripped away, carefully. His left leg looks like the product of a slaughterhouse, mangled from the hip down. The man is awake, miraculously, and he wants to see what happened to his body, but he does not have the strength to sit up and see the carnage. Oddly, there is little bleeding; the impact of the train wheel compressed blood vessels. Most of his leg, from above the knee down, is flat on the table; a bone in his thigh is pointing upward. Bone fragments scatter to the floor. Doctors and nurses work, speedily.

IVs are connected. One doctor talks to the man while others work busily.

"What happened? Do you remember?"

"I'm not sure. It hit me and knocked me down," the man says, "but I'm not hurt."

"What is your religion?"

"Catholic."

"Have you ever been in a hospital before?"

"No."

"Do you have any allergies?"

"No."

"Are you diabetic?"

"Yes."

Several of the nurses around the table seem visibly pale, unnerved, despite their experience. The Trauma doctor, supervising, shouts, "Get him ready for the OR. Fast."

Oxygen is hooked up. Spencer, helping out, attaches an EKG unit. A Foley catheter is inserted into the man's penis, to measure kidney function, check the urine for blood, do a diabetes test. The Catholic chaplain arrives, an older priest with white hair; he holds the man's hand and prays. A nurse covers the dangling leg, held to the thigh by a thin strip of skin, and the mangled stump, with a sterile cloth; a weathered work shoe protrudes on the lifeless foot.

The Trauma doctor shouts, "Let's go, let's go. Let's get the

X-rays and go." An X-ray machine is beside the table; the technician goes to work.

"God, there's nothing left to save on that leg," one EW nurse whispers to another.

The patient is wheeled out to a waiting elevator, on his way to the OR. Spencer, who has stayed through it all, looks shaken. "God, I'm glad I'm in one piece," he sighs.

When Spencer returns to the AES, it is after 9 P.M. and fifty-six patients have been checked in. Another nurse is slapping the OD. "I'm up, I'm up," the woman replies, angrily.

In one of the examining rooms, a young black man tells a black nurse's aide that he's going to kill someone unless he gets psychiatric care. The aide steps out and tells a nurse, who scrawls on the man's chart, "PAO [Psychiatric Admitting Office] desired."

At 10 P.M., an ambulance brings in a policeman who fell down a flight of stairs pursuing a fugitive. He is in severe pain.

A policeman brings in an attractive, chic young woman; he walks beside her but does not touch her. She had been working late, alone, in a midtown office when two men knocked on the door, asking for change of a $5 bill. When she reached for her purse, they pulled guns.

She tells the story to the triage nurse.

"They took my money and then they told me to undress, so I wouldn't be able to chase them. But when I undressed, they raped me. Vaginally and anally," she says, speaking slowly, deliberately. The triage nurse calls for the on-duty GYN resident, Bob Nachtigall; he gets to the AES in a few minutes, sees the woman, examines her, gives her medication and sends her home. As she leaves, she seems calm. "In a day or two, that's when she may realize what happened," Nachtigall says. Walking out of the AES with the policeman, the woman smiles and says, "It's all finished. All finished."

At 10:30, the family of the railroad worker arrive: his wife, their grown children. They sit in vigil in the waiting room. "He *must* know he lost his leg," a son says. The mother weeps. "You can go up to the Surgery recovery area," a nurse tells them, "and wait for him there." The family files out.

The patient count at 10:40 is sixty-two. By 11 P.M., it has slowed down. A medical student sits behind the back desk practicing suturing on a piece of flannel cloth. A resident leans against a wall, smoking a cigarette like a man awaiting the firing squad. A nurse adjusts her hair. Spencer keeps walking, peering into examining rooms, talking to patients on beds. He removes an IV line from the OD, wakes her up in the process. "I was sleeping," she hollers. "I haven't slept in three nights."

"What got you here?" Spencer asks her.

"What got me here? Junk got me here. I was on heroin when I was nineteen. Now both my husband and me are on methadone."

"You know you shouldn't take downs with methadone. Meth is a down in itself. Listen, I don't give drug lectures, but if you mix meth with other drugs you can kill yourself. You ought to know to be careful. Now get on your feet. You must be ready to get out of here by now." He helps her off the bed, to the bathroom. When she's gone, Spencer asks a resident, "Is she supposed to go to Psych?"

"No. She was an OD in search of sleep, not death," the resident says. When the woman comes out of the bathroom, Spencer tells her she can go home. She walks a compulsively straight line to the front door.

Her path crosses with that of a very old Russian woman accompanied by two policemen. She has the face of a peasant, weathered, unadorned, the face of a benevolent durable grandmother. She does not speak English. The police report that she was vomiting and seemed to be in pain on the street, so they brought her to Bellevue. The doctors scurry around looking for someone who speaks Russian. The old woman is placed on a bed; she is nervous, frightened, baffled, all at once. She sits on the edge of the bed, peering to her right and left, her eyes wide open, and she trembles. She speaks in Russian, softly. Down the hall, a chubby Puerto Rican nurse's aide sees her. She walks over, stands in front of her, puts her arms around the Russian and hugs her. The old woman is comforted. She continues to speak in Russian; the nurse's aide answers in Spanish. They seem like unlikely old friends, but friends nevertheless.

Spencer realizes that it is midnight, that he can go home. He knows he won't be able to sleep, immediately. He'll read or watch TV until the tension evaporates and exhaustion takes over.

THURSDAY

Nursing Service Report

Gerald Titus, gunshot wound of chest—was shot by his father, who is a retired policeman. Father Martin Titus is in Holding Area with C. O. P. D. and two 13th Precinct guards.

Mary Johnson is very depressed—was told yesterday of the death of her children. (She is in the Ground L ICU.)

James Brunning, psychiatric patient, said he swallowed a spoon and a glass. He complained of pain. Underwent exploratory surgery. Spoon and glass not evident. A radio antenna was removed. His condition is fair.

A-1—Pablo Velez, 46-year-old admitted from Willowbrook, mentally retarded, has been quiet until yesterday, when he became agitated and hit two patients and two employees. There were no major injuries. Patient was sedated and was quiet. The incident occurred at 12:50 P.M.

M-6—Alice King—at 7:30 P.M. had been taken to the chapel by the priest. The priest left her for a few minutes. While she was praying she looked up to find a man staring at her—she heard a sound of a switch-blade opening—she ran out to Administration Office—security was called—they apprehended the man and he was admitted to PQ-1. Security submitted a detailed report.

Bernard Weinstein begins his day by phoning the new Director of Anesthesia, recently hired but not yet in residence, who tells him that he wants to report to work a month earlier than planned, just a month away. Weinstein is pleased. The Anesthesia department, without a chief for months, has been a nagging problem.

He talks to the director about scheduling the operating rooms to avoid waiting; now, patients must wait until the surgical team assembles before they can go to the OR. Weinstein hopes to eliminate the waits once Surgery moves into the new hospital.

The next call is from a friend in administration at Queens General Hospital. The friend needs examining tables.

"Sure, we've got examining tables," Weinstein says. "From our old outpatient department. We bought new ones for the new hospital and we've got the old ones in storage. Just send me a request. Then all you've got to do is take some of our disposition problem cases." He laughs.

A bureaucrat at the state auditor's office calls, with a trivial question. An audit has been completed at Bellevue. Weinstein, in fact, takes such audits seriously.

"They went through here and told me we had too much tuna fish on hand. A lot of silly shit like that. *Mea culpa,*" Weinstein says to one of his associate directors, who has strolled in. His name is Felix Calabrese. He speaks Italian and he has been enlisted to help guide the mayor of Naples around Bellevue. He tells Weinstein that he's found some help, an Italian Dermatology resident.

"This resident went to school in Rome. He's an Italian Italian," Calabrese tells Weinstein. He adds that the chief of the Chest Service has volunteered, too. Weinstein makes a few suggestions, what they ought to show the mayor, stressing the new hospital.

"He's arriving at two-thirty?" Calabrese asks.

"Yes. Be there at two-fifteen."

"I'll be there at two."

Weinstein gets a call from another associate, who's been studying the engineering report on problems in the new hospital. Weinstein, who has tried to understand the report, tells the caller, "It doesn't translate the technical terms for me, so I can relate it to patients and staff and get dramatic about it." The associate promises a translation.

Weinstein talks to the chief of Pediatrics for his opinion about a neighborhood child health station and a community group that seems to be competing with Bellevue to take it over. Weinstein knows that the Bellevue community board wants Bellevue to run the child health station. The neighborhood group proposal to run it, which Weinstein has read, does not seem to supply services as comprehensively as Bellevue can, and offers only a small role for Bellevue, providing psychological testing.

The chief of Pediatrics urges opposition to that alignment.

Warren Schubert, the well-fed, earthy, unpretentious Director of Food Services, shows up to escort Weinstein on rounds of several wards. It's a mission designed to find out what patients and nurses think of the hospital food. A dangerous mission.

"That's a sharp jacket you're wearing," Schubert tells Weinstein.

"I've got to keep up with my staff," Weinstein says.

In the background, they overhear an elderly woman volunteer peddling religion to a zonked male patient who keeps nodding off as she repeats, "Can I give you some nice tracts to read?" She is one of Bellevue's volunteers, who travel the corridors regularly.

The days of working as a hospital volunteer out of a sense of noblesse oblige are almost gone. Bellevue's volunteer program, which was begun sixty-five years ago and complements the Auxiliary, is headed by a professional, full-time chief, Mrs. Luise Davidson, who recruits constantly by writing letters. Bellevue's more than five hundred volunteers come from the hospital community, from the outpatient population, and from high schools and colleges. Volunteers donate time, most of them a half day per week in most of the areas of Bellevue, from the Home Care program to the clinics, libraries, labs, admitting offices, the AES and the recovery room, wards, and the thrift shop on the Upper East Side. Some are even trained by the Red Cross to assist nurses in taking temperatures, blood pressure, respiration rates and in moving patients and feeding them.

While this woman volunteer obviously prefers spiritual treatment, Weinstein and Schubert shift to more pragmatic matters as they head toward one of the wards they'll survey. A little farther on Weinstein stops in his tracks. A costly respirator is sitting, disheveled, next to a bulging trash basket in a corridor. He picks up a phone and calls one of his associates, to report it. He asks him to come over. The associate arrives, breathless, a few seconds later.

"Am I right?" Weinstein asks. "This is an expensive piece of equipment? Somebody should be doing something about it?"

"Yes, you're right," the associate says. "I will do something about it."

Weinstein and Schubert move on, joined by an amiable black woman, the dietitian for the wards they're going to tour.

In the first ward, when asked for her opinion of the hospital food, a nurse refers to the "green liver" they've been getting.

Schubert, sheepishly, explains that the color can change when the liver is cooked in the basement kitchen and later warmed on the ward. The same nurse indicates that an Armenian patient may not be eating what he wants to eat, because he can't speak English.

Schubert, 32, administers a staff of 565 employees in 4 master kitchens and 93 patient pantries, on a budget of $1.5 million annually. Numbers fill most of Schubert's day. That means using, per week, 108,000 eggs, 2,700 loaves of bread (white, low-sodium white, rye and whole wheat), 290 six-gallon containers of milk, 4,300 half-gallons and 4,700 half-pints. The total milk bill per month is approximately $16,000.

Two weeks' worth of meat for Bellevue includes 1,950 pounds of "Beef, Rounds, U.S. Good"; 4,700 pounds of "Beef, Chucks, Boneless, U.S. Good"; 600 pounds of "Beef, Boneless, Brisket, Corned"; 1,250 pounds of "Beef, Liver, Fresh Frozen, Style A, Sliced"; 1,050 pounds of "Lamb, Legs, Fresh Chilled, Double"; 1,020 pounds of "Butts, Boneless, Fresh"; 2,000 pounds of "Chickens, Eviscerated, 2½-3 pounds." Before Thanksgiving, Schubert orders 3,000 pounds of turkey.

Bellevue makes its own cakes, puddings, Jello and rolls. It has its own butcher shop. Food is shipped from the master kitchens to the patient pantries in bulk, then is reheated and served on the wards. The pantries stock and clean the dishes and utensils.

Schubert thinks longingly of the new Bellevue, where one main kitchen will relate to four relatively automated satellite units. The main kitchen will prepare entrees and soups only. Each satellite will be responsible for the rest and will have the staff to do it; nurses will no longer have to serve and pick up trays. Schubert walks up to an old man in bed and offers his stock question: "What do you think of the food?"

"Well, we could stand a change of menu for breakfast. From that farina and the hard-boiled egg."

"We're working on it," Schubert tells him. "Be well."

He talks to Weinstein about his efforts to get French toast, pancakes, scrambled eggs onto the breakfast menu occasionally; Schubert is sensitive to the wishes of the patients.

"Good idea. The hard-boiled egg is not too popular," the dietitian says.

In another ward, Schubert stops another nurse. "How do you find the food service? Say it like it is."

"I guess you'd say it is improving," she says. "It's on time, when the elevators are working. But, in general, the patients don't care for our food."

Schubert, Weinstein, the dietitian and the nurse amble through the ward, looking for a likely candidate to interview. They see an old black woman, slumped over in a chair. Taking a chance, Schubert leans over and says to her, "How do you find your food?"

Her head snaps up from her chest, instantly.

"Tough," she cackles, "tough. Those hamburgers are too hard and too dry. Why, if you squeezed them, you wouldn't get one drop of juice out of one. Not a drop. And that turkey. The turkey looked like they just threw it in a pot and boiled it. No kind of taste. No kind of taste whatsoever. A Tennessee bulldog, those hamburgers. You pull one way and I pull the other and the damned thing just don't break." She is worked up and Schubert is not certain just how accurate she may be. Weinstein is laughing.

The group escapes the old woman's wrath and heads for another ward, where the head nurse has an answer to Schubert's standard query.

"The patients complain every day about the way the food is cooked. They're tired of turkey and chicken, macaroni and spaghetti. Or those on a special diet, getting hamburgers and applesauce three days straight. They say they never get pork chops or steak. And some even like franks and beans."

Schubert is making notes. He tells Weinstein that a selective menu, new to Bellevue, is being developed. He hopes to have it available when the new hospital is populated with inpatients. Also, he's hoping to have it printed in both English and Spanish.

The tour ends at noon. Weinstein is due at a community board meeting in the administration conference room, but first he meets quickly with an associate, to discuss an emergency generator full-load test that is planned. If the power from Con Edison fails, the emergency generator must take over; it hasn't been tested before, so power will be turned off to find out how well it works.

Weinstein approves the plan. There's no need to run off to lunch. There'll be food at the community board meeting.

Weinstein gets to the community board meeting at 12:15. Few board members have arrived, but the food has, from a Bellevue kitchen. There is corned beef, egg salad, tuna salad, bread, cookies, hot water for tea, coffee. Weinstein makes himself a sandwich and finds a seat at the long conference table. The board members begin to arrive. Finally, there are twenty people around the table, including the Director of Social Services, the Director of Nursing, the Director of Community Relations, one of Weinstein's aides, a staff surgeon who is on both the medical and community boards and assorted board members. It is a conglomeration, representing all races and a wide age range; several of the board members have known Bellevue as patients, one of them in Psychiatry.

The meeting is called to order. One woman eats frantically, having seconds and thirds, beating a path to the food table. A man reads his mail, which he's brought with him. A woman embroiders. Issues and questions are raised.

Can Bellevue use, and fund, a program for Physicians' Associates? Although the medical board is opposed to the idea, and Weinstein knows it, the community board will study it and offer its opinion.

There's a need for more blood donors. Should the community be solicited, to bring it closer to Bellevue? What about the use of a mobile unit? Should other community groups be enlisted? Posters in stores? In clinics? In Spanish? The board discusses it, postpones decisions until more information can be obtained and reviewed.

One of the board members raises a delicate matter: the loss of the resident staff in Anesthesia due to the loss of the department's accreditation. It's causing difficulty in coverage, the board member insists. She's investigated it. It is an example of how the board, facing the administration, plays devil's advocate.

Weinstein had anticipated that the question would arise. He tells the board that a new chairman for the Anesthesia department has been hired and will be in residence soon. He's already begun to recruit attendings, Weinstein asserts.

The surgeon comments that anesthesia "is not an attractive field, despite the good pay, the regular hours, no house calls. Few American students want to go into it. I don't know why." He adds that Bellevue wouldn't need residents in Anesthesia if it could hire enough attendings and nurse-anesthetists, but he realizes that the hospital wants to continue the training program run by N.Y.U., despite the fact that it fails to attract local students. Most of those in the department are foreign. "When the new chairman gets here," the surgeon says, "he'll be the only American M.D. in the department."

"The solution," Weinstein says, "is proper leadership and talent in the department. What does the new chairman need to do the best possible job?"

One of the board members, ruffled, says, "We do have the responsibility to our patients and this is a frightening situation." Her comment ends the discussion.

The next issue: a loss of HEW funds could affect some Bellevue services, particularly crippling the computerizing of clinic records in Pediatrics.

The city must budget compensatory dollars to meet that loss, Weinstein says. Several board members agree that it would be a good idea to lean on Congressmen in the district, and on Senator Javits.

The talk turns to the neighborhood health station and the need for comprehensive medical care for the community. Various community groups seem to be competing to provide it. The best idea, one board member offers, would be to convert the Health Department's child health stations into treatment centers, in the neighborhoods themselves.

Weinstein concurs. After all, he points out, they are in all the boroughs, accessible to patients. The consensus is that mobilizing those resources would be a valuable outreach program for Bellevue to undertake. The board should seek funding from the city, working with other local groups to achieve it.

One of the board members wants to know about the program designed to train soon-to-be-retired policemen and firemen as nurses. It is a new program. "How has it worked out?" a board member asks.

Another board member, informed, notes with some sense of sarcasm that none of the fifty members of the initial class now works at Bellevue, although all were trained at the Hunter-Bellevue Nursing School. The general opinion of those familiar with the program is that the graduates weren't top-notch, but further study is ordered into what one of the board members calls "the Gunsmoke program."

Weinstein discusses the evacuation of the present old Psychiatry building, and the move, eventually, into the top floors of the new hospital. He asks for board support for the plan.

The support is there, but one board member wonders what will happen to the $16 million previously budgeted for renovation of the old Psychiatry building.

"Maybe it can be used for another purpose at Bellevue," one board member suggests.

"Not likely," says the man who has been reading his mail. He understands the tenuous nature of political promises.

"Anyway, the finishing of the top floors of the new building, to tailor them for Psychiatry, will cost more than that," another board member adds.

Weinstein promises further reports on the matter.

At this point, one woman board member challenges another for attention. Both shout "You're out of order" at the top of their voices, until one simply seizes attention by not backing down.

Should the board have access to patient records? She asks the question, waits for an answer. One of the board members, a young woman, is a lawyer. It's a tricky matter, she points out, and the HHC, asked for an opinion months ago, hasn't produced one yet.

Weinstein's assistant announces that funds have been received at Bellevue to give board members a stipend, up to $25 per month. One member, taunted by the HHC's language in providing the money, says it could be interpreted as wages, which means he can't accept it. The president of the board, not present today, will be informed.

The Director of Nursing is invited to comment on the fact that one of the board members saw an ad in the *Times* for nursing supervisors at Bellevue. Why? The board member insists on an answer.

Betty Kauffman, the Nursing Director, explains calmly and knowledgeably that there is a nursing shortage. There's a need for fifteen nursing supervisors, especially on the evening and night shifts. She's been unable to fill the vacancies from within the hospital, although Bellevue has more than seven hundred R.N.s on duty. The salaries are competitive, but she admits that the pace at Bellevue, and the physical surroundings, have led some nurses to leave. However, she insists that most of those who do leave do so because they're getting married, moving, getting out of nursing or going into some other area of medical care.

Kauffman's sober explanation seems to provoke a woman board member. She shouts that Bellevue doesn't employ enough people from the surrounding community. Several other board members disagree and challenge her assertion. She cannot meet their challenge, but she does want everyone to know that she knows poor people in need of menial work who can't get work at Bellevue.

The meeting is four hours old and there is more to be covered. The supply of corned beef has dwindled to a few wilted scraps. The coffee is cold. Cookie crumbs have invaded the top of the conference table. Ashtrays are filled with butts.

Weinstein is very tired.

Dirk Berger's day begins as usual with morning rounds. The head nurse, shuffling through notes and chart entries, brings the staff up to date.

After rounds, Berger meets one of the ward's social workers and talks to her about a former ward patient, now living at home, who is sick and won't come in. She needs medication. Berger prescribes it and sends it to her with the social worker, who borrows Berger's car for the task.

Social workers are vital at Bellevue. There are seventy-five social workers, each with a master's in social work. There are fifty-five case workers, with bachelor's degrees, nine paraprofessional social health technicians (high school graduates who have completed a forty-week training course), fourteen clerical staff members and four administrators with M.S.W. degrees.

The Social Services staff works for Bellevue rather than for any of the city social agencies. Its director is Mrs. Frances T. Poe, a black woman who has spent nine years at Bellevue and twenty-eight years in social work. In 1972, her staff dealt with 62,947 cases, including 27,761 new cases that year. Case-work interviews—talks with patients, doctors, nurses, families and others related to a patient's care—reached 223,019, most of them done in the hospital or by phone.

The activities range from caring for children at home while their mother is at Bellevue to standing in line at the Social Security office to pick up a check for an old man who simply can't stand in line for hours. Social Services is the conduit to welfare and aid programs for needy patients at Bellevue. Social workers help patients find schools, training, homes, jobs and continuing counseling service.

Salaries are modest. A full-fledged social worker, with an M.S.W., starts at Bellevue at $11,000. A case worker begins at $8,600. The social health technicians earn a starting wage of $7,000. More often than not, Bellevue's social workers take on the characteristics of zealots, like the one who was willing to take Berger's car to bring medication to one of the ward's former patients.

Berger is standing in the doorway to his office when his old friend from the Aberdeen, the chain-smoking crone, comes rushing up to him. "They'll steal my stuff back at the hotel," she shrieks.

"Yes, they steal," Berger says to her. "But don't worry. I'll take care of you and your stuff."

At 11 A.M. he joins the ward residents and several social workers in the conference room. An older, respected senior psychiatrist, gray-haired and intense, has agreed to interview, in their presence, a recent admission to NO–6, Jack McCurdy. The group gathers in the room, and before the patient is invited in, the resident on the case provides the patient's history.

McCurdy is 60. He's been on the ward for three weeks. He had been discharged from a state hospital after being there for almost two years. He had been living with his wife, but had felt depressed. He felt inferior to his active, working wife. One night he put his hands around her throat, an attempt that never went beyond that gesture. He was admitted to Bellevue in a coherent state.

Born in Ireland, he was one of eight children; the family came to New York when he was a teen-ager. He quit school during the Depression, to go to work. Eventually, he studied sales and marketing and got a job. He was married in 1948. Ten years later, he suffered a severe depression, related, he felt, to the reorganization of the firm he managed. He went into shock therapy, spent time in a private mental hospital, began to see a psychiatrist. In 1960, he became a corporation executive and held the job for more than ten years, never late or absent. He began drinking in the early sixties as well. Then, in 1969, he began to suffer pain in his right arm, an inability to use it that he recognized as psychosomatic (he remembered having it when he was very young). A few months after that he took twenty Librium, knowing he wouldn't die, but seeking attention. In 1971, he retired from his job, stayed at home. His wife worked, and he learned that he couldn't stand to be alone. He entered Manhattan State voluntarily and wanted to remain there. According to the resident, "He is a passive-aggressive, suffering from neurotic depression, and a latent schizoid."

At this point, the senior psychiatrist has been given a skeletal view of the patient's past and the patient is brought in and seated next to the psychiatrist, who begins his questioning. McCurdy is of average height, thin, with carefully combed graying hair. He is very pale. He wears a black suit, white shirt, and thin, black-and-white-striped tie. His meekness is apparent. He squirms in his chair as the first question is asked.

"You're Irish. What was your father?"

"A farm laborer."

"Did your family tend to treat you as a baby?"

"No."

"How did you get along?"

"Better with my father than my mother."

"Why?"

"My mother favored my oldest brother when he was a baby."

"Did that bother you?"

"Yes, unconsciously."

"Did the others resent it, too?"

"I don't know."

"What happened to your father?"

"He died. My mother is dead, too. Their house was occupied by my older brother and one of my sisters."

"Have you had much to do with your older brother?"

"We were never close. But there wasn't any open resentment."

"Were the others closer to him?"

"No."

"Who takes care of you now?"

"My wife. I worked for a long time. I retired because of a psychosomatic illness in my arm. I became tense and ran off the job. They recommended that I retire. I get Social Security and disability from that company."

McCurdy sits nervously, crossing his legs, uncrossing them. His answers are given in a soft, clear voice.

"Your wife has always worked. Who decided not to have children?"

"Me."

"Why?"

"I was afraid of the responsibility, because my best friend married my younger sister and died when their children were young."

As he answers the question, McCurdy begins to cry, soundlessly. He wipes his cheeks with a handkerchief. The tears continue to roll down his face. The senior psychiatrist reaches over, touches him on the shoulder.

"Your wife never resented not having children?"

"No."

"When were you married?"

"When I was in the Navy."

"Who's the boss in the family?"

"I was, in the beginning, but she struck out on her own when I needed psychotherapy."

"Why?"

"Our relationship was too close. We kept nothing from each other. We should have had separate lives, as my doctor told me then."

"What did she do?"

"She started to go to school, to museums, to read."

"What do you read?"

"Nonfiction. Biographies."

"Do you resent her?"

"No. She was doing the right thing."

"Then you drank?"

"Yes, but I was never an alcoholic."

"I didn't say that. Were there any depressions in your family? Are they a dour lot?"

"Yes" is McCurdy's answer to the question. There is a pause, a silence in the room. McCurdy looks directly at the senior psychiatrist for the first time.

"My wife is a librarian, and at times I feel like throwing the work she brings home out the window. I don't like to be neglected." He looks away.

"Why did you go to the state hospital?"

"I look back and wonder why I stayed there. But I did keep busy there."

"Okay. Thank you," the psychiatrist says to McCurdy. "And good luck."

McCurdy gets up and walks slowly out of the room, back to the ward.

"He's not a schizo," the psychiatrist tells the staff. "Infantile. Compulsive. Whatever inspired his wife to be independent hurt him badly, threw him back into childhood. He's not too sure of his masculinity. He doesn't want to be poppa. He wants to be baby. He's so passive. He got a job at Manhattan State when he was there. He was respected. He's still very depressed, but I'm sure he's never had delusions or hallucinations."

The resident who is treating McCurdy asks, "Have you seen the psych tests?"

"Yes and I dispute them. All our Rorschachs seem to find schizophrenia. Yes, he is depressed and, yes, there is a paranoid element to it. He's intact, though, with good reasoning, intellectual insight. He never grew up emotionally."

The resident notes, "Well, he *is* improving."

"Sure he is. Losing his job put him at loose ends. And his wife was working, probably overdid that independence. Said the hell with him. So he thought of killing her. He's not a manic-depressive, for sure. Not the type. Anxiety and depression, sure. The psychosomatic stuff is crap. He doesn't really believe it. He keeps his anxiety in check and his anger, too, by being obsessive. If he could be angry, he'd be better off. A fucked-up character disorder. Not psychotic."

"Would working with his wife help?" Berger asks.

"If some common activity can be found. But she needs him like a hole in the head. Oh! I forgot to ask about their sex life."

"He would have been upset by it," the resident says. "You questioned him like a machine gun."

"I had an hour. You can't futz around."

"When you press him, he gets tearful and withdrawn. You saw it," the resident says.

"The dynamics are clear. Beautiful. You have to carry him, support him for years. Someone he can talk to. He's not stupid. He never wants that tit to be taken out of his mouth. The prognosis is not good. Keep him on some minor medication for anxiety and see him every two weeks. The door should always be open for him. See what his wife can do to mobilize him. He was a child with his wife, for years. Might be well to see her, separately, find what she's willing to do."

"I've seen her," the resident says. "She loves him and is willing to do anything, but she won't give up her independence."

"Could he help her with her library work? He should get out of the house. It's very depressing there for him. And he's a nice guy, not crazy, a very reliable worker. You know, this is the kind of case you see in private practice. They *potchkeh* around. But if you get one, you've got him for twenty years."

"His own doctor has had him for almost twenty years," the resident says.

"See? But he was doing better when he was able to work. His retirement was the worst thing that could have happened. A weird family. Get him a job as a volunteer at Bellevue. He's better than most. He has a tremendous amount of ego strength. He's still holding his own, without any loss of reality. He's an unhappy baby and has been all his life. He must have been very scared when he tried to choke his wife."

The resident nods. "You could make a movie about *him,*" he says softly to a doctor sitting next to him, "starring Don Rickles."

"It must have been a shocking business for him, his most desperate cry. A scream of rage, of being ignored for years," the senior psychiatrist says. "He didn't attempt to justify it. Didn't talk about hearing voices. He apologizes. She didn't deserve it. And children would have meant competition for him. Oy! Do you know what I'm trying to invent? A tit that squirts Coca-Cola for guys like him. Any questions?"

The psychiatrist dashes out; the others disperse.

After a diet Dr Pepper lunch Berger is back on the phone. He calls the Aberdeen to find out how Johnny Rogers is doing. The word is favorable, nothing to worry about now. He gets a call from the Vietnam veteran's unhinged wife; he tells her that her husband will be released tomorrow. She can't decide if she's glad or sad about the news. While Berger talks to her, the resident on the case stands next to him and whispers, "She makes him angry."

Berger cups the phone and says, "That's what family therapy is for. Work on it."

As soon as Berger puts the phone down, the ward clerk, an

experienced, tough woman who has held the job for years, struts in. His residents, she says vehemently, must do a better job filling out patient records. Berger tells her that the patient load makes paperwork suffer, but he assures her that efficiency is just around the corner. She is skeptical, but doesn't want to pursue the conversation.

A patient arrives to see Berger. He's discussed her case with the resident working with her and wants to find out what he can for her. She is Elaine Green, a 65-year-old woman. She's lived on welfare for years. A few days ago, she took a pint of wine, thirty 5-mg. Valiums and some sleeping pills, made a unique broth of it all and drank it. She fell asleep, and when she awoke, miraculously, she felt ready to go to Bellevue.

She had been living in what she called a "fleabag hotel" on Ninth Avenue, before that in a desolate apartment in the Bronx. She learned to live "with bedbugs, roaches, pushers and drunks." She didn't know if her last husband, in a string of five or possibly six, was alive or dead. She hadn't seen him in years. A gentle, coherent, large and motherly woman, with thick gray hair, glasses, and wearing a demure print dress, she sits back, relaxed, and tells her story to Berger.

She started drinking at the age of 15, Scotch. She was married at the same age to a man three times her age, a lawyer. She remembers that "We had champagne for breakfast. Those were the days." She drank a quart of Scotch every day for twenty years. Then the money ran out and she went to beer, then to cheap wine.

"But I've never been drunk," she insists.

"I have a daughter who is forty-six and a son who's twenty-five. I see them when I go to see them. It's a long trip and it's expensive and I won't ask them for carfare. I write to them."

Berger encourages her to tell him more about her life.

Fifteen years ago, she was sent to a state hospital. "Mother and I had a verbal row. And Mother said I threatened to kill her. I just *wished* her dead, that's all, and said every mean thing I could think of."

She remembers being in a private sanitarium when she was 20, for drinking; her mother placed her there. She says she has not had any trouble in fifteen years, not until this year.

"I was vaguely unhappy with the way I was living and I saw a doctor. He thought I had lost too much too quickly. My son got married, my mother died and my dog died and I couldn't pay my rent."

Berger asks her about suicide.

"I don't see anything wrong with suicide. A person has that right. The pills I took didn't kill me and I'm glad they didn't. I just fell asleep. But, you know, all my friends have died or moved. I was desperate. I had nothing to eat. I was dispossessed by Welfare. Not one check arrived for weeks. I went down there and tried to find out. No luck. I wonder how many people commit suicide because of how Welfare treats them."

"You're right about that," Berger says. What other problems has she had?

"Well, I've been taking Dexedrine for thirty years. Fifteen mg. once a day. It's the best drug ever invented."

Berger leans forward in his chair. He is surprised. The resident had not known about the woman's Dexedrine habit.

"I do feel that I did a damned fool thing. But it did some good things for me. I've decided to become a Roman Catholic. I have met this wonderful doctor here who has given me hope, inspiration and cheer."

Berger suggests she might want a room at the Aberdeen.

"I hope I can live there, because I've heard that they don't have troublemakers there. But I do need my Dexedrine."

"Not from us," Berger says.

"Well, then, there goes my food money."

"It's expensive on the street now."

Mrs. Green smiles at him knowingly. She seems to know how to get her pills when she needs them.

"Let's make sure that Welfare doesn't screw up again. They almost killed you. Before that, you survived plenty of trouble without wanting to kill yourself."

"I can get a job as a cook and go up to Needle Park," she tells Berger, calmly, confidently. "After all these years, Dexedrine can't hurt me."

"It's hard to pep up on no money," Berger tells her, "but we can talk again soon about that."

Mrs. Green gets up, still a proud woman, and walks gracefully out of Berger's office.

As she leaves and disappears into the corridor, Berger sighs, "Jesus, a sixty-five-year-old speed freak!" He doesn't have much time now to think about that. A resident, a social worker and a patient are waiting to see him. They file into his office.

The patient is a 50-year-old Peruvian-born woman, married, with two married daughters. She entered Bellevue a month ago, when her husband sent her to the Psychiatric Admitting Office after she had withdrawn and had not eaten for a week.

Today she seems composed, friendly, tells Berger she is feeling better.

Berger asks her if she's ever had a problem like this before. Never. What does she think about what happened?

"You know, as you grow older you do go through change of life. You get nervous," she says. She is placid, composed, able to relax. An attractive woman, she is well dressed, clean, friendly.

"Do you remember feeling sad?" Berger asks.

"No."

"Did you have trouble sleeping?"

"Yes, a little bit."

"For how long?"

"Months."

"Do you remember feeling bad in the morning?"

"I feel good all day. I keep busy. I shop. I cook. I like to relax. Then I can work better."

"Do you sleep okay on the ward?"

"Well, I have some trouble. The noise keeps me awake."

"Do you drink?"

"Beer makes you fat. Whiskey does, too. I like tea and coffee. Coffee is my thing."

"Remember that you couldn't remember things when you first got here?"

"I did feel strange. It was hard to adjust."

"Scared?"

"No. It just wasn't like sleeping in my own bed."

"You want to go home?"

"I'm waiting for my doctor to tell me," she says, smiling at the resident.

"Something brought you here. You were different then," Berger says.

"I know I was wearing the wrong dress for here. I wasn't expecting to go out in a long dress. I didn't even know I was going out."

Berger tests her memory, her perception, with several verbal tests. Can she define a proverb? Yes, she does, with relative

ease. Can she repeat a story he tells exactly as he tells it to her?
Not so well. Berger stares at her. She is smiling at him.

"You'll be getting a weekend pass," he tells her.

"Fine," she says, getting up and walking out. When she's
gone, the resident tells Berger that she had paranoid delusions
for a week preceding her admission. When she arrived, she
wasn't making any sense. A brain-scan test seemed to indicate
"decreased uptake, left side," an abnormality that can indicate
a minor stroke. There is a tic on the left side of her face, almost
inconspicuous. Other tests are being done.

She is not hysterical, Berger says, and she does have some
classic menopausal symptoms, including the kind of fear that
can pose as paranoia.

"I agree," the resident says. "Maybe she needs tincture of
time, along with some support from us."

The meeting breaks up on that note. There's another ward
community meeting. Again Berger presides, but the patients
are the speakers.

An old, dignified black man insists that patients should pick
up their own dishes and bring them to the kitchen after meals.
A second man agrees with him. A third says that it must be done
in an orderly fashion or the kitchen will be in chaos.

The chubby woman is scribbling poems on a pad. She reminds the staff that she fought for Kool-Aid instead of ice water
at the last meeting. "Now I ain't gettin' either one," she says,
laughing.

One patient wants the dormitory doors left open during the
afternoon, for naps. Another wants them closed, because someone has been mussing up his bed after he makes it in the morning.

One man whispers to another. The latter speaks for him:
patients shouldn't put out their cigarettes on the floor. It makes
a mess.

An old woman, withered and deluded, turns to a young black
man in a large Afro and asks him for a cigarette. "I'll pay you
back," she snarls. "You don't have to give it back, Momma," he
says, a wide smile on his face.

Berger's old friend from the Aberdeen wants everyone to
know that she knows that someone is carving up the soap in the
women's bathroom, and throwing it into the toilets. "What the
hell are they trying to do?" she asks. "Make a boat?"

When the meeting ends, Berger tells the staff, at a brief conference, that it was "a healthy meeting, less psychotic." One of his clinic patients is sitting in the hall, waiting for him. He is chatting with a nurse until Berger sees him. "I'm too sick to work. I'm a nut," he says to the nurse. Berger clasps his hand, puts his arm around his shoulder and leads him into his office. The patient is young and deranged, managing, barely, to exist outside the hospital after several stays within it. Berger continues to keep an eye on him.

After their session, Berger could go home. He won't. Tonight he must lead a group therapy session of discharged patients from NO-6. Familiar faces, familiar psychoses, unpredictable behavior. It may keep him at Bellevue until 8 P.M. After that, and the drive home, he can have the first solid food of the day, and a glimpse of his children before they go to bed.

The case of the teen-age Haitian girl, begun yesterday at the teaching conference, continues on Thursday. Ken Kirshbaum attends, as usual.

Her case, the psychiatrist in charge says, is one of moralism versus materialism. The girl's mother is middle-class and moralistic, which leads her to deny, or fail to recognize, her daughter's feelings. Tempted by materialism, the girl is caught in a value struggle and is saddened and depressed by it.

"Her view, in extreme, is polarized. She will kill herself or kill her father. That value problem is common to adolescents. In this case, she chooses the same sort of man her mother chose, sees herself unhappily married as her mother was, and fears the future."

From the age of 2 to 5, he points out, she lived without her mother or father around regularly. "She must have felt rejection and accumulated her anger later. Also, she was unable to choose between the models set by her parents. Her father was excessively strict, while her mother was passive."

According to him, "We must assume that her relationship with her father was mutually seductive, judging by the men she sees now. Her hostility toward her mother was another component. She's more like her father, but her expectations resemble her mother's."

One of the residents says that it is extremely common for parents to be blind to their children's behavior until it is too late. This girl, he says, has a neurotic conflict with familiar symptoms, a depressed achiever, the sort of person who feels worthless.

She seems motivated for treatment, another resident points out. She did show up at the clinic on her own.

The presiding psychiatrist suggests that her dreams be studied, that her conflict be discussed with her, that she be made to understand the dependency-anger-self-image-rejection pattern. Her choice of men, her confusion over ideals are signs, he says. "Find out what is behind them. And when you do, remember that she will need support in order to verbalize her fears."

A resident uses the term "blame" in assigning responsibility to her parents for her plight. "You can't blame the father, the mother or the daughter for that moment that led the father to attempt incest. Legally, the father is guilty. Psychiatrically, it is far more complex," the psychiatrist says.

In his opinion, he continues, the mother is more central to the girl's problem than the father. It is imperative to get the mother into treatment, too. When the daughter is 18, she shouldn't simply flee. For best results, mother and daughter should be treated, to salvage that important relationship. "The prognosis for the girl, with intervention, is good," he concludes.

Kirshbaum goes to visit his clinic supervisor, a short, plump woman with clipped brown hair. She is middle-aged, wears a prim yellow dress trimmed in lace, and harlequin glasses.

Kirshbaum has come to see her to discuss a case that he finds elusive. The patient is a middle-aged woman who first came in to see him to tell him she felt she was losing control of her emotions at home. She's fine at work, but her relationship with her husband is strained. He has been bedridden, and her dependent needs are being exchanged for his, which has unnerved her. Her life needs organizing, and if her husband is too sick to do it, or does it in an overbearing way, she would prefer that Kirshbaum do the organizing for her.

"Something is not kosher there," the supervisor says.

Kirshbaum recites the story, in detail, and the supervisor interrupts with her own comments:

"Look at how damned hostile she is without even recognizing it."

"She doesn't think that any of her nastiness is showing."

"Ken, you must ask for clarification."

"She'll slip through your fingers all the time unless you are concrete with her."

"On account of you," she says to Kirshbaum in a motherly way, "she can be hostile to her husband and you get the blame. You're going to be used that way. She wants you to believe that she's taking care of the whole world.

"With this patient, stay with the here and now. Don't go plumbing. She is so concrete. A thinking disturbance. She is showing you she can't abstract. So don't you do it either. Watch her. I'm beginning to think you must be more direct with her without telling her what to do. Pull together what she says. Don't tell her to leave her husband or to stay. I'm ready to say she has psychotic breaks, minute thought breaks. She is not all there. Localize her. Structure her. If you dive in, she'll give you a rationalization or she'll get sick as hell."

Kirshbaum, enrapt, listens. It is advice he needed to deal with the patient. He is grateful. When he gets up to leave, the supervisor wants to talk to him about a case that's troubling her.

One of the residents she advises has a suicidal patient. She's discussed the case with the resident and is worried. The patient, Maureen Barnes, is a 29-year-old woman, will be 30 within a few days and has threatened to commit suicide on her thirtieth birthday. She has told the resident how she plans to do it: pills and slashing her wrists. What to do? The supervisor thinks the woman should be hospitalized immediately.

"You can't keep her in forever, of course," she says, "and we know that she has slashed herself before and taken an overdose. If she lives, the resident can enter her delusion, tell her the birthday has passed, the signs of death are gone, and try to help her. But waiting is a risk. I say call the guards," she says. Kirshbaum shares her concern; he'll think about it.

He doesn't have time to linger, however. He walks briskly to meet with the psychiatrist who ran the morning's teaching conference; he wants to talk to him about an adolescent he's treating, again a search for informed advice.

It is the teen-age Puerto Rican boy who has threatened his family with a knife. Kirshbaum tells the psychiatrist that the boy is "destructive, aggressive without an awareness of the consequences. The mother is a chronic paranoid-schizophrenic. The boy has no impulse control. If he gets angry, he acts. He can't read well and has trouble with simple math. When I asked him to subtract seven from a hundred, he said, 'Ninety-eight.' He sits in the chair, numbly, and doesn't speak unless he has to. He has few friends. They've treated him in Medicine, for asthma and fainting spells. I just don't see the potential here for long-term, insight-oriented treatment. This kid doesn't have the resources to deal with intensive treatment."

The psychiatrist asks if there's been a neurological work-up done on the boy.

"Yes, two years ago. And psychological tests three years ago. He could have an organic problem, I suppose."

"He must have trouble in school. If not, if he can control his behavior, you've got to explore that. Find out more about his life at home." He urges more tests, a call to the boy's school. "You know, maybe he'd be better for one of our activity therapy groups than for individual therapy."

Kirshbaum tells him he'll do more checking and will talk with him about the boy again soon. He heads to Medicine to do a consult on a ward patient with a psychiatric history.

If Lanie Eagleton sits at home listening to Noel Coward records, reading Hemingway or watching *Gunsmoke* reruns, no one at Bellevue knows about it. At Bellevue, Eagleton is all business. For him, the work ethic dominates. Since the Chest Service is not filled with life-or-death emergencies, Eagleton's methodical style, however unlike Marcus Welby's, is appropriate. There is more hard work on the Chest Service than there is excitement, and Eagleton prospers on hard work.

This morning he got up early, to do a bronchoscopy at 8 A.M. He is stifling a yawn when he gets to the 9 A.M. staff conference, but perks up immediately when he studies the X-rays on display.

A young, bearded, intense resident presents the morning's cases. The first is a former coal miner, "a Polish gentleman who is eighty years old. His respiratory system has deteriorated over the past few months."

Staring at the X-rays, Eagleton points out that "if his condition is chronic, it could be a tumor. If it's acute, it could be one of a number of things."

The second patient is a 41-year-old woman who had been Eagleton's 8 A.M. appointment. She claims to have had asthma since she was one year old, says she had a lung operation at age 15. "Her trachea looks good to me," Eagleton says. "Her bronchi are small, bilaterally. Some edema. Looks like a very extensive pleural disease, but she can't give us a good history. She just remembers taking an antibiotic for a year once, but no accompanying antituberculous drug."

At the end of the conference, he announces that there will be a meeting with delegates from Surgery this afternoon, to resolve possible surgery on several patients, one of them Sarah Morgan, the psychiatry patient. Eagleton thinks she has a tumor and he supports surgery. The surgeons think she might have an enlarged pulmonary artery and are reticent. Yesterday, Eagleton has found out, she had a pulmonary angiogram, a test that involves injecting dye into the pulmonary artery and under fluoroscopy watching it flow from the pulmonary artery to the vessels of the lungs. The results, and the possible debate, will highlight the afternoon conference.

As they all move out of the meeting, Eagleton is preoccupied by the case of the psychiatry patient. He talks to a resident about it. "She's been tested exhaustively," he says, "for tumors elsewhere in her body. The single lung tumor may not be cancerous, but as I see it, it is an abnormality justifying surgery." He hopes to convince the surgeons.

A group of residents tags along as Eagleton walks through the wards. The patients are, for the most part, old men and women. Many of them are alcoholics. There are few young patients. The problem, as Eagleton explains it to the residents, is that the service does not get its patients soon enough.

"We should see the sick at an earlier age, not wait until they're clearly ill," he says. "What good does it do to wait until someone is terminally ill? If you can admit a patient earlier, the stay is shorter and you do the person more good."

Eagleton doesn't need rhetoric to make his point. He halts in front of a bed. In it is a gaunt man in his fifties, an alcoholic. He is getting a 5 percent dextrose solution IV and has a drain in his side. His skin contains the shadows of years of dirt. The nurse on duty is attempting to instruct him in the use of a toothbrush and mouth wash, but the man is not paying attention to her.

"I've come to change the tubes at Buckingham Palace," Eagleton tells the nurse. The patient is draining pus into bottles, via an Emerson postoperative pump, an electronic machine which draws out the fluid which has passed from the man's lung, through a large hole, into the pleural space. The lung has partially collapsed.

On hearing Eagleton's announcement, the man begins to grimace and groan. "What hurts you?" the nurse asks. The man does not answer. He has been sedated, to combat the DTs, which can in itself be fatal. In alcoholics, the use of sedation can ease withdrawal, controlling it within a week.

Two nurses lift the man from his bed and put him into a chair-toilet. "Have your bowel movement while you're sitting down," one of the nurses tells him. His face shows pain.

Eagleton replaces the tubes and bottles with a new set. Throughout the process, the patient is unquestioning. As Eagleton leads the procession of residents out of the ward, he tells one of them that he's not optimistic. In the old days, a man in such shape probably would have died. Today therapy and time can be effective, but this man is "full of infection and is not in good physical condition. He won't heal, I'd guess." As Eagleton leaves the room, he can hear an intern talking to a nurse nearby. "The guy is getting woy-ser and woy-ser and woy-ser," the intern is chanting. The man, like so many others Eagleton has seen, may go right back to drink and neglect.

"Does that frustrate you?" a resident asks Eagleton.

"I've managed to forget moral judgments like that," he answers. "If we get an alcoholic with a disease, we treat his illness. If we succeed and he goes back to drink, I can't allow myself to care. I once did, but now I must patch my own sense of morality just as I patch our patients."

It is time for lunch.

In the doctors' cafeteria, Eagleton shares a table with doctors from other services; he doesn't know them. A young woman resident says, "I'm having so much trouble with the nurses. They get snappy and I get snappy, too." She sighs. She doesn't want trouble with the nurses. Two residents from Africa, bearded, whisper to each other and laugh. A prominent psychiatrist, surrounded by residents, does not speak to them. He glares at his meal, hastily downs his food, preoccupied. The room is full of young men with long hair and beards, in white jackets, and women with long straight hair and white jackets.

The 3 P.M. surgical conference on the Chest Service is well attended. Eighteen doctors fill the Chest Service library, including residents and attendings from both Surgery and Chest. Several cases are presented. Lanie Eagleton listens.

A first-year resident in Medicine is there to present his own case, a 78-year-old white woman with a mass in her left lower lung. All studies so far are negative for other causes, so the resident assumes it is cancer. He has ten X-rays on the viewer.

The surgeons seem willing to operate, using the fastest possible procedure to "wedge it out," as one surgeon indicates. The resident from Medicine is worried about the patient's ability to withstand surgery at her age. "True. She could outlive her tumor," says one of the Chest Service attendings.

"Look at it; if you want her operated on, we'll operate," says a senior surgeon, an attending who looks like a former football player. Dr. John McClement, the chief of the Chest Service, adds his voice: "It is possible that cancer in old patients can be less malignant, that the patient can live on without surgery."

The surgeon, growing increasingly interested in the case and his role in it, points out that such an operation can be done in less than two hours "if the mass isn't too tricky to reach." He decides to see the patient himself before making a final decision.

A Chest Service resident presents the second case: an alcoholic in his fifties who was brought to the Emergency Ward by the police. There is a cavity in the man's lung visible on X-rays. He is not close to death, but he may be a candidate for a pneumonectomy (removal of part, or all, of a lung). The surgeon is willing but not enthusiastic; he suggests trying to heal the man's lung with anti-TB therapy first, waiting a month and reconsidering surgery then. "Looks to me like a rupture of a tuberculous cavity into the pleura," Dr. McClement says. The consensus is to wait and see.

Eagleton presents Sarah Morgan's case. A routine X-ray revealed a lesion, he points out. Extensive tests didn't show much more than that, the presence of the mass. Eagleton is literal, unemotional; he wants to convince the surgeons to do exploratory surgery. She is a prematurely old woman, sad and lost, and he does not want her to succumb to the miseries of her psyche *and* the pain of her body.

The surgeons stare at Eagleton while he runs down the case. One of Surgery's chief residents is there. He is not convinced by Eagleton's presentation.

"Explore or not explore? Risk or no risk? That's our choice.

I want someone to tell me there is something there," he says. An attending surgeon, older than the others in the room, says, "I get the impression that there *is* something there, but I can't tell if it is marginal."

Eagleton admits, under questioning, that the lesion is the only one he could find. But, he suggests tactfully, that may be enough. He does not push his opinion, become aggressive.

"I suppose," one of the surgeons says, "that it should be considered as carcinoma until proved otherwise."

The husky surgeon indicates that "We could operate without seriously inconveniencing her, to see if this is nothing, if it is her pulmonary artery, if it is cancer. If it is cancer, we can expand the surgery immediately to pneumonectomy, not waste any time, go right ahead, if that's appropriate. If it is a case of doing something or doing nothing, I'm inclined to have a look."

That opinion is the crucial one. The room is now silent. A resident's wristwatch alarm goes off; he jumps out of his chair. The others laugh. The surgeons will "have a look" at Sarah Morgan's lesion. When the conference ends, Eagleton calls Dr. Berger in Psychiatry, to tell him that it looks like the surgeons will cut into Mrs. Morgan.

One prolonged event dominates Diane Rahman's day in Obstetrics. It is the case of Jenny James, the teen-age black girl who had left school when her membranes ruptured and had come to Bellevue for help.

When Rahman gets to the ward, she is told that, overnight, there were signs of fetal distress. When Jenny had contractions, the fetal heartbeat slowed. The contractions were minor, insufficient, complicating matters, and Jenny had a slight fever, indicating the presence of infection.

At 8:30 A.M., Jenny is moved into one of the labor rooms and is hooked up to a fetal monitor. In the labor-delivery area, a feeling of tension is accumulating. Doctors confer.

The consensus is that the team of residents on duty will have to be ready to do a Caesarean section. As the residents discuss the facts of the case, Jenny is screaming, in pain. A nurse urges her to stop shouting, to breathe deeply. She is given oxygen. A blood sample is taken and speeded off for analysis. On the IV pole beside her bed there is a handwritten sign: "Upon delivery, please call her mother." A phone number is listed.

Rahman goes to Jenny's bedside. She repeats "Easy," softly, over and over, hugging the girl. The fetal monitor is beeping. A nurse comes in, to shave Jenny's pubic hair. While she's doing it, Jenny screams again, then sighs, "I'm sorry. Really, I'm sorry."

The chief resident is concerned. She goes to a nearby phone and, with Rahman on an extension, calls Jenny's mother.

"Your daughter ruptured her bag of water," she tells the mother. "But she hasn't gone into labor. She had a fever last night. We had to stimulate labor, but now she's having labor on her own. But the baby is suffering inside. Maybe the umbilical cord is around the baby. We don't know. We want to do a Caesarean, but we need your approval. Dr. Rahman is on another phone to witness it. Okay? Fine. Thank you very much."

Within less than twenty-four hours, it has become clear that Jenny's natural contractions won't be enough. An IV Pitocin drip was tried, to induce birth before any infection spread, but when the fetal heartbeat slowed with each contraction, the drug was discontinued. When she was taken off the drug, Jenny's contractions slowed down.

The chief resident is edgy, pacing. A nurse reminds her that when the mother arrives, she must sign a form approving the Caesarean. The chief resident assembles a crew of nurses and tells them to scrub for a Caesarean. "Have everything ready," she tells them.

She's still not convinced that a Caesarean is the proper choice. Cutting means risks and assures future Caesareans, too. And fetal monitors are not always definitive. She decides to try Pitocin again; either it will quickly accelerate the contractions or it won't. If it doesn't, a Caesarean will be done. "We'll have to move fast," she says to Rahman, who has remained near her, to do whatever must be done.

The fetal monitor continues its beeping. The baby's heart is beating. However, the range is disturbing, from a relatively satisfactory 120 beats per minute to a troublesome 60. In normal births, the heartbeat can slow down during a contraction, but resumes its rapid pace once the contraction is over. Not so in this case. If the heartbeat remains at a low level, there is danger. The chief resident is undecided. She phones an attending physician for help.

Rahman returns to Jenny, who is complaining of feeling "tingly."

"You're breathing much too fast, so you're feeling tingly all over. If I breathed that fast, I'd feel tingly, too," Rahman tells her.

A nurse injects ampicillin, an antibiotic to fight the infection. Jenny screams, howls wildly. More Pitocin is administered.

It is 9 A.M.

The African resident arrives and quickly changes into a scrub suit. The anesthetist arrives, followed by the anesthesiologist. Jenny's screams echo through the hall. Rahman examines her.

"Her cervix is dilated, but not enough," she tells the other residents.

Jenny shrieks.

"When you scream like that, the baby's heart goes down," a nurse says. "Just breathe," she tells her.

At this moment, a patient arrives to see Rahman in a nearby examination room.

"I'm here for an abortion," she says. Apparently, she has managed to bypass the abortion clinic. She is sloppily dressed and is covered with a thin film of dirt.

"There just aren't any beds available on the ward today," Rahman tells her.

"Jesus. It ain't easy for me to find a baby-sitter to get down here," the woman says, irritated.

"I suggest you see someone in Social Services. They'll help you with that. And give me a call in two days, for a bed."

The woman pivots without answering and, cursing, plows down the corridor toward the elevator.

Rahman returns to Jenny. The Pitocin doesn't seem to be effective. The flow is cut off; the contractions slow immediately. An epidural needle is placed in Jenny's lower back, ready to provide anesthesia if the Caesarean goes forward. The chief resident phones for blood-test results, for signs of infection. They're not ready yet. She is frustrated, nervous. Two residents and a medical student study Jenny's X-rays. At 9:35, the mother arrives.

The chief resident takes the mother aside and tries to explain what's going on. She tells her that there is need for an epidural because they don't want to use general anesthesia for fear of harming the baby, already in a "stress situation." The mother nods, her face a blank.

The phone rings. It is the senior resident, whose presence comforts Rahman. He hopes to be there soon, but his car has had a flat tire. He'll do his best to rush. Another phone call: the attending the chief resident called minutes before says he may not be able to get there in time. "We may have to go in quickly, in minutes," the chief resident tells him.

At 9:50, the senior resident arrives; he changed the tire himself. While the doctors assemble in Jenny's room, another woman, whose membranes ruptured at twenty-eight weeks, is moved into an adjoining room.

The anesthetist tests the epidural. When it is needed, it must numb the body from the waist down. Jenny's mother watches, then kisses her daughter and walks out, to pace in the patients' recreation room on the ward itself. On a TV set at peak volume, a doctor in a soap opera is melodramatically troubled by his wife's illness.

"The fetal heartbeat is holding steady at 130," the African resident announces.

The delivery room is ready. Only sealed packages of sterile instruments remain to be opened. However, Jenny's labor has slowed. So does the pace of those involved in her case.

At 10:10, her temperature is taken: 98. The infection may be under control.

The phone rings again. The attending hopes to arrive in twenty minutes; he asks that everyone be scrubbed and prepared. A few minutes later, a second attending arrives; he calls the first and tells him not to bother. The chief resident is happy to see the attending; she explains the case to him. He talks to Jenny's mother, then, at 10:45, he decides to wait, again to attempt to induce labor. The Pitocin drip is resumed. It is the last chance for a conventional delivery. There is evidence that the cervix is dilating increasingly.

At 11 A.M., the chief resident decides to wait for some sign of fetal distress on the monitor—a slowdown of the heartbeat—or a failure to go into labor, fully, within an hour. Then she'll make the decision. If the baby's life is at stake, she'll do a Caesarean. A nurse checks Jenny's blood pressure and temperature (99). Jenny's contractions resume, more frequently. She is screaming again: "I don't want this. I can't take it."

At 11:15, Rahman examines her again. She is responding to Pitocin and the fetal heartbeat is sound. "It may be a case of the fetus leaning on the umbilical cord, then sliding off of it," the chief resident theorizes.

Nurses and residents are encouraging Jenny to "push." She is screaming, almost incoherently, in pain. The chief resident is pacing, saying, "Patience. Wait. See. Give it time." Rahman reaches in to feel the fetal head.

"Whoever has to go to lunch, go to lunch," the chief resident says. She continues to pace, debating the merit of a Caesarean aloud.

"If the compression of the cord can be eased, perhaps, by letting the woman rest without encouraging contractions . . . But if improvement is not evident on the monitor and the labor is insufficient to expel the fetus, then . . ."

At 11:30, suddenly, the fetal heartbeat drops drastically, below 60 beats per minute. The doctors and nurses in the room watch the monitor, then quickly go into motion.

There is no time for anesthesia. Everything must be done in seconds. The contractions are working. Jenny's bed is wheeled into the delivery room. She is shouting again. The anesthetist and a Pediatrics intern come running down the hall. Everyone goes into the delivery room. Within seconds, Jenny gives birth, on her own.

It is a girl, small in size, with the umbilical cord draped around her shoulders. The cord may have been tight and loosened later. It is impossible to know now. The baby is not breathing properly; oxygen is given. The baby is given antibiotics, to avoid the possibly lethal danger of respiratory infection. A placenta culture is rushed to the lab. The baby is taken to the Premature Unit in Pediatrics, listed as "critical."

Jenny is taken to a nearby room, to recover. The doctors straggle out of the delivery room.

"I didn't hear anything for fifteen to twenty seconds. Not a heartbeat," Rahman tells the senior resident. He shrugs.

Diane Rahman's afternoon is anticlimactic after the furious pace and tension of the morning. The birth of Jenny's daughter has drained Rahman. She gets through the afternoon, preoccupied by the events of the morning, and falls into bed at 8 P.M.

In GYN, Bob Nachtigall has the feeling that today may be free of astonishment, full of ritual. After an easy night—only a rape case in the AES—he's on the GYN wards at 8 A.M., making rounds, moving from patient to patient, asking questions, looking at notes taken by the night nursing staff, examining patients.

In checking a batch of charts, Nachtigall notices that a nurse's aide has indicated "20" as the respiration rate for all the patients. Nachtigall wonders if she ever bothered to check the rates at all. He suspects that someone once told her that 20 was normal. He summons a nurse and raises the matter, adding, "I have only a slightly greater confidence that the temperatures are right."

Beside the bed of the woman who wants to go home to allow her husband to return to his job—he's been caring for their newborn child while the mother has been battling a post-partum infection—Nachtigall sees a note on her chart, a note from the chief resident. The chief examined the woman last night; she can go home today. Nachtigall is pleased; it is an endorsement of his judgment.

Back in GYN, he's confronted by a rape victim sent up from the AES. He's seen many of them. He does not treat them casually. After he examines this one, he talks to a medical student about it.

"They come in invariably upset, but most of them are outwardly composed. Most of them have stories about being out with a guy, willingly, and having it get out of hand. Just incredibly poor judgment in men, some of the time. Occasionally, one has had the shit beat out of her, but many of them have been driven home after the rape.

"I don't like to come on like the stern doctor with them. I tell them that I'm sorry I have to do this, but it is a legal matter. I try to get their stories without doing that awful number, 'And then what happened? . . . And then?' The cops are often sort of asensitive. They don't abuse the women or laugh at them, but they're thankful when I'm done and they can get the hell out.

"My job is to check for signs of violence, forced entry and the presence of sperm. The truth is that a woman with half a brain won't resist. A vagina is tough. It'll take a baby's head. So I've never really seen what might be called forced entry, severe lacerations. I do a thing when I have a rape case to check. I remind myself what it might be like if I found myself in prison. I wouldn't last fifteen minutes untouched and that's a terrifying thought. Think of it this way. A woman is raped by a man and brought by other men to a male doctor. He shoves a metal cock, a speculum, into her, recapitulating it all. I suspect they must think, 'Here it goes again.'

"I look for sperm, but it doesn't prove rape. The only real service I can perform is to give pills to prevent VD and morning-after birth control pills.

"It's a legal problem with plenty of psychiatric overtones. These women need medication, not an elaborate and horrifying work-up.She needs another woman to talk to, to get out her anger and her frustration. It is a helpless feeling, like being pinned down by a bully when you're a small boy."

The medical student has not interrupted Nachtigall's monologue. When it is done, Nachtigall shuffles through some papers. One abortion case has been admitted; three others, expected in today, have canceled. Nachtigall remembers that he is on duty tonight and is due in the operating room in the morning.

A young woman stalks into the GYN examining room while Nachtigall is there. She walks up to another resident and says, "Listen to me. *Listen.* I have to have this abortion today. I said *today.* Or he'll beat me to death. We have sex all the time and we don't want any kids." The resident asks for more information. Nachtigall eavesdrops. She tells the resident that the man she lives with is 65 years old. She appears to be in her twenties. The resident suggests that she come back tomorrow for a full examination. Reluctantly, she agrees. As she leaves, one of the nurses says, "Wow! I wish *my* husband was like that."

As the woman leaves, another enters. She is tall, good-looking, chic, black. She has been sent to GYN by the receptionist in the main waiting room at Bellevue, by mistake.

"I've got this terrible pain in my stomach," she tells the resident. Nachtigall is still on the phone, waiting for a lab report; he watches the black woman as she squirms in front of the other resident. He explains to her that he can't treat her until she goes to the AES and is admitted; if she's got a GYN problem, then he can take care of it. Or she can go to the GYN clinic.

"It's a rule," he says.

"Let me get somethin' straight, baby," she says, her anger rising. "You are tellin' me that I have to go through all that bureaucratic bullshit even though I'm in pain and that pain might just get worse?"

"Exactly," the resident says. He is not intimidated by her.

She does an about-face and stomps off.

The resident turns to a medical student and says, "Let me tell you about the red tape at Bellevue. And you pay good attention to me."

For Nachtigall, it's been a quiet day. He hopes it will be a quiet night, too.

Over coffee, the night-duty resident reports to Bruce Mack about developments and Mack reports them to Dr. Randt at their morning meeting. The middle-aged woman who was rushed from the EW to Neuroradiology for an angiogram went downhill rapidly. The angiogram was done; it indicated extensive bleeding, a large clot, a large aneurysm, swelling and distortion of the brain. The neurosurgeons couldn't operate on her. At 8 P.M., she had a cardiac arrest and died.

The prisoner from the city jail who had attempted suicide was unruly, disruptive, he insisted he did not want his head wound sutured. The resident on duty gave him Valium and summoned a Psych consult. The Psychiatry resident told the Neurology resident that Psych wouldn't accept the man with an unsutured wound. The two doctors agreed that they would await secondary healing of the wound—healing itself without stitches—before taking any further action. The patient was transferred to the prison ward, from which he can go to Psych or back to jail.

During the early morning hours, police brought an attempted suicide into the AES. The Neuro resident told Mack that the man had jumped onto the subway tracks in the path of a train. He was hit, but, miraculously, was not killed or even seriously injured. He suffered a head trauma, but no brain damage. He will lose several fingers and one of his feet was lacerated. "He looked a mess," the resident reported to Mack. Mack, in turn, tells the story to Randt.

"I remember a similar case," Randt tells Mack, "in which an accident victim was examined by a resident who noted 'He's a mess' on the man's chart. Later, that resident had to go to court to explain that seemingly flippant notation." Randt asks Mack to tell the resident to insert only specific medical information on patients' charts.

After his meeting with Randt, Mack has an hour to work on

his paper. He shuts the door to his office and writes until 10:30, when the Neurology residents stroll in for today's conference with the attending.

"I was called to see this guy in the AES," one of the residents tells Mack. "When I get there, I found this weird-looking guy who informs me that he's the King of Sardinia. Fine, I said, and I started to examine him. He stops me and tells me again that he's the King of Sardinia and tells me to show him some respect. You won't believe this, but I had to bow before he would let me examine him."

"The AES. Sure. I remember one day when I was there and they brought in this woman who seemed to have been beaten and sodomized," Mack says. "When they took off her clothes and turned her over, they saw written in Spanish on her behind the words 'THIS BELONGS TO LEFTY,' with an arrow pointing to her rectum."

The attending arrives, interrupting the exchange. The first case to be discussed is that of a 42-year-old black prisoner who has been in Bellevue for ten days after complaining of being dizzy and weak; he says it is the result of a beating he got from prison guards. Tests have been negative.

"No one is ever beaten in prison," the attending instructs the residents, sarcastically. "He fell down the stairs no doubt. They're always very slippery."

The attending checks an EEG done on the man, sees nothing disturbing and tells the resident on the case to discharge the man.

Another resident presents the second case on the agenda. Another prisoner, held in the hospital prison ward, killed his wife by stabbing her, then shot himself, not seriously, in the head. He has told the resident that he doesn't remember any of it, and denies being a drug addict or alcoholic. He insists he is an epileptic and adds, gratuitously, that he is "well read."

"He's certainly well read on epilepsy," the attending suspects.

All neurological tests on the man were negative. The resident thinks he is feigning a sensory defect, numbness on his left side, to avoid returning to prison.

"I doubt that temporal-lobe epilepsy is causing his aberrations," the attending says.

"The nurses say he's irritable," the resident offers.

"His wife certainly found that out," the attending says. "He probably planned to say someone killed his wife and then attacked him. He never thought that 'someone' wouldn't use both a knife and a gun."

"There's one good thing about him," the resident says. "He's the first patient I've had whose stockings I could take off without passing out from the smell."

The group leaves Mack's office for the EEG lab, to study several EEGs done on the patient.

Two early EEGs, analyzed by the attending, show a slight abnormality, nonspecific and minimal. "Not clinically significant," the attending says as he shuffles through the graphs. The latest one is normal.

Next stop: the prison ward. In the ward, a large cluttered room filled with beds and men in blue pajamas guarded by Department of Correction officers, the two patients are tracked down. The attending examines the prisoner who asserts that he was beaten by guards. He is tall and silent. He does not speak during the examination, which shows nothing of concern. The attending instructs the resident to discharge the man, which simply means authorizing his return to jail.

The wife-killer appears next, a stocky, overweight black man wearing aviator sunglasses. He complains immediately to the attending of a numbing sensation on the left side of his face, pain in his head and the fact that his left eye tears "for no emotional reason." The attending examines him thoroughly. He asks him to move his eyes; he studies the eyes closely. He tests sensitivity to pinpricks. He applies pressure to both of the patient's outstretched arms, lifting himself up in the process. The prisoner, proud of his strength, says, "I used to box. I'm obese now, but I'm still a little in shape."

"I used to run," the attending sighs, then dismisses the prisoner.

"The inconsistencies are obvious," he says to the residents.

"Is this hysteria or malingering? The findings certainly aren't indicative of anything organic. And it's hard to distinguish between hysteria and malingering at times." Whatever the case, the attending feels, there's little that can be done for him; he orders him discharged, too, back to prison.

The doctors disperse after their visit to the prison ward, the attending back to his private practice, the residents back to their chores on the wards and in the clinic.

Mack decides to forget about lunch. He can use the time to work on his case presentation. He finds an empty office with a typewriter, dumps his notes on the desk. He decides to pass up a Neuropathology conference this afternoon, because it could be dull and he needs the time. He puts a piece of paper into the typewriter and stares at it.

Several hours later Mack remembers that his wife must be double-parked in front of Bellevue, waiting for him. He runs down the stairs to the main floor. He has a day off tomorrow and he and his wife are taking advantage of the long weekend. Their luggage is in the trunk. They're driving to the New Jersey shore for a few days. It may take a day or two to rid his mind of the work and frustrations this week has brought, but he knows that it will all resume on Monday.

In Surgical Pathology, the interns and residents share copies of the *Times*. These tend to slow down the awakening process. Eugene Fazzini, at his small table and microscope, tries to counteract it.

Fazzini announces some of the cases to be considered this morning. Among them: a cyst in a pharyngeal wall, a pair of gall bladder specimens, an inflamed foreskin postcircumcision, a tissue sample from a hand, a lipoma of the neck, an appendix, two warts and an ovarian cyst.

Fazzini tells the group that the cyst in the pharyngeal wall was discovered in a woman who had swallowed a chicken bone and thought *that* was her only problem. The comment inspires several residents. They perk up. Another keeps reading the *Times*. Another glances hypnotically at a book, *The Baroque Concerto*, by A. J. B. Hutchings. Fazzini glares at the resident reading the paper; the resident is threatened and abandons the paper. To compensate for his faux pas, the resident asks a question about the cyst in the pharyngeal wall.

"I answered that before," Fazzini snarls. "When you were reading the *Times.*" His stance is that of the proud academician, reprimanding a lazy student.

Undaunted, Fazzini again tries to cut through the early morning fog. The resident reading *The Baroque Concerto* gently puts it down, his eyes on Fazzini.

Fazzini refers to the tissue from the hand. Two residents offer that it must be a burn.

"It looks like a second-degree burn, doesn't it?" Fazzini says. His size, his presence, his intelligence make him formidable. The residents nod approvingly.

"Well, it isn't," Fazzini says. "It's trauma. The guy was run over by a train." The rest of the residents are now alert, listening carefully.

The warts aren't warts at all, Fazzini tells them. They're papillomas from the breast of a nursing mother.

The ovarian cyst was discovered when the surgeons, removing an appendix, spotted it.

Fazzini goes through the slides, commenting, encouraging the residents and interns to reach their own conclusions.

One resident is in an adjoining area, flipping through Pathology reports in a file cabinet. When specimens are sent to Pathology by other services, they get prompt attention; the origin of the specimen and Pathology's evaluation of it are noted in a formal report.

For example, a 9-year-old girl stuck a "foreign body" into her ear and came to Bellevue. All such objects, once removed, must be forwarded to Pathology for study. This one was a peanut. Pathology, literal and accurate, recorded its analysis in a written report: "It consists of a bean-shaped nut in two halves with a single fragmented cavity."

The morning analysis of slides stretches almost to lunch. Eugene Fazzini has his snack, brought from home, and chats with the resident who has been delving into the Pathology reports file. Fazzini has scanned the *Times* and, checking his watch, realizes it is time to conduct a GI conference. He collects his illustrative material and walks over to the general hospital.

Fazzini takes his show on the road often in the course of the week. The expression is appropriate; his presentations are aspects of the teaching function at Bellevue and, at the same time, essential to the diagnostic process.

In the dark room filled with GI residents, the slides projected brightly seem like a series of abstract paintings. In fact, Fazzini has considered enlarging some of them and displaying them as art. The slides are of many colors, depending upon the stains used, and it is possible to produce hundreds of such slides from a single tissue specimen.

The conference ends in midafternoon and Fazzini returns to

his office. He finds a batch of mail waiting for him. It includes a small mailing tube containing slides; a small-town hospital wants his opinion on a serious case. There is a letter from a pathologist at a California university and a paper from a member of the Pathology department at another New York hospital.

Fazzini puts the slides onto the microscope and peers at them. Minutes go by. He shifts the slides around under the lens, looking for patterns, signs he can recognize and define. It takes time for a pathologist as skilled as Fazzini to come to a firm conclusion. It is sometimes possible to reach them quickly, but in many cases Fazzini's intense concentration and encyclopedic memory are what lead to a diagnosis.

By the time he's studied the slides to his own satisfaction, Fazzini's day at Bellevue is almost done. He writes a letter to the pathologist at the small-town hospital, giving his opinion. It was not difficult to reach; Fazzini has seen thousands of specimens. Theorizing is his discipline.

When Lori Chiarelli gets to the Emergency Ward, before 8 A.M., she confronts a weary resident, who has been up all night. He is the resident who initially treated the man with acute bacterial endocarditis and he has been following the case over many hours. He tells Chiarelli that the patient was taken upstairs for the cardiac catheterization, which confirmed the aortic valve problem. However, it was discovered that the man had diffuse intravascular coagulation (blood-clotting problems), and the surgeons were wary of operating, for fear of massive bleeding in the OR. The resident, speaking slowly, tells Chiarelli that he argued with the surgeons.

"Any delay would bring him closer to death, I told them," he says.

The surgeons prevailed. The patient was returned to the EW late last night. According to the resident, "We hit him with every drug we could find and he showed some improvement. There's a chance that he might make it, if he's still around when they're ready to do the surgery." There is bitterness in his voice. The patient, he tells Chiarelli, was moved out of the EW again, at 6 A.M., shifted to the Coronary Care Unit. The resident moves sluggishly toward the door, to get some sleep.

Chiarelli spots a notice on the EW bulletin board; several nurses are hosting a bring-your-own-bottle party tomorrow night. It supplements Bellevue parties, drinking sessions, usually at the end of the work week, held on various services. The hospital page will, from time to time, announce "liver rounds" on a specific ward; it is code for an off-duty respite.

Chiarelli surveys the ward and counts six male and three female patients. She walks the length of the ward, flipping through charts, transferring the information to the Board she maintains.

The hospital page announces that "there will be mass at 8:30 this morning in the Catholic chapel." There are chapels and chaplains for all the major faiths at Bellevue; patients and troubled relatives take advantage of them.

Medical residents have begun to drift into the EW. Eleven of them gather around the bed of the black man who came in with what doctors thought, initially, was kidney stones. They have done many tests on him and have emerged with a new diagnosis: cancer, evident in several organs. The man is 30.

There are two men, one black and one white, with stab wounds. Both were superficial wounds, so the surgeons could treat them in the EW; had there been severe blood loss or internal damage, they would have been taken to the OR.

A young woman with abdominal pain, fever and a rigid abdomen is visited by a GYN resident, who feels that she has PID, pelvic inflammatory disease. A black woman in her thirties took sleeping pills and chased them down with liquor. A middle-aged man with massive GI bleeding has been given units of blood all night.

There are three old people from the streets: an 82-year-old woman in a coma, an old man with pneumonia as well as likely TB, and an old man with fluid in his lungs and a fractured clavicle.

The woman in the coma is visited by a Neurology resident, who decides she isn't a Neuro patient but belongs to Medicine. "A toxic metabolic problem," he says.

The old man with pneumonia has a GU (genitourinary) complication. A medical resident discovers it when he tries to insert a Foley catheter into the man's penis. There is a block; the man's prostate is the size of a grapefruit.

The GI bleeder demands attention; several doctors confer at

the foot of his bed. He has a duodenal ulcer and rectal bleeding. He is getting phenobarbital, Maalox, penicillin and blood. Residents move in and out of the ward.

At 10:30, the ward is silent, except for the padded sound of the nurses' footsteps and the ubiquitous presence of the cardiac monitors' beeping.

The old man with the fractured clavicle is moved out, to a Medical ward.

A psychiatrist appears to interview the latest OD. It is the same woman resident who interviewed the Puerto Rican OD yesterday. She walks over to the woman's bedside and speaks softly to her. After several minutes, she confers with the Medical resident on the case and tells him, "She's not psychotic, but she is a terribly unhappy person who has cyclical depression. This was a serious attempt and I'd like to see her come to the clinic but that might take years. Maybe the best thing to do is to transfer her to Psych when she's stable here."

There is a mild commotion several beds away. Three residents and a nurse are struggling with the old man with pneumonia and the enlarged prostate. He squirms, bellows, grabs, claws, as they try to insert a tube into his nose, to drain his stomach. He is a spindly old man, but he has strength. His skinny legs, with toenails that seemingly haven't been cut in years, flail and he grabs a nurse's stethoscope and holds on. Eventually, the collective strength prevails and, despite his bleating, the tube is in place. His bed is wheeled to a GU lab for a cystoscopy, to discover what sort of obstruction exists in his urinary tract; it may be more than the enlarged prostate. To do that, the resident assigned to the case needs the man's written consent. They have not been on the best of terms while grappling over the tube. The resident puts a pen in the patient's hand, holds the hand while it traces an "X" on the permission form.

As the old man is wheeled out, there is a friendly but firm debate between the GYN resident and a surgical resident about a diagnosis on the young woman with abdominal rigidity and pain. The GYN resident defends his view that it's PID. The surgeon feels it may be an appendix close to rupturing, but he isn't sure. They agree to wait, to see if antibiotics effect a dramatic change. If they do, the gynecologist will win. If not, the surgeon can reserve OR time, to explore.

After lunch, Chiarelli continues her perpetual effort to keep her Emergency Ward records up to the minute. The mood is calm; the ward is silent.

In a split second, the mood and the silence are shattered.

Two residents come rushing in with a stretcher-bed, from the AES. It bears an old man in cardiac arrest. Quickly, residents and nurses surround the man. One doctor pumps his chest, another intubates him to facilitate breathing, a third takes a blood sample.

"We don't know anything about this man," an AES resident tells the others. "Nothing."

The man is given oxygen through a hand-held Ambu bag, pumped by a resident. A needle goes into the man's neck, for IV use later. The EKG is on; it reveals wildly irregular lines when the chest is pumped manually and a flat line when the pumping pauses.

"Excellent blood pressure," says one doctor.

"Good rhythm," says another.

"Somebody pump. Let's bang him well."

Chiarelli has the defibrillator ready. "Everybody away from the table," she says, and applies the two circular metal plates to the man's chest. Another nurse turns on the current, jolting the man with the sudden surge of power.

"Good pulse."

"We need another jolt."

Chiarelli tries again, but this time the machine doesn't work.

"Circuit breaker," she says. Another nurse rushes to the back of the unit, searching for it. Chiarelli finds it first, clicks it.

Another jolt hits the man. A blood-gas sample is rushed off for analysis. A catheter is inserted into the man's penis. A resident continues to pump the man's chest; he is alternating at it with another doctor, because the process can be exhausting.

While the group continues to work on the man, a police siren is heard approaching the driveway outside. The siren means trouble; it is kept on only when the case is a clear-cut emergency. Several EW nurses run outside.

A few seconds later, the doors to the EW come flying open. A young girl is on the stretcher. A young policeman is alongside.

"She's just thirteen and she was trying to get off a bus and her foot got caught in the door when the bus driver drove off," he says. He is shaking.

The girl's arm and hand are badly mangled; her hand is like a claw, frozen in a deformed position. Skin is ripped away, revealing bone and tissue. She is pale, quivering, but she is awake and alert.

Chiarelli moves in, rushing over from the old man's bedside; another nurse replaces her there. Chiarelli gets the girl's name and address and her mother's name. The policeman rushes out to find the mother. Doctors come running, while Chiarelli and another nurse work rapidly.

"Blood pressure 120 over 80."

"Pulse okay."

"Trauma. Plastics. Pediatrics." The call goes out for help from other services.

A catheter is in place, an IV line, oxygen.

An X-ray machine is wheeled in.

"There's a clot on her butt," a nurse tells Chiarelli. There is a large red blotch on her buttocks. All her clothes have been stripped away.

A Surgical resident, Trauma doctor and Pediatrics resident arrive, in seconds. The surgeon yells for "tetanus, Hyper-Tet and antibiotics."

"X-ray the pelvis, too," the Pediatrics resident says.

"There are two lines in now. Urine's clear. Temperature 99.8"

Chiarelli is stroking the girl's forehead, talking to her softly. The girl is in pain, but she is answering questions precisely.

"Wiggle your feet, your toes," a doctor asks her.

She does.

"Follow my finger," he says, passing it across her face.

She does.

"What hurts?" he asks.

"My back," she whimpers. She is frightened, naked, in pain and in a strange place, surrounded by strangers.

A collar is placed around her neck, so she won't move and aggravate any injury that might be there.

Down the ward, another team works on the old man. A doctor is still pumping his chest. The defibrillator jolts him again.

"Shock again."

"No pulse."

"Again." Another jolt lifts the man off the bed.

Suddenly, the group around the man seems to relax together,

as if they sighed in unison. The EKG graph is flat, a straight line. "It's three-thirty," a doctor says, looking at his watch. "That's it." The doctors and nurses walk away. A nurse covers the body and pulls a curtain around it.

A plastic surgeon has arrived to check out the 13-year-old girl. A nurse has replaced Chiarelli at the head of the girl's bed and is talking to her, soothingly. Despite the trauma and the shock and the terror of being surrounded, the girl remains coherent. The plastic surgeon, studying the girl's hand, says, "First, we've got to evaluate the bones and the circulation in that hand."

X-rays are back, minutes after they were taken. There is a lumbar fracture in the lower back. "L–5," Chiarelli whispers to another nurse: the fifth lumbar vertebra. Bad but not dangerous.

The doctors confer beside the girl. There is extensive damage to nerves, tendons and compound fractures in the hand. The plastic surgeon wants to know more, and says to the others, "Let her rest for a few hours. Watch her belly for rigidity, pain, tenderness. I don't want her up in the OR yet, not until we know what we've got. Her hand is not as bad as it looks."

It is 3:45. The girl's mother has been driven to Bellevue by the police. A surgical resident meets her, outside the EW.

"Your daughter had an accident on a bus," he tells the woman. "So far she doesn't look too bad. She injured her left hand."

The woman looks at the doctor intently. She is Hungarian. She doesn't speak English. The doctor realizes it, says "Oh, no" and runs off to find a doctor who can translate. The woman is not much bigger than her daughter. She is thin, short, neat, composed. Her eyes are wide and full of fear, however, as she sits, politely, almost daintily, and waits for the doctor to return.

Chiarelli seems involved in this case. She lingers to look at the girl, get opinions from various doctors, while the evening nursing shift arrives. There is no disruption; as they arrive, the day shift exchanges information and moves out. For Chiarelli, it is time to leave. She does it reluctantly. She can find out tomorrow, if she has the time and can find the doctor on the case, what happened to the girl.

The radiologist welcomes the Medical residents, interns and medical students to the morning's 8 A.M. X-ray conference: "Welcome to the breakfast club." Behind him, a series of X-rays are illuminated.

"How old is this lady?" the radiologist asks.

"Eighty-two," says George Feldman, sipping coffee from a paper cup.

"Incredible how much stamina she has," the radiologist comments. He has seen the patient. Now he's confronting the problem for which the X-rays were ordered. He says, happily, that "the likelihood of carcinoma lurking here is minimal."

At 8:40, Feldman arrives at the ICU, where three of his old women patients remain. One, an old Puerto Rican woman, is febrile and hypertensive.

"Have you given her medication by mouth?" Feldman asks the intern assigned to the case.

"She can't swallow," the intern replies, alluding to the congestion which has troubled the woman and which, until today, had kept her on a respirator.

"Have you heard of a tube?" Feldman says without raising his voice.

The group moves on to an old woman with possible tracheal bleeding. "Has ENT come to see her yet?" Feldman asks.

"I've tried to get them for three days," the intern says. "They're always busy."

"I'll go off and drag one up today," one of the medical students volunteers.

"Disgraceful," Feldman mutters.

The old woman who has had both a stroke and, later, a cardiac arrest rests almost lifelessly in bed, breathing heavily through a trach tube.

"How is she?" Feldman asks one of the medical students.

"Stable," the student answers.

"So why is she here?" Feldman asks. "She might be better off on a ward."

"Anyone on a trach needs intensive medical care," the intern on the case intervenes. "If you get a hard time about the bed, I'll defend keeping her here. There's an empty bed over there if we need it."

At 9:15, the group visits the ward. Six old women occupy one of the rooms. As they move from bed to bed, Feldman orchestrates the conversation. What are we doing for this patient? What should we be doing? He sustains the dialogue as part of the perpetual teaching process at Bellevue. Although the patients' welfare is foremost in his mind, he does not disregard that responsibility.

As he moves into the male ward, Feldman notices that one of his patients, an old black man, is dressed and ready to go home.

"Stay away from alcohol," he tells the man. "Your liver can't take it. You're in the process of killing yourself."

"Oh, yes, indeed. Yes, indeed, Doctor," the man says. He pledges that alcohol will not touch his mouth.

"It's been nice having you here," an intern says to the man. "See you in two weeks in the clinic." The man glides out, smiling.

"Think he'll show up?" a medical student asks the intern.

"No."

Feldman's group keeps moving. The ninety-pound old woman is walking around, smiling, her large belly protruding in front of her.

"She should be in bed and stay in bed," Feldman tells the intern. He has seen, in her chart, that she lost another pound yesterday. Diuretics will be continued, to try to reduce her fluid content, and more liver tests will be done. She has cirrhosis.

The young Puerto Rican mother's bed is empty; she is off to have her angiogram.

A new admission is a 52-year-old black woman with a history of hypertension that has resisted drug therapy. She had a stroke five months ago and has congestive heart disease. She is now on five different medications.

At 10, the young attending shows up and Feldman and an intern describe a case to him. As they begin, Feldman's beeper goes off. He dials the number the beeper provides and discovers that the chief of Medicine is ready to discuss one of the cases Feldman is working on. The meeting with the attending is postponed until the afternoon and Feldman heads to meet Dr. Saul Farber, the head of Medicine at Bellevue, as well as head of the department of Medicine at N.Y.U.

Dr. Farber sits behind a desk, surrounded by medical students, interns and residents. One of the medical students, nervous, voice cracking, quickly outlines the case for Dr. Farber, while Farber flips through the patient's chart. It is a case of an old woman with heart disease and a hiatal hernia, who came into the hospital complaining of shortness of breath.

Feldman contributes what he knows about the woman, then the entire group goes to the ICU to see the woman. Dr. Farber talks to her. "I lost my breath," she repeats several times in response to his questions. He examines her, looks at her X-rays, files his findings in his head. He leads the group back to the office, passing a sign on the ICU door, a quotation from Aesop: "No act of kindness, no matter how small, is ever wasted."

The woman has pneumonia, Farber declares, caused by "aspiration of blood, and a possible secondary infection." His instructions are specific: "Keep her on one antibiotic. Don't switch from one to another, chasing organisms. Take her off it as soon as you can. Don't put any needles into her chest. Leave her alone. I don't think she has a primary hematological problem. Most important, do very little mechanically. Don't try to explain everything that happens. She's very old and will fall apart. Take it easy. Give her a brand-new mask for the respirator twice a day. She's a setup for infection. And tell her we're sure she's going to get better."

As the doctors and students file out, Feldman turns to the medical student who presented the case and says, "Well, we haven't done very much wrong."

He goes to the ICU and asks the head nurse to change the woman's mask twice a day.

"If they've got them in Supply, we'll do it," she says.

The medical student walks over to the patient's bed to transmit Dr. Farber's message: "You're going to get better."

Feldman heads back to the ward, finds an empty chair and a desk and begins laboriously making entries in patients' charts. He allots a few minutes for a hamburger, french fries and a Coke in the snack bar, then leaves to report for a tour of the new Bellevue building, which Medicine will move into, if all goes smoothly, within a few months.

Feldman's tour of the new Bellevue is conducted by a tall, attractive, articulate young woman from Administration. Few of the doctors on the tour eye her; they're far more interested in the facilities offered by the new hospital. It is in almost traumatic contrast to the complex of old Bellevue buildings. It is bright, colorfully painted, impressively equipped. For forty-five minutes, Feldman and the other residents peek into rooms—there will be no open wards in the new high-rise Bellevue—examine built-in equipment, the view of the East River, the immaculate bathrooms, the water fountains that work, the high-speed elevators.

"It'll be a pleasure to work here," Feldman says, and the other doctors agree. "There'll be a lot of problems. It *is* Bellevue, after all. But it's certainly better than the old place."

At 2:30, he's back on the ward, resuming his meeting with the attending. An intern is along, too, to present the history of a new admission.

The patient is a black man, 29, obese and listless. He's been unemployed for two years and lives with two other men. In his past, he's used various drugs, from amphetamines to LSD, with occasional hallucinations. He's been in at least one psychiatric hospital. He complains of lethargy and drowsiness. He sleeps often. He says he suffers from decreased libido and decreased hair growth on his face. Medical examination has revealed that he is hypothyroid. Treated in the Bellevue clinic for several months, he's shown no improvement. He sleeps twelve to fourteen hours a day, he says, and has gained 150 pounds in two years.

Neurological tests were normal; he has no motor defects, except for a slight tremor in one hand. His private physician, he claims, has been giving him Haldol, Dexedrine and 40 mg. of Valium a day.

"That's enough to make anyone sleepy," the attending interrupts.

The intern says that "The man's mother and her sister were both schizophrenic. His father had a stroke, followed by terminal cancer. He died when the patient was ten." The patient has told the intern that he is heterosexual, but not active; he is unable to get an erection. He drinks two to three quarts of diet soda a day.

"He seems cheerful, alert and can maintain a conversation," according to the intern. "There seems to be no evidence of hair loss. He does manifest hypogonadism. EKG, blood tests, urinalysis and chest X-rays are all normal." He has a known endocrine problem, hypothyroidism, with a psychiatric component, the intern adds, concluding that "it could be a mid-line cerebral lesion."

The attending suspects a hypothalamic lesion or a pituitary tumor. Or, he feels, it could be psychiatric. Feldman wants to see the results of more tests, including pituitary studies.

"Take him off all the medication except the thyroid medication," the attending recommends, "and watch him to see if the drowsiness is drug-induced. The clinical picture you give points to a hypothalamic basis. That is, from my broad years of clinical experience. At least three or four."

A Psychiatry consult has been requested by Feldman and at this moment Ken Kirshbaum shows up to see the patient. He knows Feldman and they chat about the case.

Kirshbaum recognizes the patient. He has seen him before in the psychiatric clinic.

"A schizophrenic. A chronic thought disorder," he tells the attending after interviewing the patient. "This man has a long history of psychiatrists. He goes from one to another, and there's a history of psychiatric disorder in his family. He has episodes of derealization. If he has narcolepsy, it's an endocrine, not a psychiatric, problem. He abuses drugs. I think he's deteriorating, heading toward psychiatric hospitalization."

The attending says, "Unless it *is* a hypothalamic lesion. That, of course, could aggravate any psychiatric condition."

Feldman has run off to another conference. The Renal Fellow involved in the debate over the young Puerto Rican woman yesterday strolls in looking for him. He hasn't time to wait, so he leaves a message with one of the interns.

The angiogram was done on the woman, he tells the intern, and the finding was: normal arteries and a small kidney, not renal artery stenosis as he had suspected. No need for surgery.

"Tell Feldman he can discharge her," he instructs the intern, "and we'll see her in the clinic."

When Feldman returns to the ward, on his way home, the intern spots him and gives him the message. Feldman listens, without comment. As he walks out the door, there is a smile on his face.

Sol Zimmerman spent the night on the Premature Unit, getting to sleep at 2 A.M. At 6:00, he was awakened by a phone call from an intern. The 16-month-old child he had treated in the past, a child he had visited on a Pediatrics ward earlier in the week, had died of congenital bile duct obstruction. The parents, suspecting the end, had spent most of the evening with the child. It died a few hours after they went home to get some sleep. The intern called them, he tells Zimmerman. It is the sort of news that prevents Zimmerman from going back to sleep even if he felt so inclined.

At 7:30, he is in the ICU, to discover that one of the twins is arresting and revives it. Zimmerman returns to the Premature Unit, in time to receive a lab report on the baby with persistent fever and diarrhea.

He reads the report carefully and is surprised by it. The baby has Group D strain salmonella, a bacterial infection that can kill a small child if untreated, but can easily be defeated by an antibiotic, ampicillin, less harsh than the one that had been used on the child, gentamicin. Now Zimmerman can attack a specific disease; the child's condition is no longer a mystery. When three stool cultures in a row are negative, free of salmonella, the baby will have triumphed.

However, it is important to Zimmerman to trace the source of the infection. This baby can be cured, but others could have been infected. A carrier should be found and a plan formulated to prevent the spread of the disease.

Babies who were in the nursery area with the one who has salmonella must be checked. The baby was transferred from the nursery to the Premature Unit, where it was kept in isolation. Mothers of babies in that room in the nursery must be examined, too. Nurses must be tested. Zimmerman calls Bellevue's chief epidemiologist and the investigation is set into motion, including the scrubbing of rooms and equipment. To complicate matters, the actual carrier may be asymptomatic; only a stool culture will be indicative.

At 10 A.M., Zimmerman makes rounds with an attending in the ICU and the Premature Unit. One baby in the latter has pulled out her feeding tube five times in a day; the intern is anxious about it. Another baby, with an enlarged heart, may need corrective cardiac surgery, but the surgeons won't operate until the baby weighs thirteen pounds, double its present weight. The baby is having trouble keeping down its food, compounding the problem. Zimmerman, up much of the night and now into his second day on minimal sleep, looks tired. He gets through rounds with the attending, then wearily sits down. An intern approaches.

Zimmerman looks at him, emptily. "When I get home in the afternoon after working all night like I did last night," he says, "my wife may not be home yet. I just fall into a coma and when I wake up the clock may say 6:15 and I think it's time for us to have dinner. But then I realize that the sun is out and it's morning and I have to go back to the hospital."

After lunch, Zimmerman returns to the nursery to examine a jittery baby whose mother has been an addict.

"The baby doesn't look so bad now, but these babies can go into withdrawal a month after birth," he says to a nurse. He explains that it takes between ten days and a month to taper such a baby off its inherited habit, using carefully administered doses of phenobarbital. In this case, to worsen the situation, both baby and mother have positive VD tests, so the baby must be transferred out of the nursery to a ward where it can be observed and treated. Babies needing antibiotics are moved out of the nursery.

Zimmerman responds to a page, a call from the infectious-disease consult, who tells Zimmerman that the mother of the baby who was in the bassinet next to that of the salmonella victim has been cultured and found to have salmonella. She must have touched the baby while visiting her own in the nursery. Oddly, her own baby has not shown signs of the disease. Other mothers, who shared the ward with her in OB, and their babies as well, must now all be tested.

Zimmerman sits down in a chair at the ICU nursing station. Another resident walks over, sits down beside him. Neither doctor seems to have the energy to get up. They talk about their efforts to help the twins survive, the possibility of a "miracle." It inspires Zimmerman to tell the resident a story.

"Once we had a teen-age Chinese boy here in the ICU. He was in a coma, with meningitis. We were giving him penicillin, plenty of it, and we didn't seem to be winning. It looked like he would die.

"One night his parents, two little Chinese people who didn't speak much English, showed up to see him. The mother asked me if I'd mind if she did something. I asked her what she had in mind.

"She wanted to put hard-boiled eggs under the boy's pillow

and put some hot quarters—you know, coins she would heat up with a match—on his neck and back. I guess it was some sort of ritual those people knew about, and I thought for a minute and said, 'Sure, why not?' and they went into his room and put the eggs and the quarters all around, then they left.

"I didn't know what to say, but I guess if you pushed me I would have said that they were weird or crazy. But, what the hell, I left the eggs and the quarters there all night.

"The next morning when I got to the ICU, early, the boy was awake for the first time in days. No more coma. He was, in fact, obviously getting better. Don't ask me if it was the millions of units of penicillin or the eggs and quarters. Who cares?"

There are some nights when a surgeon on call can relax for a few hours. They do not occur often. Last night, Mary Williamson managed to get to 5.45 A.M. At that hour, emergency surgery was necessary on a 70-year-old man with serious, persistent GI bleeding.

He had needed ten units of blood to combat his loss. At 9 A.M., he is doing well as the surgeons, led by Williamson, try to uncover his problem. He is not in shock, fortunately, despite his age and the bleeding. In fact, mysteriously, the bleeding was not evident when the surgeons opened him up. They decided to perform two procedures: a pyloroplasty and a vagotomy. The former enables the stomach to empty faster by repairing the opening from the stomach to the duodenum. The latter is the cutting of the vagus nerve, the pneumogastric nerve, to reduce acid production and protect the duodenum from ulceration.

The work that began at 5:45, jolting Williamson from her nap, continues. Still no evidence of the source of the bleeding. Williamson comes out of the OR to phone an attending for advice.

"It's very disconcerting," she tells him. "The man's liver is cirrhotic, but there's nothing engorged in his stomach. His blood pressure is okay. He's putting out urine. There's a scarred ulcer bed, but no bleeding."

She tells the attending that they've done a gastrotomy, an incision that allows them to study the stomach, but haven't found anything yet.

There may be something to be found in the esophagus, she

tells him. She is very tired and stares into space as she speaks. Ironically, this is a day on which she was not scheduled to operate. It was her day to attend conferences. This operation is chewing into time she had hoped to give to other purposes.

"We haven't done anything to help his situation, no matter what it was," she tells the attending on the phone.

She decides to call for an endoscopic examination of the man's esophagus. Through an illuminated tube, the esophagus can be seen and evaluated. Within a few minutes of peering into the esophagus, she sees a large clot or lesion, high up on the esophageal wall. There is some bleeding. There are marked varices, dilated and tortuous veins. She can't tell if what she's seeing is a clot or an ulcer base or a cancerous growth.

She phones another attending, one she has relied upon in the past.

"I feel like I'm running home to mother," she tells him. "I need your help." She tells him she can close the incision she's made or proceed. "I think the man needs more than what we've done. Do you have any suggestions? I'm usually very gutsy about this, but in this case I just don't know."

She tells the attending that the patient has had radiation therapy for cancer of the larynx, not far from the erosion she's just seen, but the more she thinks about it, the less she thinks it resembles cancer.

She listens to the attending, then decides to proceed as planned, ligating enlarged veins if they're found. She won't hazard entering the esophagus. She returns to the OR and is joined by another attending, who scrubs in to help.

In the corridor outside the OR, a New York City policeman guarding a patient in surgery has cornered a resident.

"She was such a bitch. You know what kind of a bitch that broad was? Let me tell ya. She was such a bitch that she woke him up to throw the lye in his face. He jumped up and he pushed her head into the fan. Killed her. You can believe that. And he beat the rap. He beat the rap. You can believe that, too," the policeman tells the resident.

The resident stares at him, smiling uncomfortably.

At 11 A.M., Williamson is still in the OR.

A surgeon at the nursing station is canceling a scheduled operation he had hoped to do this morning.

"Can you believe it?" he says to the head nurse. "He wasn't

supposed to have breakfast. Okay? We knew it. Fine. So a nurse's aide on the ward brings him breakfast. She tells him to eat it, that it's good for him. He tells her he isn't supposed to eat. She says, 'Eat, eat,' so he eats. Well, we'll do him tomorrow if they leave him alone. It's the third time this week that's happened to me."

At 11:30, the attending comes out of the OR. One of the surgery residents loitering in the hall asks him about the operation.

The attending tells him that they still don't know why the patient was bleeding or where he was bleeding from. A senior resident, who has walked up to join them, comments, "There'll be a sequel to this story. You can bet on it."

Now, the pyloroplasty and the vagotomy are completed. The patient has held up well. He is not bleeding. He emerges from the OR at 1:15, on his way to the recovery room nearby, with Williamson alongside. He is wheeled into a room with three other patients recovering from surgery, and Williamson goes off to write her chart notes. She tells a senior resident about a busy evening recently, while she writes her notes.

"I just don't envision another night like that, going from case to case. I could psych myself up for it, I suppose, but . . ." Her voice trails off. She explains to the resident that the source of the bleeding in the last patient could be that lesion seen in the upper esophagus, near the larynx, but it's in an inaccessible place. The entire procedure in the OR, she says, "was very unsatisfactory. We spent most of our time trying to find the right thing to do."

She sits back in her chair and sighs.

She says that if the bleeding recurs, a thoracotomy may be the only move left: cutting into the chest wall to get at the source of the bleeding.

"This attending came. That attending came. And the patient was stable throughout, a rock. He might turn out to be a rose. But there's no reason to think that anything we did will improve him dramatically."

While Mary Williamson is talking to the resident in the recovery room area, a nurse rushes in and tells her that she thinks one of the patients is in cardiac arrest. Williamson gets up and walks over to the patient's bed. A first-year OB-GYN resident, a woman, was passing by when it happened and she is giving manual heart massage, pumping the patient's chest. He is in his twenties, swathed in bandages on his head and abdomen, the victim of a car crash.

The nurse tells Williamson that she was instructed by the surgical resident on the case not to revive the patient if he arrested. The resident felt that the brain surgery had left the man unable to function, "a vegetable." A neurosurgeon, who had done the brain surgery, arrives and confirms the instruction to the nurse, not to revive the man. The surgical resident who gave the order shows up, too. A nurse is moving a defibrillator toward the patient's bed. The surgical resident waves her off. He tells the nurse that he left a chart note with his instructions. The nurse flips through the chart and can't find it. The OB-GYN resident who helped now feels like an intruder and slinks away.

The patient seems dead, although the respirator he is on continues to expand his lungs and his chest continues to move. The surgical resident, surveying the scene, growls, "Everybody reacts emotionally to these things," and leaves. Williamson, who has observed it all without comment or action, moves on to see the patient she's just worked on in the OR; his blood pressure is dropping and she is worried. The nurses go on to other chores.

A young nurse goes over to the auto accident victim's bed and notices that the cardiac monitor shows that his heart is beating. She takes his blood pressure. He is alive. She tells the other nurses, who resume caring for him.

Williamson is done on the OR floor for the day. She changes into her white skirt and jacket and goes on quick rounds with other residents and an attending. As they walk through the halls, from ward to ward, one of the residents asks her if she'll miss Bellevue once she's out of it and in Africa.

"I'll remember it as Mother Bellevue," she says. "Maybe not as a woman exactly, but as a kind of all-providing, warm, living being for all of us who ever worked here.

"Maybe it tries to do too much and maybe it does some things poorly. But the Bowery people get help here. The poor get fed. There is a warm spirit at Bellevue. It's a hospital that never says 'no' to anyone. It's never too much. That's the attitude I found here. I know it means learning to work under any kind of conditions, too. The idea that it's better to do something than to do nothing. There may be a lot of slipshod stuff here, sure, but there is that spirit that has characterized this place for years and years."

At 4 P.M., Williamson and dozens of other residents and attendings gather for the weekly Mortality and Morbidity conference, known as M&M and presided over by the chief of Surgery, Dr. Frank Spencer.

A mimeographed series of sheets are handed out, giving the details of cases to be discussed. Some are stories of medical successes; a few are about patients lost.

Spencer is an internationally known cardiac surgeon, head of the department of Surgery at N.Y.U., as well as Bellevue's chief of Surgery. An ingratiating man with a high tenor speaking voice and a slight Texas drawl, he is well known in and out of Bellevue and is remembered with particular fondness by many medical students because he always managed to know their names shortly after meeting them.

At this conference, he dominates; although he is a slim man, not physically imposing, his knowledge commands the respect of the doctors in the room. Other attendings, several almost as well known as Spencer, offer their comments, too.

In explaining one case, a surgical resident tries to explain how a tube came out of its original placement, inside a patient. He can't offer a reasonable explanation, he admits.

Spencer turns to him and, without a trace of anger, says, "You've got to have an explanation. Invent one. The guy just didn't spring a leak. You can't say 'Beats me' and stop. You've got to come up with the best intellectual explanation you can."

The subject of tracheostomy (creating an opening into the trachea, to assist breathing) comes up, one that inspires debate among doctors. It can save. It can damage. Spencer says, "You may kill someone trying to avoid doing a tracheostomy. I'd trach someone with chronic lung disease the first time he sneezed."

Carefully, with humor, Spencer teaches the residents by giving his own opinions on the cases presented. The conference room, an old and musty one, is filled from the highest row down to the front table and blackboard with attentive doctors.

Midway through the conference, an ambulance siren is heard approaching the hospital. Several residents perk up, move to the edge of their seats. The siren comes closer. Finally, it is outside the room, pulling up to the AES entrance. Four residents leap up and out of the room. The conference resumes.

One of the cases deals with a 69-year-old man with both coronary trouble and carcinoma of the rectum. He was given a triple coronary artery bypass first, then low anterior resection for cancer. Why? "We would have killed him the other way around," Spencer tells a questioning resident.

The case given the most time is that of a 73-year-old woman. She was taken to the OR for surgery and was found to have "a necrotic gall bladder enclosed in an inflammatory mass of hepatic flexure, duodenum and omentum. The gall bladder had perforated and sealed against the duodenum."

The gall bladder contained stones. In an effort to do as much as he could, the attending on the case went beyond the point at which some surgeons would have stopped. He attempted to solve the entire problem in a single operation. The patient died.

The surgeon, who is present, feels obliged to explain.

"The surgeon is counted on for his judgment," he tells the audience, as if he feels that he is on trial. "How far should one go?" he asks. "I felt obliged to go on with this operation and that is what may have killed this woman."

"You can't stop if there's something to fix and you don't fix it," another attending says, supportively.

"After all, she was a frail old lady," another attending offers consolingly.

The residents in the room are avoiding a possible debate. An older attending does not.

"I would see no crime in backing off," he says. "Just drain the duct and get out. Leave the stones for later. You can go back later if you've got a live patient. If you do more, you may not have a live patient."

The issue remains unresolved, except in the minds of the listeners. Each doctor can study the case, as it is outlined on a mimeographed sheet, and reach his own conclusion.

It is 5 P.M. and the doctor and the medical student are sitting in the doctor's Bellevue office. It is a characteristically cramped office, lined with books: *The Life of Sir William Osler* by Harvey Cushing, *Platelets and Their Role in Hemostasis, Tumours in the Human Body* and the 1965–66 Harvard University Catalogue.

This doctor, a full-time attending at Bellevue, is known as a maverick. His opinions are not necessarily endorsed by the

A.M.A. or the HHC or the powers at Bellevue. He is known for not being reluctant to express them. Students know this, and when they're trying to figure out which hospital to do their residencies at, they go to him for advice.

"What you see in Bellevue is the end of the two-class system —private medicine and charity medicine," he says. He has been at Bellevue for more than twenty years and has seen it change.

"Today we ought to be committed to private care for all patients. The trouble is, they don't come to Bellevue expecting it. The prevailing theory is that charity patients can be treated differently, medically and socially. That's the old belief. It's not one doctor taking care of one patient. The patient is the key In our system, the doctor benefits. The patient may not. If you come to Bellevue, you usually see residents, not attendings, and without much supervision. You could see a different resident every time. And there's no follow-up when you leave the hospital.

"There ought to be public practice of medicine the way private practice used to be."

He talks about the role of the resident in a teaching hospital. It is a system, he says, that came into full flower after World War II, when teaching programs provided education and training. Hospitals set up residencies to get good doctors. That very effort, he feels, has made the resident the in-hospital doctor.

Attendings, getting rich and lazy, won't get up at night, so the residents assume the burden and the responsibility, even without the experience to do so. The need of the resident for training and the need of the hospital for service are not always compatible, he says.

"And we're training people we'll never need. There are twice as many neurosurgeons in the pipeline as we'll need. So what will happen? There will be unnecessary operations. Or they'll have to go into practices they're not trained for. Or the competition will be cutthroat. We are training residents without regard for the medical needs of the country.

"Residents should be trained under very close supervision. To protect the patient's best interest. At Bellevue, the chief resident has unlimited, unsupervised privileges. Bad medicine isn't good teaching. It's wrong.

"So you get the rationalization that for 'certain patients' the system is okay. For those who can't pay, that's who. The two-class system all over again. And the resident doesn't learn more just by doing more. He makes more mistakes. I don't think that residents should teach each other the mistakes they've learned along the way.

"I want to decide when a resident needs help. There are some things an experienced attending should do, always. There can be a team including the resident, of course, which works under the supervision of a senior attending. And there is that transitional time, when the resident must make decisions, but he must have someone to consult before he etches in flesh and blood."

He stays at Bellevue, he says, because he feels a commitment to the public system in New York. He was trained at Bellevue. It has a new plant and the money it needs to run it. The trouble, he feels, is in the intrusion of politics, the power manipulators, the health-pimps. Problems of patronage and mismanagement plague public hospitals. It should be changed, he tells the medical student.

"We need neighborhood centers without waiting time, without lines, with full-time doctors. At the large hospitals, we need salaried, full-time chiefs of service, not men who are around part-time and have their own private practices. We need basic core staff, paid adequately, to carry on both teaching and care, with the patient coming first.

"We need a national health-care system for ambulatory care. Ninety percent of our patients are ambulatory, so we need preventive-care programs in the neighborhoods. Good care. I know of a case in which a patient came to Bellevue for two years with rectal bleeding before it was diagnosed as inoperable cancer. Do you know that there isn't a good burn center in all of New York City? A place the size of Sweden.

"The affiliations with medical schools give the schools the power to direct the hospitals. They get programs the school wants, not programs the city may need. We need a city medical school to staff city hospitals, with free tuition in exchange for public practice later, for students who can't get into medical schools now. We've got to train doctors to go out into the communities. Now we're training too many specialists, not doctors who can handle general practice in the city.

"But then, I'm thought of as a maverick."

He has made a speech without intending to, and the student

has sat, motionless and attentive, through it all. The doctor gets out of his chair, reaches across his desk to shake the student's hand. As the student leaves, he realizes that the doctor did not once urge him to serve his residency at Bellevue. He has heard, concisely, a voice of dissent.

At 3:35 P.M., two hospital policemen are playing gin rummy in the security office near the front desk of the AES when Tom Spencer gets to work. He takes a quick walk around the place; there are six patients on stretchers, three resting in the Observation Unit. The day-shift head nurse tells Spencer what he will inherit.

"See that little old lady sitting in the corner back there? She wanted to end it all. Know how? She took a bottle of Sominex. Yes, Sominex. Saw too many television commercials and thought it would do the job. You may want to have someone talk to her or get a psychiatrist to do it.

"There's a big black guy who was mugged. His head is badly lacerated. And a man about forty-five, in a gray suit, who came in with a fever of 105. The resident thinks he has pancreatitis, wants to give him a shot, some pills and an appointment at the clinic. Back there in bed, there's an old lady with a fractured hip. She's not happy here, wants to get out to go to a private hospital. And there's a nice-looking woman, middle-class I'd say, who apparently fell out of a fourth-story window. She told me, 'My friends will never believe I fell. They think I'm nutty.' That's about it. It's your problem now. I'm going home."

Before Spencer can do anything about what she's told him, an ambulance siren shatters the silence. Spencer joins several other nurses and two doctors in the dash toward the front door. It is an old woman, ashen-purple, in cardiac arrest. They rush her into the Emergency Ward. Spencer pumps her chest; another nurse gives her air by hand through an Ambu bag, more effective than mouth-to-mouth resuscitation. Four doctors and three nurses surround the woman.

An EKG is hooked up, studied. Blood samples are taken, IV fluids initiated. The woman looks on the verge of death; her pallor deepens. A defibrillator is wheeled up; everyone backs away from the bed except the nurse who holds the plate to the woman's chest. The current is turned on; it jolts the woman, moving her body momentarily up off the bed. The electrical heart stimulation may have helped. Doctors resume pumping her chest manually. She is a fat woman, and as they pump waves of fat course across her stomach. Within ten minutes, she is beginning to respond. Her color begins to change, turning to a healthy pink. The EKG reveals that her heart rhythm is moving closer to normal. She will make it. Spencer returns to the AES.

A black man who has been mugged awaits him. He is a large, muscular man who must have been assaulted by several men; he looks more than able to handle one other man. His upper lip is bulging grotesquely. His nose is broken, his right eye swollen shut. He wants to speak, but he can't get the words through the swelling. Spencer does an EKG on him and is not pleased with the results. On the man's chart, which will be picked up by a resident on duty, Spencer notes that the EKG needs further analysis, that the man must be seen by one of the Trauma surgeons, an oral surgeon, an ophthalmologist and held overnight, at least, for observation.

In the background, as ever, things are happening around Spencer. An ambulance brings in a filthy alcoholic wearing putrid, discarded clothes and an abandoned golf cap. Another alcoholic sticks his head out of an examining room and slurs to a passing doctor, "I need ten million dollars. Got a cigarette?" The doctor glares at him with barely veiled disgust and says, "Man, you're drunk as a skunk. Sober up and I'll get you a clinic appointment." A few feet away, another resident, surly, shouts, "Jesus Christ, Psych sends over a guy who's complaining of a sore throat and it turns out he's got metastatic carcinoma."

It is 5:10 and the pace is slow. A Medical resident talks to the woman who fell out of the fourth-story window. "It's all so silly," she tells him. "I was trying to retrieve my cat. I didn't make it."

"I've got bad news for you," the resident tells her. "I've looked at the X-rays. You've got a fractured rib and a broken back. Two fractured vertebrae. It will become very painful. The best thing is for us to admit you to the Trauma Service here. You can be in bed and we can watch it. The bones will heal by themselves, but you'll have to be in traction. It'll be okay, as long as the bone fragments don't get to the spinal cord."

A man, a friend, has joined the woman in listening to the

resident's appraisal. They are atypical, well dressed and articulate, obviously educated types, rare to Bellevue. The resident anticipates trouble and gets it.

"I really don't want to stay at Bellevue," the woman says.

"That's right," her friend adds.

"Why?" the resident asks.

"Well, simply because it's Bellevue," she answers.

"What's wrong with Bellevue?" the resident asks.

"Never mind," the woman's companion says.

"Take my word for it," the resident says, his voice becoming louder, "you won't get better care at any other hospital than you will get here. And you shouldn't be moving around with a broken back."

The woman sighs. The resident walks to the back desk, to arrange for her transfer to a ward. He turns to Spencer, who has been eavesdropping, and says, "Tom, that lady will be complaining of back pain the rest of her life." A black prisoner, accompanied by two police guards, sits sullenly in one of the examining rooms. He was kicked in the scrotum in a jail fight six weeks ago; a clot developed and is still there. A Genitourinary specialist is on his way to see him, from the innards of Bellevue.

At 6 P.M., Spencer and his male nurse friend head to the neighborhood McDonald's for dinner. Inevitably, they discuss experiences at the AES. The friend teases Spencer about his reputation for being retiring, gentle, despite his size. "I remember one evening when a very well-dressed man, in his sixties, came in, looking pale and sweating and complaining of chest pain. He certainly looked the part to me. I mean, he looked respectable and all that. And just as the doctors were getting to work on him, you walked in, took a look at him and screamed, 'You're a liar.'"

"You bet I did. I remembered that guy. He was a Demerol freak. He'd go from hospital to hospital describing cardiac symptoms and he'd get Demerol from each place. I threw him out that night."

"Reminds me of the night I was on and there was this pompous, hostile guy demanding attention. The resident who went to see him was wearing a yarmulke, and the guy took one look at him and said, 'I don't want no Jew doctor.' I threw that son of a bitch out myself, and he probably didn't even know I was

Jewish." The friend rubs his hands together in retrospective satisfaction.

As Spencer and his friend walk through the front door of the AES, the police are bringing in a Puerto Rican teen-ager with a stab wound in the side. "This place is fantastic," one of the policemen says to the clerk at the desk. "If something happens to me, I want to come here."

A few minutes later one of the hospital volunteer workers, a middle-aged woman, comes in, hysterical.

"I was walking to my car, just a block away, just a block from Bellevue, when I saw this man carrying a stick. I noticed him, but I didn't think much about it. Then he got to me and hit me over the head with the stick and just kept on walking, not even running." She is in pain and fearful. Spencer assures her that a doctor will see her, agrees with her that the streets of New York are perilous, and she stops crying.

Spencer strolls from room to room. Everything seems to be in order. Nurses are working; residents are scattered throughout the AES. Again, when matters seem under control, the unexpected intervenes. An ambulance drives up, with a 26-year-old black woman who has been shot three times with a 22-caliber weapon.

A doctor and Spencer take a quick look at her and decide that she can be treated in the resuscitation room, rather than wheeled directly into the EW. Several policemen are with her and a white woman, who says she's her neighbor. "Somebody she knows shot her," the neighbor testifies. "Somebody she knows very well. I saw it. She just shot her and then ran out of the hotel we live in, jumped in a cab and was gone." The hotel is a seedy one in the East Twenties.

The black woman is howling. On the table, she jumps up and down, screaming. There is a bullet hole in her cheek, another in her foot and a third in her shoulder. A Trauma surgeon treats the wounds, expertly. X-rays are taken, quickly evaluated. Her jaw has been shattered; there are bullet fragments scattered around in it. Metallic bits are visible on X-rays, in both foot and shoulder.

"I'm going back to the hotel," one of the policemen announces. "She'll come back. They always do. And I'll be there."

Spencer requests a page for an oral surgeon to look at the woman's jaw. Surgery to remove the bullets can be done later.

The woman has stopped screaming. Now she moans softly. Her neighbor holds her hand, chants that she'll be all right.

Within minutes, another pair of policemen arrive, with another gunshot wound case. This one is an angry man in his early thirties, chubby and gross. His clothes are grimy. He mumbles to the police, speaks Hungarian to his mother, who has come with him. He had been in a gunfight in the West Village and had taken a bullet in his right shoulder; there is a large entry wound, but no exit wound. The police want him to tell them what happened, but he won't.

"We found six bullets in your pocket," one of the policemen says to him, gripping his healthy shoulder.

"They were planted on me," the man mutters, then will say no more.

"Where's your gun?" the policeman asks

"I don't have none."

"Where's your identification?"

"Gone. In my wallet, with my fucking money, $987."

"Who did it?"

"Never mind. I shot the guy once, but that wasn't enough. There'll be one dead body tomorrow. I'll take care of it myself."

His mother is crying. "He knows who did it. He *knows*," she says in broken English, "but he won't tell me."

The external wound is treated by a resident and Spencer, and he is sent to X-ray, to define the location of the bullet, information that will be passed on to the surgeons who will later remove it.

The uniformed policemen leave and are replaced by two detectives. They attempt to question the man, but he stares grimly into space, plotting his revenge. They question the mother, without success.

Through all this, the mugged black man has been stirring on his bed in the corridor. Spencer sees him and walks over.

"Man, I'm a really hungry dude," he says to Spencer. His lips are ragged and thickly swollen.

"Can you eat?"

"Bet your ass I'll try," he says.

Spencer gets him a carton of milk, a straw, and a sandwich, which the man breaks into small bits and forces through his lips.

At the front desk, a young, colorfully dressed black man tells the triage nurse that he has a corn on his toe.

"Try Freezone," she tells him.

At 11:35, the patient count is fifty-six, the lowest this week, and doctors and nurses have time to talk to each other. An old man stumbles in; he's been mugged. Spencer listens to his story; the two detectives on the gunfight investigation listen to it, too, and fill out a report.

Spencer turns the mugged old man over to one of the doctors, then conducts his nightly narcotics count. Two codeine pills are missing. Spencer, relentless, asks the other nurses about the missing pills. One suddenly remembers: she gave them to a patient, on a doctor's orders, but forgot to register them.

A young Oriental woman, holding a Chinese-English dictionary, talks to a resident about her problem. "You have nothing to worry about," he tells her, as she flips through the dictionary trying to keep up with him.

A visiting businessman from Peru is on a bed, groaning; he is suffering from severe back pain and from a longing to be back in Peru. Spencer taps him on the shoulder and offers to call a friend for him, if he'll tell Spencer whom to call. He does, and Spencer places the call. The night shift has arrived and Spencer waves to several of them. When he's given the Peruvian's friend the necessary information, he hangs up, leans against the wall and takes a deep breath. Then he heads for his room.

Ken Kirshbaum got his dinner at a quiet neighborhood restaurant. Strolling back to Bellevue afterward, he is stopped by a young man, a demented monologist who can't possibly know that Kirshbaum is a doctor. The man, with long hair, an Army fatigue jacket, jeans and a conspicuous Band-Aid over his right eyebrow, tugs at Kirshbaum's sleeve. He tells Kirshbaum, without pausing, that he has been on methadone, has been in jail, is being evicted from his apartment, has been drinking and taking pills. Kirshbaum listens patiently. When the man is done, he tells him to come to the walk-in clinic tomorrow.

"You a doctor? Wow," the man says, stumbling off down First Avenue.

At the PAO, there are two registered nurses, several nurses' aides, a young social worker and a weary resident on duty when Kirshbaum arrives. The resident will get some sleep now that

Kirshbaum is there and he'll return at midnight to relieve him. Normally, the PAO is frantic. Each night between twenty-five and thirty people wander or storm in. They are led into the corridor, with offices on either side, beyond the decaying registration desk and waiting area. There are doctors' offices, a nurse's station and an emergency treatment area for patients who need a secure setting and whose problems can be dealt with within forty-eight hours. There is a waiting room for patients, with a television set perpetually blaring.

The first patient to greet Kirshbaum is a toothless, cranky old man who has checked out of his nursing home and been turned away from the Men's Shelter for being disruptive. The Shelter sent him to Bellevue.

The old man is neat. His shirt and shoes are new. He is carrying his belongings in a large plastic bag and carries a cane. He is somewhat deaf.

"I don't want to be in Bellevue," he snarls at Kirshbaum. "I'm not drunk. He just wants to find a park bench for the night. He knows the correct date, and when he's asked who is the current President, he shouts, "Richard Nixon, you asshole." He is an angry man, but not a psychiatric patient. He tells Kirshbaum that he can support himself by panhandling. Kirshbaum gives him a subway token and wishes him good luck.

A 19-year-old woman walks in. "I'm depressed. I just don't feel like I used to," she says. She doesn't want to stay at Bellevue. Kirshbaum gives her a mild tranquilizer and urges her to see him in the clinic tomorrow.

The phone rings. A troubled voice defines its owner as "a psychosexual retard" and adds, "I want to know why women won't ball me." Kirshbaum ends the conversation. The phone rings again. "I'm in a phone booth and I'm going to blow up Manhattan," a man's voice says. Kirshbaum recognizes it; it belongs to another resident. As they chat, a slim, clearly disturbed young black woman walks through the front door of the PAO.

She is wearing a plaid cap, clean white bell-bottom pants, a red T-shirt and a raincoat. She is either hysterical or drunk, or both. A policeman, who has been staring at her, walks away.

"Why do you turn your back on a black woman?" she screams at him. "I had a baby thirty days ago. You don't know what it is to be sick." A nurse sits her down and talks to her, calms her.

She walks out of the PAO without asking for help.

Another old man arrives, a transfer from another hospital. Bellevue hasn't been notified in advance, a gripe that Psychiatry residents voice repeatedly. It is the ship-the-dregs-to-Bellevue theory. Annoyed, Kirshbaum sees the man. He is wearing blue hospital pajamas, has a black eye, a swollen and lacerated leg, is unshaven, dirty. He is a destitute, chronic alcoholic. His chart, which Kirshbaum is studying, reveals a history of psychiatric hospitalization. He talks about taking his own life, but he is lively, not depressed, about it.

"Don't give me no razor blade or a knife," he tells Kirshbaum. "I jumped into the East River today. It was salty, stinky, full of crap. A cop took off his belt, jumped in and dragged me out. Down by the docks. I have a terrible headache." He speaks rapidly, with an incongruous amount of uneroded confidence. Kirshbaum doesn't try to interrupt.

"I also cut my wrists once and I've jumped in front of a subway train. Four times this year, I've tried." He smiles, moronically.

"The way I see it, if you're cracking up, you should get off the street. The nurses here are terrific. The doctors are hilarious at Bellevue. I'm not unhappy at all to be here," he says to Kirshbaum, who isn't quite sure what he means by "hilarious." He suspects the man only wants a room for the night. It's a familiar ploy at the PAO, by alcoholics who want to get off the street. However, the man's leg is in tatters. Why?

"I threw gasoline on myself, that's why. But not enough of it. I lit it, but a cop put it out with his jacket. Once I had a fractured skull and didn't even know it. Didn't even know it. It took me a long time to regain my balance." Throughout his breathless recitation, he is cheerful.

"You know, I was drinking my father's home brew, for God's sake, when I was nine. I've been drinking for fifty years. I can't even commit suicide successfully. I'm a failure. I want you to fix my head. I've had wine and Thorazine and Bennies today. They're fifty cents a pill on St. Marks Place. Then I jumped into the river at noon today. I lost my clothes in the river."

Kirshbaum believes most of the story, but he has doubts about Bellevue's ability to help the man, who belongs, he feels, in an alcoholic treatment center.

"One thing for sure," the man says, "I won't get a drink here.

It's a miracle I'm rational right now. My wife died last week. I called the kids, and they told me never to call again, that she was dead."

"Are you on welfare?" Kirshbaum asks.

"Welfare stinks. They mug you for your check. I make more money singing."

"Okay, here's what I think," Kirshbaum says firmly. "Bellevue isn't for you. You can go to Manhattan State, talk to the social worker here to get some lodging for the night, or come into the walk-in clinic tomorrow. Take your choice."

The man's cheer vanishes.

"I'll never go to that nuthouse," he says, referring to Manhattan State. "And I can't walk on the street like this," he adds, tugging at his pajamas. "I don't want to hear any more of your bullshit, you asshole," he screams.

"You just want a rest, a square meal and lodgings," Kirshbaum tells him, flatly.

"If you're a psychiatrist, I'm Jesus Christ Superstar," the man yells.

A nurse whispers to Kirshbaum that this man tried to get into Bellevue last week, but was not admitted. Kirshbaum tells her, "He really is an alert, manipulative guy. A truly suicidal man would be sad, depressed. He isn't. A psychiatric hospital is not his answer."

While Kirshbaum is getting ready to get rid of the man, his phone rings. Kings County Hospital in Brooklyn has a teen-age girl who has given an upper Manhattan address. Properly, she should go to Harlem Hospital if they have a bed available, Kirshbaum tells the resident at Kings County. "If they don't, send her here," he adds.

"What's the use?" he says to the nurse. "They send everyone here whenever they can."

Kirshbaum tells the old man he'll resume the conversation in a few minutes. He wants to visit Ward NO–6, to see an old woman he has treated when he was working on that ward, months ago.

The ward is almost silent. He finds the woman, who tells him that she hopes to be out soon and will come to see him in the clinic.

A few patients pace. Others sleep, fitfully. The sound of jazz comes from the radio in the nurse's station. The ranking staff member at this hour is a practical nurse. One of the psychiatric technicians is not feeling well. Kirshbaum checks her blood pressure and pulse and urges her to go home.

He's back in the PAO at 9 P.M. and immediately gets into a polite confrontation with the young social worker on duty. The social worker feels that the old man, the alcoholic, needs help. They debate the sort of help he needs and Kirshbaum agrees to send the man to Central Islip State Hospital, where an alcoholics program exists, in the morning. He can stay at Bellevue tonight and catch the bus for Central Islip at 9 A.M. The social worker informs the old man, who tells Kirshbaum, "I apologize for blowing up. You should have punched me in the mouth." He is pleased to be going to Central Islip. Kirshbaum does a physical examination on him: eyes, throat, the glands in his neck, blood pressure, pulse, chest, abdomen. When Kirshbaum prods his abdomen, he winces. Liver trouble. Possible alcoholic hepatitis. Kirshbaum writes out a prescription order, medical instructions. A tranquilizer to calm him down. Fluids, vitamins, cold compresses for his black eye. Medication for his leg. On his chart, Kirshbaum notes, "If he refuses to go to Central Islip in the morning, discharge him."

The next patient walks in to see Kirshbaum.

He is a 35-year-old black man who weighs almost three hundred pounds and has a glass eye. He towers over Kirshbaum, but his manner is not hostile. He is well dressed. His story is that he came to New York from Indiana to work at Bellevue. He has told the nurse that if he can't work at Bellevue, he'd like to be boarded at the hospital. The young social worker has seen him, too; he was told by the man that he had been in various mental hospitals, therefore had compassion for patients and could be a trusted employee. When the social worker sends him on to Kirshbaum, he says that the man is "too ill for outpatient treatment." Kirshbaum will make up his own mind about that.

The man walks into Kirshbaum's office, sits down in a chair that's not quite large enough. He squirms into it.

"Look, man, I need a place to stay and a job at Bellevue," he says. "I understand these people because I was crazy myself. Anybody can go batty, man. I'm writing a book about it. I just got to New York. Wow, this is some place, baby. I've never been here before. I did stop in Philly, on my way, with a lady."

Kirshbaum asks him simple, direct questions about his psychiatric history. The man turns hostile. He insists he is applying for a job.

"Okay, I smacked my wife, man, and she had me sent to a hospital for a month. Then I smacked her again and I went in again. In Indiana, I'm a bad risk, but, you know, I've got enough intelligence to get a job, a big car and a house."

"Do you have any trouble with thoughts you can't control?" Kirshbaum asks.

"Hey, man, you're far-out. I'm not suicidal. I'm homicidal. You hit me, I'll hit you back."

Kirshbaum's expression, solemn, does not change.

"I have money back in Indiana. My clothes are there, too. Wow, baby, this is *some* trip. I'll just go back to Indiana. I was going to work here, sure, but I haven't seen enough of New York yet."

"You just need a place to stay?" Kirshbaum asks.

"Yeah, man."

"I'll give you some medicine."

"Man, I'm trying to kick that shit. I don't rob or steal. I want a job, baby, that's all. Ooooooweeee. Wow."

"You don't have to be in a hospital."

"You a doctor, man? Wow. I thought you were a social worker."

Kirshbaum escorts him to the social worker's office. He feels the man is sick but functional, and doesn't need a bed on a ward. The social worker disagrees, but can't overrule Kirshbaum.

The teen-age girl from Kings County arrives; obviously, Harlem Hospital didn't have a bed. Two policemen found her asleep on the grass in Prospect Park and have accompanied her from hospital to hospital. They look weary, and fall into chairs while Kirshbaum sees her.

She is in her mid-teens and beautiful. She is tall, thin, a model's body, with large breasts. A great deal of make-up freezes her face. She tells Kirshbaum that she simply fell asleep while waiting for her boyfriend in the park. As she continues her story, the phone rings.

A hospital in Brooklyn has a girl with no place to stay. Can she be sent to Bellevue? Kirshbaum asks about her symptoms. "She's a little neurotic," the voice on the other end says. He transfers the call to the social worker and turns to the teen-age girl. He smiles. Let the social worker deal with *that* one. Kirshbaum is annoyed at him, for spending too much time with patients, for attempting medical diagnoses, for being impractically idealistic.

"Why are you here?" he asks the girl.

She uncrosses her legs, stares into space, turning her impeccable profile toward Kirshbaum. "The police brought me here," she says, yawning. "I was waiting for my boyfriend. Someone called the police thinking I was running away from home, because I had a shopping bag."

"Does your mother know you're here?"

"No. I've been staying with friends because I don't get along with my mother. I just spoke to her once after I left."

She tells him that she's a high school dropout whose only job in months was baby-sitting. She admits, when Kirshbaum presses it, that she did spend a few weeks in a state mental hospital a few months ago.

She moves her body slowly from side to side. Her breasts move at their own tempo; she is not wearing a bra. Her manner is seductive, secretive.

"I had a nervous condition," she says. "I went in by myself. They gave me pills that help my nerves. They're better now. I have very bad nerves."

She tells Kirshbaum that an aunt is willing to take her in. "She knows I'm coming, but she doesn't have a phone."

Kirshbaum is suspicious.

"If we send you to your aunt, will you take medication?"

"Yes."

"How much is one hundred minus seven?" he asks.

"Ninety-four."

"And seven from ninety-four?"

"You can't do that, take seven from ninety-four," she says.

He asks her what the proverb about people in glass houses means. "People should care about each other," she answers.

"Who's the current President of the United States?"

"George Washington."

"Who's the President *now*?"

"Nixon. I don't know all the Presidents," she says.

Kirshbaum asks her to draw the face of a clock. She does, awkwardly, erasing it several times. He tells her to set the hands for 10 after 10. She draws them in: 10 after 9.

"I'm very sleepy now," she says, stretching.

"Do you take drugs?"

"No, I drink."

"Do you think you ought to go to a clinic?"

"No. If my mother wants me home, I'll go home."

Kirshbaum stares at her chart. On one page, she has indicated a phone number for her mother. Kirshbaum dials the number. It is not her mother's. It belongs to her aunt, who tells Kirshbaum to "keep her, she ran away." She gives Kirshbaum the mother's number after he tells her that "running away is no reason to keep her here." He gets the feeling that the aunt, at least, wants the girl dumped at Bellevue and forgotten. The mother lives in a suburb of New York. Kirshbaum starts to dial her number, stops, starts again. He feels he must talk to her and begins to dial the number. At that moment, the girl's sluggishness, her primitively exotic style, vanish. She shows signs of being agitated.

"Can't I just go somewhere for tonight?" she asks.

Kirshbaum completes dialing. The mother is home and ready to talk to him about her daughter.

"I don't want to be committed here," the girl begins to scream, to thrash around in her chair. "I've been in too many mental institutions."

Kirshbaum listens to her, listens to her mother at the same time.

While talking to the mother, Kirshbaum mentions the name of a mental hospital outside New York.

The girl begins to weep, sobbing, screaming.

"I don't want to go there, I hate it there. My mother throws me into mental institutions all the time. I make mistakes, I know, but it's not fair because I'm not crazy. No. No. No."

She grabs the phone from Kirshbaum's hand. She is wild. Her face is red, through the make-up. Her cheeks are covered with tears.

"Mommy, you can't do this to me," she screams into the phone. "I'll kill myself. Please don't send me there. I don't touch drugs now.

"I'm *not* bullshitting you. I don't like being locked up in mental institutions. It doesn't get me better. I'm not perfect, but don't lock me up. I don't like to live like that. You send me there and I'll run away again. I'll keep running the rest of my life. I *need* you. I need my sisters and my brothers, not mental institutions. I need a lot of attention. I've been staying with people. I've been managing okay. It doesn't solve anything to lock me up. You just don't understand me, that's all. What am I going to do tonight? I'm not staying here. I'm not."

Kirshbaum is staring at her, intently.

"Maybe I am nervous and confused, but I'm *not* crazy. I do good in school. I'm smart. And you tell the doctors I'm stupid, Mommy, and psychotic. I'm not. I'm not. Just because I take drugs I'm crazy. Well, I don't take drugs any more, I hate to tell ya. I don't want to be treated like a little baby."

She is getting wilder and wilder. One of her sisters has taken the phone from the mother.

"Everything I do gets thrown in my face," she says to her sister. "You do a lot of things wrong. I'm the worst? I'm a juvenile delinquent? I don't like living like a bum. When I fucking come home, my own family ignores me. I don't need anybody."

Kirshbaum has to ask for the phone several times before she relinquishes it. He talks to the mother and learns that the girl has a three-year history of running away, prostitution, vagrancy, drugs, learning problems in school. There is a history of mental hospitals, clinics, doctors. The mother sounds reasonable, intelligent. She tells him that her daughter has just run away from the hospital.

Kirshbaum tells her that the girl can stay at Bellevue for the night, then catch the morning bus to the suburban hospital. It is not one of Kirshbaum's favorite mental hospitals, but the family does not live in Manhattan and he cannot legally have the girl committed to Bellevue for treatment. He tells the mother to cooperate with the doctors at the other hospital, to "raise hell out there so they'll know you give a damn." He says that the girl needs a good psychiatric evaluation and thorough testing. She shouldn't be released casually.

The two policemen who have been with the girl for six hours are lolling outside the door, eating ice cream cones, eavesdropping. The girl is taken away by nurses, to have her clothes changed for her overnight stay. Kirshbaum gives her a physical. She seems healthy. She says nothing to anyone now, resuming her stupor. She's taken to a ward. The police leave.

Kirshbaum, drained by the intensity of the meeting with the girl, would like a few minutes' rest. He can't have them. A skinny, unshaven man, an itinerant waiter and chronic drunk, stumbles into his office. He's come to the PAO on his own, asking to be detoxified after twenty years on alcohol.

He is suffering from anxiety and hallucinations. He admits to having had three six-packs of beer today, which to Kirshbaum means more than that.

The fumes of alcohol on his breath are overwhelming. He's been in Bellevue before and is a candidate for the alcoholics clinic.

"Put me back in shape. It'll take about two days," he slurs.

"We have only a few alcohol beds in the hospital," Kirshbaum says, "and tonight they are all filled. I can give you medication, but I think you ought to consider going into the alcohol program at Central Islip. There's a bus out there in the morning, express service. That's my recommendation."

"I get scared. But okay. I'll pack my bags, give them to a friend and make that bus tomorrow."

"Fine. Let's get some medicine for you. But remember, if you take the medicine, don't drink tonight. You could wind up in the morgue." He escorts the man to the nursing station.

The social worker is standing nearby. Kirshbaum spots him. The social worker nods. "The Central Islip alcohol program is a good one," Kirshbaum says to him, "but there's very little opportunity for follow-up. Frankly, if I see a patient who is sufficiently motivated to stop drinking, and that's the key, I'll find a bed for him here. I haven't found one yet."

Throughout the evening, Kirshbaum has been filling out forms, reading charts, keeping records, as he talks to patients. He goes back to his office to do more of that now. It is 11:30 P.M.

Outside the office, near the admitting desk, a huge black woman, in a wheelchair, sits clutching her belongings in a large plastic garbage bag, waiting for a doctor to see her. A young black man, barefoot and wearing a headband, mumbles about being at the PAO a few weeks ago. He is filthy. A security guard and a nurse chat, idly. With city police usually around, the hospital police, unarmed, are content to look menacing when that's required. A nurse sits at the nurse's station, reading Ken Kesey's novel, *One Flew over the Cuckoo's Nest*.

Kirshbaum, done with the paperwork, phones NO–6 to find out that the technician is feeling better; she took his advice and went home. A nurse comes in, to tell Kirshbaum that a 75-year-old woman, homeless, is being brought in by the police. Kirshbaum notes it, to tell the resident taking over at midnight.

The barefooted black man walks into Kirshbaum's office. He tells Kirshbaum he's an artist and asks for food. He speaks in a West Indian accent, lilting singsong, but he is so tired that he is half-asleep in the chair beside Kirshbaum's desk.

"I'm hungry and I'm tired and I want to sleep," he says.

When Kirshbaum questions him, he answers the questions with lists of food, delicacies, dishes, meals he's enjoyed, menus.

"I love myself," he says, with a sleepy smile on his face.

"You've gotten the maximum benefit from Bellevue," Kirshbaum says to him, sternly. "Your hospital now is Manhattan State, for longer-term care. Stay here tonight and you can go there tomorrow."

"As long as I get food there," the man says.

"You'll get it."

The man signs a voluntary admission form for Manhattan State and is taken off for a snack and a bed. On his chart, Kirshbaum writes, "Physical exam postponed pending a bath."

It is midnight. The resident reappears to relieve Kirshbaum. "Relatively slow night," Kirshbaum says to him.

In truth, Kirshbaum did not have an idle minute; he was able, simply, to spend more time with each patient than he would have on a truly frantic tour. As Kirshbaum gets his jacket and coat, the resident is talking to the large black woman. She's complaining of kidney trouble and tells the resident that she's been on the psychiatric wards at Bellevue before. As Kirshbaum passes the two, the resident whispers that he doesn't think the woman should be admitted. Kirshbaum tells him to do what he thinks is best.

FRIDAY

Nursing Service Report

Mary Johnson expired at 4 A.M.

Norman Goldman (34th Street shooting, gunman killed by police), gunshot wound of right leg. His leg is in traction—no dorsalis pedis or popliteal pulse and a temp of 101.

Harold Brown (14th Street explosion, bank bombing), fracture of left tibia and fibula—pulse is felt in leg.

Ground M—Alberto Cuevas (14th Street explosion), laceration of forehead and also is a drug addict.

Two others were treated and released (14th Street explosion).

Chan Lee Kung—stab wound of abdomen and expired in OR at 4 A.M.

The disaster bus went out at 8:15 P.M. to a subway accident and returned at 9:30 P.M. One patient treated and that patient went to Fordham Hospital.

Member of UN delegation from Asian country admitted to I-4, human bite of scrotum. His condition is fair.

Bernard Weinstein's secretary, Rose LaMarca, one of the most valuable people in his life, waits for him to come through the door. She usually greets him with a typed agenda for the day, which includes phone calls he must make, matters to deal with by the end of a given week, matters requiring follow-ups, and appointments. A special category covers "new building items."

She took a temporary job at Bellevue in 1949 and has been there ever since, serving several executive directors ("One of the women I worked with when I started had come to Bellevue in 1909," she remembers).

Weinstein arrives at 9:55 A.M., later than usual, because he stayed in his office last night to catch up on accumulated work. As he enters his office, his secretary, on cue, summons the members of his immediate staff, for a morning meeting Weinstein has requested. The staff files in, sitting at the large table behind Weinstein's desk. They are relaxed and so is Weinstein. With them, there's no need to seem to be omniscient, no reason to be defensive. He trusts them all.

The agenda is informal. They discuss Doris Lesser's "General Outline of Patient Move Plan," the document that will develop into a detailed plan for moving inpatients from the old to the new hospital.

Her list of priorities includes: alterations, cleaning, communications, construction, demolition, equipment, evacuation plan, keys, lockers, procedure manual, priority renovations, security, supplies, systems, phones, training-and-orientation and unions. It is a potential maze of details.

Weinstein reports on meetings he's attended this week, gripes he's unearthed that should be dealt with promptly. He assigns such problems to each one present. His assistant will confirm the assignments in writing.

He tells them what he's been doing; they tell him what they've been doing. At 11:25, the group dissolves into a larger staff meeting, the entire administrative staff, in the conference room.

There are twenty-eight people present and Weinstein permits each one to raise any issue they wish to raise. In a hospital that has thirty thousand admissions a year, coordination is vital.

One associate tells everyone that medical records will be moved into the new hospital this weekend. Deputy Director Madeline Bohman tells the group that next week the evaluation of the new hospital's operations will begin, to find problems and correct them. Lesser announces that there'll be a test of the emergency generator next week. The Director of Social Services notes that there will be two lectures of interest at the N.Y.U. Medical School. She complains about too much paperwork.

Jim Walsh, the Public Relations Director, tells them that Channel 7 will be doing a feature on emergency medicine and will be shooting some footage at Bellevue. There is mumbling and laughter; a previous Channel 7 news spot on Bellevue stressed the thriving rodents in the basement.

Ed Stolzenberg, the Psychiatry administrator, says that the dedication of the renovated courtroom in Psychiatry went very well.

Weinstein smiles and says, "I don't know why we renovated that courtroom, why we dedicated it, why I gave the judge a gavel, but it all did seem to go well."

Weinstein reports on the Employee Advisory Council executive board meeting, recites the problems that arose: methadone patients loitering in the lobby, parking, security, improved patient clothing.

He announces that the HHC approved the allocation for an interim location of the prison unit.

He discusses the competition between Bellevue and a neighborhood group to run the child health station. "It is the most confused case of health-care planning I've ever come across," he says.

He announces that the mayor of Naples will be a visitor, "if anyone is interested in shaking his hand."

One of the associates says, simply, "He's a chest man."

Weinstein laughs, looks at the associate, who is oblivious of the implication. "What did you say?" Weinstein asks. The room fills with laughter.

Weinstein points out that a doctor who surveyed Bellevue for accreditation purposes said that he found a better *esprit de corps* at Bellevue than at any other hospital he reviewed.

At 12:10 P.M., the meeting is turned over to Richard Miller, the architect, to present the Bellevue master plan. His presentation is similar to the one he offered the medical board: demolition, reallocation, construction, Bellevue in twenty-five years. It is his "Gestalt view of some of the world's prime real estate."

When he finishes, the audience applauds.

It is 12:45 and time for Weinstein to go to lunch in the doctors' cafeteria. He sits with some of his associates and talks about Bellevue to them.

"You know, a hospital is only as good as its medical staff, and I don't mean just technical skill. Verve. The drive to make the institution better and better."

He sees Dr. Joseph Ransohoff, the Director of Neurosurgery, and asks him what he thought of Miller's presentation to the medical board.

"Like smoking marijuana," Ransohoff replies. "Terrific. Except we can't get the money to tear down an outhouse."

When Ransohoff leaves, Weinstein is reminded about what Ransohoff represents. "This hospital would be medically and intellectually in trouble without a strong medical-school affiliation. And I consider N.Y.U. a strong affiliate, even if I do have disagreements with them because of differing objectives. I'd rather work those out than do without the affiliation."

That affiliation, and a strong Nursing department, make his job easier, Weinstein says. "This hospital grew and grew and what was missing was management. That's what I've tried to do, building on the strengths we had, the dedication that was here despite the resources that were missing. Resources the staff could have found in other hospitals. But they didn't leave."

Bernard Weinstein is back in his office by 2 P.M. He dictates letters, places and answers phone calls, meets with a former member of the community board who has a medical problem and wants his advice. He calls a member of the community board to affirm the board's support for his stand on the child health station issue, that Bellevue should participate strongly in it. He gets the support. He's already gotten the support of the chief of Pediatrics, so he knows where he stands. He has an interview with a woman in a mink coat wanting a staff job; he meets with Doris Lesser, to discuss again her report on the move of inpatients into the new hospital.

At 3:30, a young black Psychiatry administrator, Marvin Smartt, and the chief of Housekeeping, Lou LaBruyere, accompany Weinstein to Psychiatry for rounds. They're joined by an Associate Director of Nursing.

They begin by walking through one of the employee locker rooms. The lockers need painting. The room does, too. There is a pungent, offensive odor. They leave quickly. As they do, a Puerto Rican employee stops Smartt.

"You please do somesing about de pussycats in dere. I want to leev a few more years," he says.

The group proceeds to PQ–5, the adolescent ward. Smartt unlocks the door. A patient is asleep on a bed in the corridor.

"He hasn't slept in four days," a nurse whispers, "so we're not bothering him now."

Most of the adolescents are in the Psychiatry hospital school. A few linger, talking to visitors. A patient, a teen-age boy, is beating an activity therapist at Ping-Pong. The therapist is not trying to lose and is taking the trend of the game seriously.

The next stop is NO–5, an adult ward. A patient approaches the group, spreads his feet, glares at them.

"I dare any of you to face fifteen minutes with me," he shouts. They pretend not to notice.

On NO–4, the Associate Director of Nursing says, "This ward is the banc of our existence. There's a total lack of harmony here because it is so overcrowded. We need more staff. Inertia, that's what it is."

Weinstcin and Smartt take notes.

In PQ–4, the ward is newly painted. The inevitable TV set blasts away.

"It is hard to get our patients involved," the ward nurse says. Most of the patients look zonked. A few are busy in the activity room. Several others are sleeping. One works on a jigsaw puzzle, in slow motion. Three others play cards.

On NO–3, a ward devoted to drug research, "behavior modification" and alcoholic detoxification, the atmosphere is one of activity.

There is a patient government, the doctor in charge tells Weinstein, and a ward newspaper. Some patients cook for themselves. Some are encouraged to go out on passes and to return prepared to talk about any difficulties they had. Multiple-family group therapy—patients and their parents—is practiced.

"But there's a lot of work left to do," the doctor says.

On PQ–3, the room devoted to shock therapy is locked, unused today. The rest of the ward is populated. One patient, a young man, articulate and seemingly hyperactive, walks along with the group as it moves through the ward.

"You are Mr. Weinstein, the Executive Director of the hospital, I'm told," he says. "Well, can I see you in your office one of these days?"

"Whenever your doctor says so," Weinstein replies, hesitantly.

NO–2 is the prison ward in Psychiatry; the security is heavy. Department of Correction men are everywhere. Several accompany the group as it tours both wings of the ward (for men only). One patient saunters up, watched closely by a DC officer.

"This is the best hospital in New York State," he shouts at Weinstein.

"It's not a palace, but it is better than when I first saw it five years ago and better than it was a year ago," Weinstein says to the DC officer in charge of the unit.

PQ–2, another adult ward, is the next stop. Weinstein sees a small boy, perhaps 12 years old, transferred from the adolescent ward for fighting with the other boys.

"Is that good, to put him with adults?" Weinstein asks the ward nurse.

"Oh, yes, in this case it is. They love kids here and they are very protective."

The rounds end at 5:15 P.M. Weinstein tells Smartt he'll return soon, to see more of Psychiatry. He is back in his office at 5:30. He signs his outgoing mail and makes some phone calls. He calls a senior vice president of the HHC, to tell him that he is opposed to the building of a bridge from Waterside, a new, elaborate housing complex across the East River Drive from Bellevue, to the hospital side of the drive, except at Twenty-seventh Street. Weinstein has supported construction of a bridge at Twenty-seventh Street because it would tie Bellevue to the resources of Waterside directly. The builder's proposal for a bridge would have it at Thirtieth Street at a point where a direct link, Weinstein feels, would be useless. He tells the HHC executive that he's spoken to the corporation counsel's office and has gotten their support. He is an administrator who understands the value of amassing such support.

He phones another hospital executive director and winds up sympathizing with him. The hospital has been attacked in the press and on TV after a child died hours after being refused admission at the hospital (the doctor who saw the child thought it could be treated at home).

Soon, it is 6 P.M., but Weinstein's day cannot end yet. He plans to spend several more hours, at least, in his office. He wants to catch up on his dictation, study various memos, map strategy and, if there's time, work on his article for the professional journal.

Last night, just as Dirk Berger was leaving the ward, one of the male patients came up to him to tell him that his wife had been hospitalized. Could he get out of Bellevue to visit her? Taking the risk, Berger gave him permission, on the promise that he'd return this morning. When Berger gets to the ward at 8 A.M., the man is already back. Berger thinks of it as an omen for a peaceful day.

At rounds:

One patient seems to be in control of the ward television set, because he ripped off, literally, the knob that turns it on.

An old woman paced all night, talking about the "old days, Jimmy Walker and Jack Dempsey." The nurse thinks she is deluded. "Not a chance," Berger says. "She *remembers* those people."

The surgeons have agreed to do exploratory surgery on Sarah Morgan. The pressure applied by Berger, the resident on the case and Lanie Eagleton, the Chest Service's chief resident, has persuaded the surgeons. Mrs. Morgan does not know yet. Last night, she got up every fifteen minutes to go to the bathroom, run the water and return to her bed.

The fat woman poet is given a pass to the outside world, preparation for her discharge next week, if she continues to improve.

A nurse reports that one of the young men has been "playing with his manhood."

"Enough D. H. Lawrence," Berger says. "He was jerking off."

When rounds end, he sits in his office with a social worker. As they talk about the nuances of the patients' problems, Berger sees another ward patient, a woman who had been agitated all week, walk by his office. She is walking briskly, alertly, looking better. Berger sees that as another sign that today could be a good day.

At 11 A.M., Berger's entire ward staff meets. There is talk about the nursing shortage and plans for a patient outing. Then, one by one, they talk about their grievances, revealing what it is like to work in Bellevue Psychiatry.

The activity therapist who celebrated her birthday yesterday talks about the need for more activity therapists, to get patients involved and out of lethargy.

One of the residents says that budget increases for the hospital and the department never seem to mean more supplies. Why are some supplies so difficult to get?

A nurse asks, "Where's the air-conditioning?" Psychiatry has none, except in a few private offices, and in summer the building boils, agonizingly.

"The place ought to be renovated," one of the residents says.

"Less depressing facilities would make it less gloomy for the patients."

Another resident, his sights set more realistically, suggests that the ward get another cat, to combat the mice.

The water fountains don't work, a complaint heard in every corner of Bellevue.

Berger points out that the Psychiatry building wasn't designed for psychiatry when it was constructed four decades ago. There ought to be fewer patients per room. One of the residents tells him that the new Bellevue building, now partially open after years of planning and slow-motion construction, will do that; the largest room has four beds. Berger points out that Psychiatry will probably be the last service to move into it, three or four years away, because of a bureaucratic argument between city and state over the size of the Psychiatry facility on the upper floors of the new building.

A social worker says that she abhors discharging patients without adequate follow-up care. "We make a good effort," she says, "but it is hard to keep up." She feels that there ought to be more halfway houses, where homeless patients can be supervised, helped to find responsible places in life.

"The Aberdeen is useful, but I know it is tokenism," Berger says.

Again, he leans on the nursing problem. The best kind of care can't be achieved unless the nursing staff is expanded. Most nurses don't want to work in Psychiatry.

A resident says that the other services in the hospital seem less than cooperative when Psychiatry is involved. They may resent the attention that Psychiatry gets. It is true that many New Yorkers believe that Bellevue is only a psychiatric hospital.

The Welfare Department, a social worker notes, ought to have an office right in the hospital. It does not. Too much time must be spent on the phone straightening out welfare messes for patients. Then, the patients have to wait in long lines for their checks.

The young head nurse bemoans the lack of in-ward training for nonmedical personnel, those involved in some way with patient therapy. There's no way to expand their knowledge of treatment techniques. She adds that there's a need for personnel on all levels during the evening (4 P.M. to midnight) and night (midnight to 8 A.M.) shifts. At present, during those hours, the staff available can only serve a maintenance, not a therapeutic, function.

The meeting ends just before lunch, with clusters of doctors, nurses, social workers, aides going over the points raised. Berger slips out to have his diet Dr Pepper and catch a cab to the Aberdeen.

At the Aberdeen, the case worker on duty tells Berger that a tenant has pulled out his hair, punched the wall, broken his glasses. Berger, openly concerned, tries to find the man. He can't. The man has run off, vanished. Berger tells the case worker to let him know if the guy turns up later.

Berger's presence at the Aberdeen is announced, somehow, and after he is there a few minutes a line of patients has formed, simply to greet him, to mention a problem, to ask for medication. He sees them all. The visiting nurse tells Berger that she's worried about a young black woman who spends most of her time in her room, moody and anxious. Berger goes to see her.

Betty Manning is 29, overweight but not fat. She is wearing sunglasses, watching television when Berger comes in. She is solemn. She turns off the TV and sits on the edge of her narrow bed. The room is strewn with cosmetics and movie fan magazines.

"I don't know who I am, what I'm here for. I don't like to go out and I don't have any friends in this hotel," she says.

"If you're alone a lot, you *can* get depressed," Berger tells her.

She tells him that she's been waiting for a man she knew to get out of jail. She heard from him recently and learned that he's home and doesn't want to see her.

"How long have you been feeling bad?" Berger asks.

"It comes and goes. I can't sleep. I'm twenty-nine. I haven't done anything with my life. I had a baby and I gave it up."

She tells Berger that she's never been involved with drugs or alcohol. She was raised by a series of relatives. Her mother died and she never knew her father. She has lived in every borough in New York and has spent much of her life on welfare. She's worked, from meaningless job to meaningless job. At 16, she gave birth to a daughter, and stayed on, in the psychiatric ward of the hospital, for three months, immobilized by depression. She hadn't wanted to give up her daughter, but a woman from a social agency had urged her to and they had fought about it.

"I remember I was sad and cried. That's the story of my life. Sad. There must be something else. I just can't understand. If there's a God, there must be a reason for living."

She cries, quietly, the tears running down her cheeks from under her sunglasses.

"Sure, your life is boring and you get depressed," Berger says. "Can you have the patience to see someone regularly?"

"I'll go, but not two or three times a week."

"Just give them a chance to learn something about you." He recommends the walk-in clinic. "Have you thought of killing yourself?"

"Yes. I tried it twice. With aspirin. If I did try it again, I'd use dope. It is easy to get and there's no pain."

Berger doesn't comment. He isn't worried about an aspirin overdose. He is worried about heroin.

"Death must be peaceful. Better than pain and loneliness."

"It's okay to be alone. But you're alone *and* sad."

"I have no one to go to, to talk to."

"You feel left out. But trust that someone like me will make a commitment to you. We've never met, but here I am. I'm here every week. And you reached out to see me."

"I know I need help, but I don't know what I need help *with*. All I have are daydreams, you know, being happy in a field of grass."

She is a simple, baffled, quietly anxious woman. Berger recognizes the pattern. He tells her he will check on her again next week. He refuses to give her sleeping pills. He tells her she'll have to visit the clinic first. She accepts the bargain.

Berger returns to the hotel office, where he's greeted by a young woman in a fluffy polka-dot dress. "Please, Dr. Berger, give me some more pills," she pleads. "I won't give you as much as you want, but I'll give you something," he answers. She is pleased and turns to a shaggy young man with her and says, "A social worker at Bellevue saved my life. Did you know that? I've been out a year now. Excellent psychiatric care there. Excellent." Her manner is rigid, stilted, her speech pattern is rapid and clipped.

As Berger writes out the prescription, a neat old lady passes by and nods to Berger.

"Taking your pills?" he asks her.

"That Thorazine makes me sleepy," she says.

"Drinking?"

"Not much."

"What's not much?"

"Just two or three shots a day."

The range of patients Berger has seen reflects the way the Aberdeen can serve Berger's needs. It offers a home, a refuge, for chronic patients if they're stabilized. It won't work for those who need protective care or for homicidal, suicidal, violent, retarded, brain-damaged patients. It won't work for drug addicts, prostitutes or what the staff jargon defines as "unmotivated alcoholics." There is a need for the Aberdeen, however, within the definition that Berger enforces. That need is evident in today's visit. Berger has seen more than forty patients in three hours. After a brief staff meeting at the hotel, to improve the record-keeping there, Berger heads back to Bellevue.

At 4:30, he's back on NO–6, seeing a clinic patient, a student who does very well in the classroom and badly outside of it when he has time to think about his inadequacies. When the student leaves, Berger is confronted by the fat woman who writes poetry. She's been told that she'll be leaving NO–6 soon and she's written a poem for Berger to celebrate. It is in her own handwriting, legible, ordered. He thanks her, and when she leaves, he reads it:

> Across the river,
> along the bank,
> There's a land,
> that is never
> old or plain.
> Someday, I'll cross,
> that river,
> sip at the stream
> eat at dawn
> and drink in a dream
> across the river.

Berger stares out the window, toward the East River. It is a gray day. His secretary has gone home. The day shift is gone, replaced by the evening crew. The patients are quiet. He is alone.

He wonders about Sarah Morgan, her surgery, her fate. He

wonders if the biology professor will be sent back to his job, his cats, his desolation, better than he was when he came to NO–6. Mrs. Green, the oldest amphetamine addict he's ever seen, is enduring a life without speed. He hopes she can keep it up. He's not certain, but there are pragmatic battles to be fought, to get her out of NO–6 and into a room that won't make her claustrophobic, to make the Welfare Department serve her properly. And McCurdy, the personification of the meek. There are thirty-two patients on NO–6 when it is full and Berger contemplates the census. When he stops, it is time to go home. He gets up, wearily, and walks to the ward door. As he unlocks it, a patient calls his name. It is McCurdy. He smiles at Berger and waves, gently.

Ken Kirshbaum got up in darkness, so he could visit his wife, who has stayed overnight at her parents' place, before getting to Bellevue in time for an 8 A.M. appointment with a patient.

It is the woman he discussed with his supervisor yesterday: the dependent woman married to the man who is ill. She informs Kirshbaum, immediately, that she has decided to leave her husband and move in with her mother. She wants Kirshbaum's approval. He refuses to guarantee the results; he suggests that she come to her own conclusions. He gives her some medication to help her through the crisis.

When she leaves, he does some checking on the suicide case his supervisor raised yesterday. It is not his case, but he knows the resident involved. The woman is coming in at noon today, and the resident tells Kirshbaum he will try to persuade her to become an inpatient. The day she's announced as her last is a few days away.

Kirshbaum calls the PAO on the status of the teen-age runaway he saw last night. She refused to go to the suburban hospital this morning. The attending psychiatrist now on duty in the PAO won't send her there without her mother's approval. He has asked for it.

The barefooted starving artist caught the bus to Manhattan State.

In his office, Kirshbaum greets a new patient. He is a middle-aged black man whose welfare checks go largely to satisfy his desire for alcohol. He's been an alcoholic for more than twenty years, but he claims he's been on the wagon for the last three years.

Kirshbaum skims his chart. It reveals that he lost several relatives in a fire a few months ago and at the time was anxious, troubled and tempted to drink again. He has been to the clinic in the past, but not in the last year. The man has come to the clinic today accompanied by his daughter. She is tall, well dressed, with an enormous Afro. Her front teeth are missing.

She tells Kirshbaum that she lives with her father and that he has been drinking again and needs medication. "He's been getting Valium on the street," she says.

Her father mumbles, "I can't eat. I can't sleep."

"He sees things," the daughter says.

"I don't see nobody but you, bitch," the father says, angrily.

"He might see little dots or people," the daughter continues. She tells Kirshbaum that's why she brought him to the clinic, but suddenly she abandons her recitation about her father. Her eyes are wide open, staring at Kirshbaum.

"I'm the nut, he's not," she says. "Want to take *my* case? I drink. I'd love to see a psychiatrist. If he's handsome. You know, baby, we could get down to the nitty-gritty. But I don't like your glasses. They could get in my way."

Kirshbaum inches his chair away from her. If her father has trouble, he thinks, she's got worse troubles.

He prescribes Thorazine and vitamins for the father and warns him not to mix the Thorazine with drink. He points in a northerly direction and says, "That blue building on the corner is the Medical Examiner's office. You know about that?"

"The *dead* building," the man says. The pair leaves.

A resident who has seen them leave asks Kirshbaum, "What was that?"

"Father and daughter. She's probably crazier than he is. Grandiose and suspicious. She's not really looking for therapy. Gave him Thorazine, told him not to drink with it or he'd land in that blue building. The mixture could, if abused, be lethal, he should learn. Enough of the street Valium he was taking, combined with liquor, certainly would kill him."

At 11:30, Kirshbaum joins the other residents, a social worker and two attendings at the morning staff meeting. The atmosphere is relaxed, jocular. The stories are more like anecdotes than case histories.

One of the attendings talks about an old man who comes to

see him regularly, complaining of impotence. He carries paper-back books with him, and as he reads each page he tears it out and throws it away.

"Impotence is stinginess, not giving," one of the residents observes.

"A navel operation without the loss of semen," the attending says.

A resident talks about a woman in her twenties, married, mother of two small children, who has been frightened since the death of her grandfather. She wonders if he'll come back to visit her. She's afraid of that. She thinks of her own death, tries to decide what heaven is like. At the funeral, she couldn't cry. She is depressed.

"She has good insight and is quite verbal. An obsessive-com-pulsive planner, which gives her a defense. She spends hours working in her house, taking care of the kids. She's now into planning their college lives, believe it or not. What she's had, I think, is a phobic reaction to death. Maybe it happened when she saw the dead body in the open casket. It was the first time she'd ever done that. Maybe that's when her well-planned exis-tence began to come apart."

"Every obsessive has a dirty corner," one of the attendings comments.

"She really isn't a grownup. She lost one of her husbands. Her grandfather might have been a husband figure," the social worker offers.

They all agree that her sense of loss is normal, not psychotic. They exchange thoughts on the fact that part of mourning is guilt.

"She ought to be treated for her phobias, her anxiety symp-toms, to deal with the inability of obsessive-compulsives to ac-cept feelings," an attending notes. "Tell her it is okay to neglect her house and children for a while. She can have a kind of selective regression without shame or guilt. Treat her on the basis of two intellectuals confronting a problem. Discuss the reality of death with her, not her own preoccupation with her own death. Obsessive-compulsives adore reality, so talk about it."

When Kirshbaum returns to his office after lunch, he finds his next patient waiting for him. She is in her thirties, but she looks older. She is sloppy, gritty, covered with bruises, scars, needle marks.

"I just came in to get you to sign a Welfare form for me and to get some pills," she says. Kirshbaum wants to know more. He asks her about her life.

Calmly, she recites the details. She has not worked in several years. She has TB. She lives with a man who seems to have only gay friends. He beats her. She has lived alone since the age of 15. She never knew her father, barely spoke to her mother. She's been in prison. She's been an addict, on heroin, cocaine, speed and, recently, methadone she buys on the street. Some of the scabs on her arms are from attempts she's made to kill herself. She's been mugged in her run-down neighborhood. She has few friends. Her boyfriend has threatened to kill her if she leaves him. He owns a gun.

"Do you want me to just fill out this welfare form and give you some pills, or do you want more than that?" Kirshbaum asks her. "I don't see any psychiatric reason to complete the form, to say that you can't work, so you can stay home and have the same problems you've got now and become a virtual hermit."

She does not react, does not show any sign of disappointment.

"You can perpetuate your pattern or you can change it," he tells her.

She stares out the window, without a trace of emotion.

"It's up to you. If you learn to use a blade better than you have, you won't have any worries. I think work would be therapeutic for you. It might get you out of the position you're in now. I'd like to give you some medication and have you think about all this for a week, then come in to see me. If you want to stay on welfare, you've got to shop around for a doctor who'll help you do that. Not *this* doctor. So spend a week thinking."

She says "Uh-huh" and leaves. Kirshbaum makes notes: "Classic addictive personality with a huge dependency need. Prognosis: horrible. A masochist who stays with that guy *because* he beats her up."

More patients arrive, get medication, talk for a few minutes, leave. Kirshbaum spots the resident who's treating Maureen Barnes, the suicide case. He tells Kirshbaum that he had felt ambivalent about admitting her to the ward, but finally decided to do so. While she was in the admitting office and he was distracted, she ran out of the hospital.

Two other residents who are familiar with the case join the conversation.

"Maureen's a very sick girl, a paranoid-schizophrenic," one of them says. "She has been for years."

"I don't know what this hospital can do for her," her doctor says. "I have phoned her friends and told them to call me if they find her. She's been in therapy for years, and if she wants to kill herself, she will. And now that I tried to admit her, our therapeutic relationship may be shot to hell."

"She had plans," another resident comments. "She had a present to buy, a meeting to attend, some work to do. That's not the pattern of a suicide."

"She has a job and she doesn't want to lose it by coming into the hospital," her doctor says. "My own feeling is that she won't attempt suicide. Why wouldn't she be anxious about losing her job? She may feel trapped by me now and won't come back, but she's been talking about suicide for years to get some kind of gratifying response."

Kirshbaum disagrees. "Every suicide threat is dangerous," he says. "The well-planned ones are even more dangerous. She's described the method and the time. And that's within a few days. I would have admitted her on a voluntary basis. I would have stayed with her until she got on the ward, and I'd have seen her regularly afterward, especially over those first few days. On her birthday, for sure."

The informal debate breaks up. The woman will surface, somehow. Kirshbaum hopes she surfaces alive.

Back in his office, Kirshbaum sees a young black, a former drug addict. The last time Kirshbaum saw him, he looked stoned. Today he does not.

He tells Kirshbaum that he's been accepted at a drug rehabilitation clinic. He goes there six days a week.

"I feel good, man," he says. "I feel better than I did when I was taking the pills you gave me. The Thorazine. I don't need another crutch, they tell me down at the center. I feel in control of myself now. I feel *good*. I feel that all the cats at the center are on my side. My paranoia is going away."

Kirshbaum is pleased, but worried about the center's opposition to the Thorazine he's been prescribing.

"As a buffer, you might just take a pill when you go to sleep. It'll help your nerves, too. And you won't be using it as a crutch. What I give you is not addictive."

"But the director of the program doesn't want me to take Thorazine," the man says.

"I'll give you a note and he can call me about it. If they insist,
I'll go along, but I'd like to see you take the Thorazine for just
a month."

Kirshbaum writes the note, hands it to the man as he is walking out, smiling.

It is late in the afternoon. Kirshbaum is the only resident on
duty; the others have headed for their weekend diversions.

The phone rings.

It is Peter Parker, the despondent patient Kirshbaum had
seen earlier in the week, the patient who had spent several
hours fruitlessly in a welfare line. He tells Kirshbaum that he
went back to Welfare with the document they had demanded.
This time, he waited for four hours before getting to the desk
and got only an appointment for the following week. The
bureaucratic torture might have sent him into despair days ago.
Today it did not. "I handled it," he tells Kirshbaum. "I must be
well enough to do that."

"You can handle it," Kirshbaum tells him. "See me after your
appointment down there next week. I'll squeeze you in, whenever it is. And have a good weekend."

Kirshbaum slumps back into his chair. *That* is the bare beginning of a sound therapeutic relationship. Now it is time to pick
up his wife and go home.

Lanie Eagleton worked late last night, but got up early, to
spend time on the Chest Service wards and alone, working on
his grant proposal. He surfaces at lunch. Four residents from the
service join him, but for the first time all week his mind seems
to be elsewhere while they talk about Bellevue. He has come
to grips with Bellevue; he doesn't think about it often. They are
less accustomed to its idiosyncrasies.

"The technicians. Where the hell are the technicians here?"
one resident bellows. "The patients are here. The medical staff
is a good one. But what about that whole area in between? The
ones I have to deal with seem lazy and inefficient. They're
protected by their unions, so whatever I want to say about
them, there's nothing I can do. I do my own tests because I don't
want to wait for the damned results for hours or even days for
a technician to show up, do the test, process it and get the

results back to me." He is angry, but Eagleton doesn't try to console him. It is a problem he must learn to deal with.

"All that is true," another resident adds, "but this place is still better than most of the hospitals I've ever seen. Here, at least, the residents get involved in patient care. We care for patients and we're not, as we would be in so many private hospitals, lackeys for the attendings. I've been at a private hospital. I spent much of my time in the library, because I couldn't do much that a nurse wasn't doing on the wards."

Eagleton eats and listens, but he hasn't time to listen at length. He's due at the clinic in five minutes.

For Eagleton, an afternoon in the Chest Service clinic is like answering a series of multiple-choice questions.

The first patient is a man Eagleton knows. The man had been brought to Bellevue, very sick, months ago. Eagleton had seen him, on a respirator in an ICU, and had become interested in the case. The man had diseases of the heart, lung, gall bladder and was suffering from pernicious anemia. Miraculously, he didn't die. Now he sees Eagleton in the clinic.

He is a jovial old man with a Middle European accent. Amazingly, his experience has not turned him into a hypochondriac. When Eagleton asks him how he feels, he says, "Not too good, not too bad. I have some pain, but it's probably just gas."

Eagleton checks his medication, writes out a prescription, gives him a 1,600-calorie diet plan and an injection of vitamin B-12.

"You know, when I was young, I would walk in the snow barefoot," the man tells Eagleton. "Now I stay home." His life has changed. "I used to smoke like a pig. I rolled my own. I thought I'd never quit. Now I'm away from it for a year," he says, proudly. Eagleton shares the pride. When the man leaves his office, Eagleton tells a nurse, "I've got to keep an eye on him. If he gets a cold or an upper respiratory infection, I'd better get him in the hospital quick."

The next patient is a middle-aged black man; he has been to the clinic before, for TB, but has never met Eagleton.

"How do you like the care you've been getting here?" Eagleton asks him.

"I ain't had no trouble yet," the man answers.

"Any complaints?"

"Well, sometimes I get ache-ified," he says. "I got the gouch."

"Do you cough up blood?"

"No, man."

"Has your weight dropped lately?"

"Hell, no. I've gained ten, fifteen pounds."

Eagleton checks his blood pressure, pulse, listens to his chest with a stethoscope, gives him a refill of his medication and sends him home.

Eagleton is sneezing; he may be catching a cold. He sniffles. At that moment, the next patient enters. He is in his forties. When he enters, he looks around the small office, suspiciously. He needs a shave and is dirty. Eagleton, not sure he's met him before, remembers him now. Formerly on the service for TB, he was diagnosed as a paranoid-schizophrenic as well. He kept a knife under his pillow on the Chest Service. His TB demands attention, and Eagleton must overcome the man's hostility to get him to come to the clinic regularly. He is an alcoholic, compounding the problem, and when he stops drinking for a few days, he suffers what he calls seizures, probably the DTs. He takes medication for TB and Thorazine for his psychosis.

"I'm running out of pills. I'm running out of pills," he tells Eagleton.

"Don't worry. I can give you more of them."

"I'm tired all the time. All the time," the man says. Eagleton is not astonished; the man lives on the streets.

"Have you thought about getting into one of the rehabilitation centers for alcoholics?" Eagleton asks.

"I don't know." He is wary. His eyes cannot seem to focus for more than a few seconds on any object. His gaze flits around the office, to Eagleton, to the ceiling, to the window, to the floor.

"Come back in two weeks. We'll talk about it again then," Eagleton tells him, realizing that if he waits longer than that, the man may disappear.

When the man ambles out, a neat, well-dressed, middle-aged black woman succeeds him. She tells Eagleton that she is a diabetic; she has learned to give herself insulin injections. She has kept, meticulously, her own urine-test chart and she hands it to Eagleton. He studies it, talks to her. He has seen her before. She is, he realizes, somewhat trapped in the confusion that a large hospital can create. She had been operated on for a tubal abscess, probably bacterial, possibly TB. The surgeons removed it, but Eagleton never received an analysis of it. He was treating her for TB and wanted that added information. The specimen was lost for a month, found in an operating-room refrigerator, lost again. The surgeon's verdict in an earlier lung biopsy was that she was suffering from sarcoid, a disease marked by lesions of a tuberculous type. The treatment for that involves the use of steroids, which she has been taking. Eagleton can recognize the side effects as he looks at her.

She is weak, diabetic, has a moon-faced look and complains of possible infections. Her surgeon at Bellevue, eager to treat the sarcoid, took her off her TB medication. Eagleton is irritated by the effect the steroids are having on the woman. He reduces her intake of them, puts her back on TB medication, reducing her insulin as well. He would like to cut out the steroids completely, but the sarcoid must be treated simultaneously with the TB. As he explains all this to the woman, she does not question anything he says. As she rises to leave, he sneezes. She turns back to look at him and giggles.

A 35-year-old black man from Georgia struts in. He is very tall and very skinny.

"I been on TB pills for years," he tells Eagleton. "I'm feelin' pretty good, in fact."

"Can you run around the block?" Eagleton asks him.

"Man, you kiddin'? I ain't tryin' that."

"How about up the stairs?"

"I don't like no stairs. That's why I live on the ground floor." He tells Eagleton that he is thinking of leaving New York, to go back home.

"Can I be transferred to a hospital in Georgia?" he asks.

"Sure," Eagleton says.

"Well, I ain't ready to go yet," he answers his own question.

He is drunk and his breath seems to vaporize throughout the airless room. Eagleton suggests a new drug for the man's TB.

"I say 'yes, ma'am' and 'yes, sir' 'cause that's how I was raised in the South. You're the boss, Doc."

One of Eagleton's favorite patients is next. A clean-cut young black, he had been a ward patient, an alcoholic with lung deterioration. On the ward, Eagleton found him ingratiating, within the realm of rehabilitation. He would escort him through the wards, pointing out older alcoholics in bad shape. "Is that how you want to end up?" Eagleton would ask.

The man responded to Eagleton, took his medication regularly, got out of the hospital. Now he comes in for checkups, works as a volunteer on the ward and goes to night school. Eagleton likes to see him; they are friends. Today their conversation ends only when Eagleton realizes he has to be back on the service. The young black man leaves. Eagleton stops to talk to a nurse who has known the patient, too. "Good results," he says to her. "He really did react to what I was trying to tell him. He has the natural resources to make it all work. He is smart and he's getting over a tragic childhood—he never really had a family—all by himself." Eagleton and the nurse share a moment of gratification, then Eagleton races out of the clinic to attend a Journal Club session.

This Journal Club is for Chest Service doctors, to review and discuss articles in professional journals. Today Eagleton will present one article he's studied; Dr. McClement, the chief of the service, will present another. The meeting is well attended; the library is filled with doctors, including several visitors from other services.

Eagleton's presentation is highly technical, impeccable. He makes one joke: one mouse says to another while both are soaring in a space capsule, "Well, it's easier than cancer research." It is the only deviation from the literal that the analytical Eagleton permits himself. The doctors listen, respectfully.

Dr. McClement has done his homework, too, as thoroughly as the most studious resident. He's read a series of articles on Di-Sodium Chromo Gloculate, a drug in use in Europe to treat asthma, now released by the FDA for controlled use in America. It is, Dr. McClement points out, a treatment, not a remedy, but test results abroad are encouraging: 50 percent of those treated with it showed improvement, even better than that in children. It may have use in treating chronic bronchitis and emphysema, too.

"It stabilizes the membranes of mass cells and prevents the release of irritating substances," he says. Its effect is prolonged and there don't seem to be any harmful side effects. It could replace the use of steroids, with their side effects, in the treatment of asthmatics. But it is derived from an Eastern European herb and is expensive. Since it is taken by inhalation in powder form, much of it can be wasted when the patient swallows it.

One of the visiting doctors, from the neighboring VA Hospital, tells McClement that they have samples of it and plan to try it out soon. McClement tells the doctors that he plans to order some.

Throughout, Eagleton has listened attentively. He admires McClement's placid, understated, understanding attitude. He sees him as a first-rate teacher, and the Journal Club has been for Eagleton a true teaching experience. He has taught and he has learned. He is, at such moments, very close to his goal. When he finishes at Bellevue, he should be ready to proceed toward it.

When she completes rounds, Diane Rahman confers with the senior resident about yesterday's debate between a Caesarean and vaginal delivery on Jenny James, and she wonders what the senior resident thinks.

"I'm not the world's foremost authority, probably, but I would have done the Caesarean," he says. "Once I saw that fetal heartbeat drop and stay down for a while, I'd have gone ahead. It is possible, and we may not know for some time, that waiting produced subtle retardation in the baby." He clenches his fist, waves it in the air, sighs.

"I suppose I try to think of these babies as my own flesh and blood, not strange animals," he adds.

Rahman respects his view, but is not convinced by it. The attending was there and had urged the residents to wait and see.

Rahman is called away, to examine a new patient. The woman is seven months pregnant and suffers from thrombophlebitis. She wants to take aspirin for her pain. Can she? Rahman asks the senior resident.

"Sure, she can take aspirin, but it would be less dangerous for the baby to put the mother on IV medication for the thrombophlebitis, in a bed in the hospital," he tells Rahman. She returns to the patient and gives her the choice. The woman chooses aspirin.

A nurse tells Rahman that the Puerto Rican woman with the fetus and a tumor side by side as originally diagnosed aborted the night before. The abortion was successful. No tumor was found. The senior resident, listening along with Rahman, is pleased, for the woman's sake.

"I believe that a woman should not have to go to full-term if she doesn't want to or unless adoption can be arranged," he says. Perhaps, he suggests, she was beyond the twenty-week limit.

The tumor diagnosed by Ultrasound was illusory. It will be difficult to ascertain, and no one will try, whether the diagnosis was designed to help the woman obtain the abortion she wanted or a shadow on the Ultrasound deceived everyone.

At the nursing station, the phone rings. A nurse picks it up. It is for Rahman, and the nurse shouts her name, once, twice. Rahman is with a patient down the hall, out of range, but the nurse does not attempt to look for her. She is peeved at having to rush a urine test for Rahman only to discover that Rahman was too busy to assess the results once they were received. She hangs up the phone.

The one woman in labor on the ward, a young Puerto Rican having her first child, is having painful contractions, but the full force of labor has not yet arrived. The woman is crying. Rahman hears her and walks over to her.

"Stop crying," she tells her. "The pains come and go. Get ready for them." A medical student has crept up beside her. Rahman turns to him and says, "You have to explain to them what's going on. If they relax, labor can go better. This woman is just afraid. I'll give her Demerol and Phenergan to calm her down." She calls over a nurse who speaks Spanish, who comforts the woman in her own language.

The phone rings. A nurse answers and calls Rahman. It is her fiancé. He asks her what she'll do this weekend, while he's away.

"I'll be on duty," she says, grimly. "I'm not socializing. Not this weekend. I'm *working*."

In a few weeks, she reminds him, she'll have a month's vacation. He says something that moves her and she smiles.

The ward is very quiet. Rahman, revitalized by the call, seems less concerned about being on duty this weekend. She strolls through the ward. Babies have been wheeled in from the nursery. A Puerto Rican woman is dancing with her newborn son.

"I'm just making love with my son," she says.

Another Puerto Rican woman is holding her newborn daughter. "All that pain for just this little thing," she says.

A nurse runs past. A sink in a laboratory on the floor above is overflowing and the water is seeping through the light fixtures in OB. The nurse calls for maintenance help. Within a few minutes, three burly men with heavy equipment show up and get to work.

On the blackboard in the delivery area, Rahman's name has been entered, as it is whenever she is there, as the junior resident on duty. Today it is spelled "Rah-Rah-Man," the senior resident's handiwork.

The afternoon moves very slowly. In one sense, Rahman is pleased with the reduced pace after a demanding week. In another, she worries about being seduced by it prior to a weekend on duty. The shift from tranquillity to frenzy can be traumatic.

There is always work to be done. She escorts a patient to X-ray. She checks on a woman in labor; the woman's pelvis is small and her contractions are insufficient. Labor will be induced, Rahman learns from a nurse, and if that fails, a Caesarean will be done. The decision won't be made for hours, however. If a Caesarean is done, Rahman thinks, she hopes they save it for tomorrow, when she'll be around. The experience is valuable.

By late in the afternoon, all her patients have been checked, charts read, medications ascertained. She is left alone with a medical student. He is an intense young man, his brow perpetually furrowed, and he has decided to go into psychiatry. He wonders why she chose OB-GYN.

"I like taking care of women, that's why," she answers. "I like my patients. And in this field, you get to practice both medicine and surgery. When I was in medical school, I had a chance to work in surgery, medicine, psychiatry and OB and that convinced me. I read a lot of material in the field and made up my mind. Actually, I prefer the OB part of it. OB gets you up, keeps you awake. And these women have a legitimate reason for coming to the hospital. When these patients are sick, they recover. It's easy for me to relate to them as individuals, to help them."

The medical student listens patiently.

"It must be a good feeling to get out of here when your day is done," he says.

"Not really," she says. "I think about these patients at night, too, when I'm at home trying to fall asleep. Even then, I see them as people."

Bob Nachtigall's morning is spent in the operating room, assisting the chief resident and the third-year resident. The schedule includes a string of familiar ritualized operations; all the residents have done them before.

At 3 P.M., he is still in the operating room. In the GYN examining room, one resident is on duty. As he surveys a stack of forms on the desk, three men from India enter the room. Two of them do not speak English. One haltingly tells the resident that they are there to see a woman in the ward, his friend's wife. The Indian attempts to explain that she has had an operation.

The resident can't understand him.

"What is the patient's name?" he asks.

The Indian says it.

"Ah, yes, that one," the resident says. He believes the man wants to see the 83-year-old cancer patient, who is now in the recovery room after surgery last night. He tells them that she can be seen right now. He provides directions. Solemnly, they march out of the room. A few minutes later, they return, smiling inanely, looking as though they've been served Good Humors when they ordered shrimp curry. The resident does not interpret their expressions. America must be unnerving them, he assumes. He tells them about the patient, slowly, articulating each syllable.

"Yes. Your friend's wife had cancer," the resident explains. "She will have a large surgical bandage on for several days. She can go home in ten days."

The Indians stare at him, uncomprehendingly. They do not seem to understand what he has said. The resident is uneasy.

"What did you say the name was?" he asks. The spokesman steps forward and repeats it.

"Oh, God!" the resident shouts. "You saw the *wrong* woman."

The woman the Indians have come to see had a D&C and is fine.

The resident slaps his head and screams, "No cancer. No cancer."

The three Indians hop up and down and chant in unison, "No cancer. No cancer."

"Your wife isn't eighty-three, is she?" the resident asks.

The Indian who's been doing the talking starts to giggle. The two other Indians giggle, too.

"She twenty," the spokesman says.

"Sure. *She* can go home tomorrow. But she'll go home naked unless you bring back her clothes."

The Indians are standing in front of the resident, like some Hindu singing group, laughing.

"Bring clothes. Then she can go home," the resident repeats.

The three Indians laugh, then file out of the room to visit the woman.

The resident joins the other residents at chart rounds, in the chief resident's office. Here, with no patients to deal with face to face, the doctors can relax, or try to, in anticipation of the weekend. Nachtigall, changed out of his surgical suit, cradles his crash helmet in his hands as he enters. The chief, looking very tired, is slumped in the chair behind his desk.

"I've heard that there are a dozen ladies left on the West Side with their uteri intact. Where are they?" he asks, wearily.

He alludes to the vaginal hysterectomy he did today, on the Finnish woman. It didn't go as planned and he needed help from an attending. It took four hours instead of the customary two, and her bleeding was heavy. After that experience, the next procedure, a laparoscopic tubal ligation, didn't go smoothly either, and he had to make an incision. He tells the residents that he got only one operating room today, instead of two, forcing him to postpone several operations. "They were short on staff and had emergency surgery needs, so we paid," he says.

At that moment, a chubby drug salesman in flashy clothes enters the room carrying a large jug of cheap sangría, plastic glasses and a large bag of pretzels. While the refreshments are shared, he gives a recorded speech about the merits of his company's products. "I'll be back on Monday to make sure you follow through," he says as he leaves.

The chief turns to the resident who will be on duty tonight. "Get plasma ready for that Finnish woman and call me about her condition tonight. She lost between fifteen hundred and two thousand cc. of blood up there."

He wants the same resident to check the tubal ligation case, too. "We had that difficulty, so see what her belly looks like."

The sangría is vanishing slowly. "If you're lucky," Nachtigall says, pointing to the bottle, "you'll get nauseous and throw it up."

A foreign-born resident offers an alternative. He brings out a bottle of Old Krupnick, Polish honey liqueur, 80 proof.

"How can you go to a liquor store and ask for a bottle of Old Krupnick?" one of the residents says. No answer.

The chief wants to talk about the Finnish woman, not Old Krupnick.

"You clamped it, it bled," he says. "You didn't clamp it, it bled. A lot of blood. We were finishing the repairs when upstream, in the vagina, red stuff started to come down. We stopped the repair, with the blood just coming, despite our stitches. In waves. The anesthetist wanted to know what was going on down there. It was a matter of what to do. It became a matter of calling the attending, so I called him.

"His secretary told me that he had started his weekend. I told her I had a lady on the table bleeding. He came right up."

"Licking his chops," Nachtigall adds.

"He gets there and he tells me, 'I'll do it from the side, you sit right there.' We finally found the bleeder, an honest to God pumper, clamped it and tied it. We looked around and saw no more bleeding. 'Make believe I don't exist,' he said to me and left for his weekend.

"I guess we were too cautious and he wasn't. The man did nothing more than we could have done. That bothers me. More than the bleeding. Getting psyched out in the OR. 'Schmuck,' I could say to myself, 'you could have done the same thing.' Experience."

On the laparoscopic tubal, the scope seemed dirty.

"I cleaned it and I still couldn't see," the chief says. "I pulled it out of the patient, used another scope and got the same clogged view. I couldn't see a fucking thing. After that other operation, it was getting on my nerves. I finally realized what it was. The scope was into fat. We could have stabbed her again with the scope or pulled it out and done an incision, in the abdomen. There was no reason to insist on being heroic. We did the incision."

He tells Nachtigall and the others to reschedule the canceled operations for next week. The abortion patients can go home for the weekend and come back next week.

One of the residents tells the chief that one of the old cancer patients is "crapping in her bed and when she walks in the hall. She doesn't seem to care."

The chief looks at him and says, simply, "She is going to die."

The 83-year-old woman looks fine after her hysterectomy, the chief reports. "She pulled out of surgery like a fucking rose," he says. Her strength surprised him, but the outcome, he suspects, will not.

The chief asks one of the residents to call the recovery room for a status report on the Finnish woman. "Very good" is the message.

The chart rounds are almost over. The chief looks drained, the residents eager to head out of Bellevue for a weekend. One final word:

"As far as I'm concerned, we've done enough vaginal hysterectomies. I'd like us to do more abdominal hysterectomies. The more often you do a procedure, the more comfortable you'll feel."

His operating experience depends upon the residents' skill in finding and admitting patients for him to operate on. Each of the residents present will make that same demand when he has seniority.

With the final bit of instruction noted, the chief sips a few drops of Old Krupnick and adjourns the meeting at 6:30 P.M.

Nachtigall's feet, calves, thighs, back, arms all ache now. He is ready to recuperate. With his crash helmet under one arm, he turns to the chief, waves and runs to his Honda. He is not on duty this weekend.

The 8 A.M. Surgical Pathology conference presided over by Eugene Fazzini finds the usual sleepy contingent of residents and interns peering at the *Times,* their plastic cups of coffee and an array of slides. The latter include skin samples, prostate chips, bone marrow, multiple nodules.

On the blackboard someone has noted that today is Domenico Scarlatti's birthday. The radio blares a work by Corelli.

As Fazzini and the others move from slide to slide, from case to case, the researching resident is again digging into the filed Pathology reports.

Although pathologists do not confront patients, the reports in the file cabinet provide sketchy outlines of the crises in people's lives. One report, one of many like it, makes that point.

An old black woman, in her late sixties, came to Bellevue complaining of sensations ranging from discomfort to pain in her breast. This Pathology report indicates that the surgeons made their clinical diagnosis: carcinoma of the breast. They sent an excisional biopsy specimen to Pathology for analysis. The official Pathology diagnosis followed:

"Carcinoma, clinically from left breast. Note: the frozen section and the permanents of the frozen section showed no carcinoma. The carcinoma was found in the remaining unfrozen material." There are two signatures: the pathologist who did the study and an attending who approved it.

The woman, who couldn't have known the work the pathologists were doing, almost emerged unscathed, until the cancer was finally found. The Pathology report, sent back to Surgery, will mean a radical mastectomy for the woman.

While the resident flicks file folders, the rest of the doctors in the room move at Fazzini's command. As usual, he tempts them with leading questions, inspires them to be inquisitive, provides authoritative answers, firm diagnoses. They do not have his experience, but they are learning.

Fazzini leaves them to their slides and undercurrent of chatter. He retreats to his office, to analyze slides for his own purpose. The radio is sending out Khachaturian sound waves. Fazzini studies his slides, but is distracted by the music.

"They were right, the Russians," he says. "It is decadent."

A resident walks in, comments wryly on the state of Fazzini's desk.

"Someday, perhaps, we'll get it all on a computer," Fazzini tells him. The resident reminds Fazzini that it is lunchtime. Fazzini, too busy and too absorbed, had not noticed.

Later, the phone rings in Fazzini's office, ending his lunch-hour respite. It is a friend from medical school who is now a pathologist at a small hospital in upstate New York. The friend had forwarded some slides to Fazzini, for his opinion. Does he have that opinion now?

"That's a sweat gland tumor, benign, I think," he says. "I waxed and waned about being more specific about these tumors. On the other case, that's a big problem."

He listens to his friend, who tells him that the problem has been solved. As Fazzini listens, he realizes that his colleague's view is one he shares.

When he puts down the phone, an attending walks in, just to talk with Fazzini. It is the end of the week and the two seem to declare a moratorium on diagnoses. Two pathologists making small talk is like two coin collectors comparing old favorites. It can easily lead to a monologue.

"We had a man who had difficulty swallowing," Fazzini says. "They had examined him radiographically and had done an upper GI series, then concluded that there was a mass in his esophagus. They did a biopsy, found a mass and thought it was a benign tumor outside the esophagus. They sent a frozen section to us. We called it a malignant tumor, type not determined, and waited for permanent sections, to confirm it. We got them, and the surgeons did a resection in which we found a malignant melanoma of the esophagus. It's not exactly unknown—there have been thirty or forty cases reported before—but it certainly was unexpected. A rare malignancy."

The attending is intrigued. Has Fazzini had any other odd cases lately? Yes, Fazzini tells him, and he's writing a paper about one of them.

"This woman had a rock-hard mass in her rectum," Fazzini begins. The attending leans forward attentively.

"The surgeons were certain it was carcinoma of the colon, clinically. We were certain it wasn't. It turned out, when we were done, to be a benign solid teratoma of the broad ligament of the uterus, which had perforated into the colon.

"The surgeons saw it as a firm mass growing out of the rectal mucosa. To us, the tissue looked like perfectly benign skin, although not in its normal place in the body. They did a resection of the colon, including a hysterectomy, because the ligament that supports the uterus was attached to the mass. But had it been carcinoma, they would also have had to remove the anus, a mutilating procedure. We're not sure there's ever been another case like it, a benign solid teratoma of that ligament in which it presented as an intrarectal mass."

Fazzini smiles at his own triumph. He and his colleagues will account for their findings, in specific pathological detail, in the paper he hopes to present at a conference in a few weeks. The case makes a point central to his existence: pathologists must deal reliably with the familiar, but solving the puzzles of the unfamiliar is where the excitement lies.

It is after 5 P.M. Fazzini and the other attending are ready to leave Bellevue for the weekend. Fazzini paws at the papers on his desk, tosses some slides into a box, flings the *Times* into a wastebasket. He's heard of a restaurant in Chinatown he's never visited before; he'll reach his diagnosis of it tonight.

At 7:45 A.M., Lori Chiarelli is alone at the far end of the Emergency Ward, copying pertinent notations from patients' charts to the Board. There are five women and four men on the ward this morning. As Chiarelli works, a resident comes up and interrupts her to give her a progress report on the 13-year-old girl who had been dragged by a bus yesterday.

She was taken to the operating room at 10:30 last night. She spent four and a half hours in surgery, to begin the repair on her mangled hand; three more operations will be necessary. The problem with her lumbar vertebra, interpreted as a fracture in one of the first X-rays taken, proved to be congenital, not traumatic. In the recovery room, the girl was visited by her mother, who asked her if she had been careless. When the mother left, one nurse told another, "I think her mother was mad at her."

At 8:30, Chiarelli escorts the nurses on rounds, telling them what she wants to stress about each patient.

The 30-year-old black man with cancer. The Italian man with internal bleeding. The old woman with a toxic metabolic disturbance. The young Puerto Rican woman with possible pelvic inflammatory disease. One of the new admissions is a 75-year-old man who complained of chest pain. His chart is thick, because he's been a Bellevue patient for nineteen years. The entries in the chart over that period indicate a consistent pattern of symptoms: tachycardia, chest pain and weakness.

As Chiarelli points to the man with cancer, one of the nurses leans toward her and asks, "Does he know?"

"I'm not certain," Chiarelli whispers.

The GI bleeder is having less bleeding, but there is blood

evident in his urine; he's been given more units of blood. The young woman with PID, Chiarelli tells the other nurses, "is getting worse and they can't confirm what's wrong with her." There are four old women with various pulmonary and neurological conditions, the complications of age and, in several cases, of too much alcohol.

Chiarelli finishes rounds; the nurses scatter. The ward seems to be in the order in which Chiarelli wants to see it. She sits down, something she doesn't do often, and chats with the new nurse on the day shift.

"I've been a nurse in the jungle and I've been a nurse in the city and I'm not sure there's that much difference," the nurse says to Chiarelli.

"The most important thing is to be a good one, to care about what you're doing, to like doing it," Chiarelli says. "A nurse is top-notch if she pays attention to detail, has good professional judgment. That covers everything. She ought to be pliable, not starchy. You know, you've got to know when to follow rules and when to break them. In the EW here, and you've seen it for a few days now, you've got to have good judgment, common sense, a sense of priorities, and know plenty about medicine."

"What about the doctors around here?" the nurse asks.

"Around here or anywhere else, certain things matter," Chiarelli replies. "It's easy to be pleasant on a quiet day. When things get rough and a doctor is still patient and does what he's supposed to do and more, that's a good doctor, assuming he knows his medicine, of course. He should be a good human being *and* know his medicine. And he should be able to say 'I was wrong' as well."

"What about keeping up with what's going on in medicine? Is there a chance to do that at Bellevue?"

"Sure, you can learn at Bellevue. It's an academic institution, after all. Doctors read and they love to talk about medicine. So pick their brains. Read the journals, too, and ask questions. Go to conferences. Very good people lecture around here all the time."

"You hear so many things about Bellevue. What's it like for you?"

"Well, for one thing, I can speak my mind freely. I can tell a doctor that he stinks. I can air frustrations and tension. We do without some equipment, you know, some of the fineries, and parts of this place are filthy, so we're entitled to scream, to say what we feel. It helps us work. And the patients here are real, unpretentious. Most of all, the nurses aren't handmaidens. That's the beauty of working with the poor. You're truly helping them. There is *need*."

"And politics, I suppose. It *is* a city hospital."

"Right. The red tape. I just can't accept it. I can't believe that if you want a blood-pressure cuff, you can't get one. It takes years to get important equipment."

"But you stay with it?"

"You bet. I guess I'll always be in bedside nursing. I won't ever sit behind a desk. I'll always need a hectic area. There are times when I wonder if I can keep up the pace.

"The public thinks that nurses marry doctors and become rich housewives. Anyway, the doctor is a myth, Superman. Some women respond to that, I'm sure. But I see doctors as men doing a job, like anyone else, but spending a lot of time at it, which isn't so good if you're married to one. Marrying one means living with a man who spends hours away from you. You better be a complete person to be able to deal with that, doing your thing when he's off doing his. Then you don't resent each other. The longer you're alive, the more you realize that a man is a man, with a quality of his own. So when a nurse matures, she gives up that mythology about doctors, and sees him as a man, as she should."

It is 9:30 and the conversation ends abruptly when the young woman with the possible PID suddenly goes into shock. Her blood pressure has dropped. She is septic: there is infection present in her blood, source unknown. Her IUD (intrauterine device) seems to be sitting in an infected area; it could have caused or aggravated the infection. A kidney dye study and abdominal X-rays seem to corroborate the presence of infection. Mysteriously, other tests show nothing of significance. The Gynecology and Surgery residents gather around her bed, joined by Chiarelli and the new EW nurse. The doctors decide to attack the infection with stronger antibiotics, to give her blood transfusions. When she's out of shock and her blood pressure has risen satisfactorily, exploratory surgery can be done.

"Surgery, after all, is scheduled trauma," Chiarelli whispers to the new nurse. "You don't do it on a patient in shock, if you can help yourself."

The doctors confer on the case. They can remove the IUD and drain the abscess they suspect is there, in the uterine wall, but that could lead to a hysterectomy on a young woman. In any case, right now they need Hyper-Tet to help battle the infection. A surgical resident goes to a phone, to locate some. There isn't much around. He manages to scrape up enough from the Pediatrics ICU and the VA Hospital.

The Gynecology resident and the Surgical resident debate their theories. The GYN resident defends his PID diagnosis. The surgical resident wonders aloud. Is it a perforated gall bladder? A perforated appendix? Whatever it is, he says, "it is an intra-abdominal catastrophe, a multisystem disease that seems localized in the pelvis."

More invasive procedures are required before surgery can be done. A test is done, a culdoscopy, in which a tube is inserted into the vagina, to the cul-de-sac (the back of the vagina) to the intra-abdominal cavity. If pus or bile emerges, the doctors will have more to go on. While they're doing the test, a pathologist appears with a lab test result, confirming the presence of intra-abdominal infection. He is positive. He joins the group of doctors around the woman's bed, trying to solve the riddle. Through it all, she has been weak, uncommunicative.

"Nobody drops the ball until we solve this," the GYN resident says.

The culdoscopy is inconclusive. No bile is detected, diminishing the diagnosis of perforated gall bladder. Oddly, no pus is detected either, rebutting the PID theory. The group of doctors is baffled. A GYN attending, summoned to contribute his opinion, says, "If you open her and find PID, she'll have a scar. If you don't open her and she has something worse, she'll be in serious trouble."

"Okay, we'll do the exploratory surgery," a surgical resident says. To confirm his view, he talks to one of his attendings on the phone first. Then he reserves OR time.

The patient, who has been awake and silent, now asks to see a Roman Catholic chaplain. Chiarelli phones him.

At the other end of the EW, a resident is taking a blood sample from the man with cancer.

"Sorry, but we need more blood," he tells the patient. "We want to do more tests."

"Why, man, why?" The man grunts. "I know I'm going to die."

A few minutes later, the man is transported by two messengers to a Medical ICU, to begin chemotherapy which could last for months.

Two surgical residents are assessing the GI bleeder. They have narrowed their diagnosis down to a bleeding colon, but now the man seems to have pneumonia. He is given antibiotics. The residents perform a colonoscopy: a lighted tube is passed through the man's rectum. No luck. There is too much blood obscuring it. More tests are scheduled, to try to pinpoint the source of his bleeding.

At 11:45 A.M., an elderly man with a head trauma is brought in from the AES by a Neurology resident. The man fell down a flight of stairs. He has a skull fracture and a large scalp laceration. When the EW nurse takes off his shoes, she discovers he's wearing two right shoes. When a resident grips the man's head to examine it, one of the patient's teeth falls out. The Neurology resident wants to do an angiogram on the man, to determine the extent of brain injury. He phones Neuroradiology; there's a woman being angiogrammed now and they'll call him when she's been done. The patient is babbling in German; it is impossible to get his version of how he feels.

"Does he have a wife, for God's sake? Can't we get her here?" the Neurology resident asks.

It is 12:30. Chiarelli, late for her assigned lunch period, rushes out.

On her way back to the Emergency Ward from lunch, Chiarelli sees the plastic surgeon who operated on the teen-age girl with the mangled hand. She waves at him. He comes over and gives her a report.

There may be some residual damage to the hand, but the girl won't lose it. Chiarelli tells him that she'd heard that three more operations will be necessary. He confirms that, but he's confident that the girl will be able to use the hand again.

Down the corridor, Chiarelli sees the Medical resident who was the first to treat the black man with acute bacterial endocarditis. They pause in the middle of the busy corridor. He tells Chiarelli that the man was operated upon, open-heart surgery. His aortic valve was indeed eaten away. The valve was replaced and the man is now recovering, although during surgery he needed 32 units of platelets, blood cells to encourage clotting.

"Amazing. Just amazing," the resident says.

By 2 P.M., the 22-year-old Puerto Rican woman whose condition has been a riddle has gone to surgery. Chiarelli turns around and sees that her bed is empty.

At 3:30, there is a report from the OR. The surgeons have opened the young Puerto Rican woman. Findings: normal tubes and ovaries, normal appendix, normal gall bladder. A surgical resident in the EW, who takes the call, shouts incredulously into the phone.

"You mean zero?" he shrieks. "Zero?" He listens, hangs up. "Can you believe *that?*" he asks. "There was nothing going on. Nothing. Very strange. And unusual in the face of what we thought we knew. The infection must not be in the abdomen, but someplace else, radiating pain from some other area." He flaps his arms disconsolately. "Either that or she'll just get better on her own and be out of here and we'll never understand just what happened."

Chiarelli spots a nurse standing nearby, listening to the resident. She walks over to her.

"Upset?"

"No," the nurse says, "just fascinated."

"Well, that's what this place is like at times," Chiarelli says. "You know, no clear-cut answers."

It is 4 P.M. The mysteries and the tribulations now belong to the evening shift. The weekend belongs to Chiarelli. She grabs her coat and purse and rushes out to greet it.

George Feldman, rested after the best night's sleep he's had in days, is alert at the 8 A.M. X-ray conference. The cases presented include two of Feldman's. The first is a series of films of an old Jewish woman with pneumonia presently in the ICU, with arthritis, TB, and other ravages of age.

The radiologist comments: "An incredible case. That's a horrible-looking lung. A lot of destruction, loss of lung. An old case of TB. Her cervical spine is strange and hyperextended, too. Her hands show advanced destruction of the bones, with erosion into adjacent areas. It's arthritis of some sort. I don't know what kind."

There's a new set of X-rays on the man with lymphoma. His fever went up to 105 last night, an intern reports, and new films were done in search of an answer. The radiologist illuminates the X-rays: "That's a tremendous, big spleen. A gorilla spleen. There's a big density in the lung, too, probably fluid. A real infiltrative process going on. No doubt about it."

As the conference ends, Feldman is told by an intern who was on duty last night that one of his patients died. She was an old Puerto Rican woman with congestive heart failure. She seemed to be improving when Feldman saw her yesterday and he is astonished at the sudden development. According to the intern, she died quietly in bed, was found by a nurse.

"The only way to prevent that is to monitor *every* patient electronically and that's a big investment for any hospital," Feldman says.

He escorts his group of interns and medical students to the ICU, to check the status of several patients there.

An old Puerto Rican woman has a swollen tongue, so conspicuous that it is sticking out of her mouth. Feldman is bothered by it. He turns to the intern on the case and asks, "Did she have a seizure and bite down on that tongue? What happened?"

"Don't give me a hard time this morning," the intern pleads. "I didn't get a minute's sleep last night. I missed a few things, okay, but don't push me."

Another intern suggests that an anesthesiologist might have injured the patient while trying to intubate her. The tube is in, with the swollen tongue around it, but the tube is in her larynx, rather than fully down into her lungs, Feldman discovers. The intern wants to remove the tube, "to see if she can breathe on her own." Feldman, irritated, tells him that if it is to be removed, he'll do it.

"This is the way people die on the wards," he says.

The group leaves the ICU to meet an attending on the ward. They visit a new patient, an earthy 19-year-old Puerto Rican girl. She's been a drug addict, first on heroin, later on methadone. She's made fifteen to twenty visits to the AES since she was 10, with similar complaints, most of them minor ENT troubles. She has stab wound scars on her abdomen. She was treated for syphilis a year ago. However, her brother had rheumatic fever, and she has both a slight heart murmur and anemia. These factors led the AES doctor who saw her to make a tentative diagnosis of SBE, subacute bacterial endocarditis.

It is a potentially serious diagnosis. If she is treated for it, she will be committed to a six-week course of medication in the hospital. Feldman is skeptical about the diagnosis. "They've missed a few in the AES," he tells the attending, "so they're being very careful lately. In this case, I think they're wrong."

The attending talks to the girl, who complains of swelling and pain in her neck, sore throat, cough, running nose, headache and fever. The lab tests are normal, but a throat culture and blood cultures are still in the works. One of the interns suggests more blood tests.

"Stop with the blood tests," the attending insists. "You'll have to transfuse her."

He concludes that she has a strep throat, to be confirmed by the culture, thrush and some polyps in her throat, which could be removed while she's in the hospital. "Normally," he says, "she could have been treated as an outpatient. Why was she brought in at all?"

"The AES thought she had SBE," Feldman says. "I'm glad you agree with me."

The attending moves on, the interns and students scatter, and Feldman walks over to look at an old Jewish woman whose X-rays were depressingly analyzed at this morning's conference.

She is 78, birdlike, her breathing sustained on a respirator. As Feldman is about to examine her, two older women come through the door to the ICU and join him at the woman's bedside. They are neatly dressed, reserved, concerned.

"Does she have a chance, Doctor?" one of them asks Feldman.

"A chance? Yes."

"How is her heart?"

"Her heart is fine. Her lungs are causing the trouble."

The three silently stare at the old woman. She is too weak to speak, to recognize their presence.

"Doctor, let me tell you something," one of the visitors says. "She is one of the most wonderful women you'll ever meet."

"I found her on the floor," the second friend adds. "She was there, there on the floor. It was so sad."

"A wonderful woman," the first friend repeats.

"Are you her relatives?" Feldman asks.

"No, we're just neighbors, that's all." The two women are weeping. They thank Feldman and leave.

"They think she's going to die," Feldman says to an intern, "and it's tough to prevent that from happening. But there is a chance. There *is*. Her heart is in good shape."

Feldman talks to the old woman, who does not respond, although her eyes, flashing her desperation, move from Feldman's face to the bed and back again. The tube bringing her oxygen is taped to her mouth, so it is not visible and she cannot easily speak around it. Her hands are tied, at the wrists, to the sides of the bed, so she won't dislodge the IV tubes providing her with nourishment and medication.

Feldman realizes that the woman will need a tracheotomy, to make suctioning her lungs easier. He explains it to her. "You'll be able to eat," he says to her, "and we'll get you a bell so you can get a nurse if you need one. You won't be able to talk with the new tube in you." Weakly, the woman signs the form permitting the procedure.

As Feldman walks away, he tells the nurse, "I hate to do it to her, but she has so much stuff down there she must be suctioned."

It is after 11 A.M. and for Feldman it is time for academic medicine. He is slated to attend Medicine's Mortality and Morbidity conference (Surgery has its own). More than twenty doctors are there, including several chiefs of service and well-known attendings. Today's conference offers residents a chance to understand the intricacies of two cases, both presented by residents who worked on the cases.

The conference ends at 1 P.M. The two cases presented were chosen because they were either rare or baffling. For Feldman, the conference was informative.

Feldman has lunch, then walks over to the Coronary Care Unit, a few steps from the ICU, to see a 44-year-old Puerto Rican man who has had a myocardial infarction. The CCU is one of the best-equipped rooms in the hospital, with equipment to monitor the condition of its patients continuously. From a large central desk, nurses and doctors can check both the blood pressure and the heart function of all the patients, electronically.

Feldman examines the man, carefully, talks to him. The man tells Feldman he's been married for seven years, but hasn't had an erection in two years. Feldman tells him that he's suffering from hypertension and, in men, the medication for it can have that effect. There is evidence that the man has arthritis, too, and may be hyperthyroid. He's had abnormal liver function tests in the past, his chart reveals; there's a history of alcoholism. This is the man's second MI.

If all goes well, Feldman notes, the man will stay in the CCU for five days, then spend three weeks on a ward. The primary sign of danger to be spotted is arrhythmia. It is an irregularity of the heartbeat that can be fatal and is most likely to occur within three or four days after the MI. Feldman doesn't have to remind anyone to keep an eye on the man; in the CCU that is taken for granted.

Feldman returns to the ward. One of the interns walks up to him and tells him he's just admitted "one of the grossest women I've ever seen. Her hair was all matted down. She had lice and scabies. Jesus."

"They should have taken care of that in the AES," Feldman tells him. "She'll have to be disinfected and all her clothes thrown away."

A medical student runs up to inform Feldman that the throat culture on the young Puerto Rican woman is positive. She has a strep throat.

Feldman strolls through the ward, finds another new admission. She is an old woman with bleached hair and make-up, plenty of it.

"Her mental status," a medical student tells Feldman, "is off the wall." When she arrived at the AES, the diagnosis was pneumonia and she was given an injection of penicillin.

"She doesn't look well at all," Feldman says. "Somebody who is this age and looks this ill should get antibiotics IV. And maybe not penicillin. We've had several old ladies for whom that was the wrong drug. You won't be treating all the disease organisms with it. Follow her sputum daily. We've been burned on that before."

The medical student makes notes in a small notebook.

An old Puerto Rican woman in a nearby bed asks Feldman to kiss her. She points to her check and says, *"Ahora."* Now. Feldman walks by. The woman stops the medical student. He walks over and strokes her arm, gently, but doesn't kiss her.

An old black woman with a head full of pink plastic curlers and totally lacking in teeth moans at Feldman, "Please let me go home. I want to go home."

"This is the best place for you," Feldman says to her. "You'll get better here."

"I can't relax knowing I'm going to die," she wails.

"You aren't going to die here," a nurse tells her.

"You'll get better here, then you can go out and solve the world's problems," the medical student adds.

Elsewhere in the room, the lice-infested woman is screaming as three nurses wash her thoroughly. The blond-haired old woman with pneumonia is having a conversation, in a shrill voice, with an imaginary friend.

"I ask Jesus to let my soul go to rest," the black woman shouts. "I ask Lord Jesus, what am I to do? What am I to do? Am I to go or am I to stay? It is so hard. What am I going to do? Will someone please get my sister and my brother?"

"Your sister is coming to see you today," Feldman tells her, interrupting the incantation.

"You're better than you were. You're going to get better every day," the nurse contributes.

"This place is getting to me," Feldman sighs. "I'm at the point where I don't want to walk into the ward."

A medical student rushes up and tells Feldman that one of the patients refuses to take her medicine. "I tried," he says. "Really, I tried."

"I'll get to it myself," Feldman says, closing his eyes, "I'll get to it."

It is late in the afternoon now. Feldman confers with students and interns, reads charts, double-checks medications.

As he leaves the room, there is a phone call for him at the nursing station. It is a friend from Boston who wants to offer him a country house for two weeks. Feldman doesn't have time to talk to him at length. All he can think about is that he's minutes away from a free weekend.

Sol Zimmerman got more sleep last night than he'd been able to get in days. He gets to the Pediatrics ICU at 7:30 ready for work. When he walks into the ICU, a resident who has been on duty all night tells him that at midnight the Infant Transport Service brought a baby in from a small hospital in Brooklyn, a black boy, born prematurely.

It had been born at 8:30 P.M. with a severe respiratory disorder; RDS is one of the most common threats to the lives of premature babies and is usually evident within the first twelve hours of life. The Brooklyn hospital, without the facilities to deal with the baby, phoned Bellevue. Bellevue makes room in the Pediatrics ICU, by preparing to move the boy-girl to the Premature Unit.

A nurse is getting that baby ready for the move, dressing it in blue socks, blue shirt and blue bonnet, to make the trip down the hall, while Zimmerman confers with other residents about the new admission. He is failing to oxygenate his blood; there is low oxygen content in it. This means that there is a serious possibility of brain damage. Oxygen is being administered.

"We were due for a disaster from the outside," Zimmerman says. "You want normal cases? Go to Elsewhere General Hospital, not to Bellevue."

In the Premature Unit a few minutes later, Zimmerman discovers that the original salmonella baby is doing well on antibiotics. However, a baby who had shared the nursery room with that one now has diarrhea.

Zimmerman phones OB for today's delivery schedule. The only one on the list is that of a Class A diabetic mother, indicating that complications are possible and precautions must be taken.

He visits the nursery. No problems there.

At 9 A.M., Zimmerman and the other residents gather in a conference room to celebrate "bagel rounds," with an attending whose month-long tour of duty will end today. There's an enormous bag of assorted bagels, two large slabs of cream cheese and coffee. There's talk about the new ICU admission and how he got there, via the Infant Transport Service. The fully equipped ambulance for such tasks is the only one in the city and is based at Bellevue. One of the doctors, who spends much of her time in the Infant Transport Service, talks about it.

The service transports approximately one thousand babies each year from sixty-nine hospitals in the city to thirty-one centers equipped to handle such emergency cases. A single phone call from any hospital in need gets around-the-clock service. The program, which began in April, 1971, depends for its success on doctors and nurses who staff the Bellevue center and dispatch the crew and ambulance. The ambulance itself is a wonder of conversion. It contains an air-conditioner, incubators, oxygen supply, suction apparatus, a heater, a heart-rate monitor, and plenty of lighting and counter space to work en route from hospital to hospital.

After the bagels vanish, Zimmerman goes back to the ICU, where another resident tells him that the burned baby, who had been crying, has stopped, looks better, is eating. But he wonders if the crying could be an indication of possible brain damage; she may have had some cerebral bleeding earlier in the course of treatment. Zimmerman doesn't think so. He thinks that the girl is ready to be transferred to a Pediatric Surgery ward. He is encouraged by the improvement she's made and how she has begun to relate to the nurses in the ICU. In retrospect, he thinks, her crying may have been due simply to fear.

In the Premature Unit, the babies seem to be doing well; Zimmerman talks to interns and residents. "On this duty," he tells an intern, "we can't talk to the patients. We *can* and we *do*, but they don't talk back. So we have to talk to each other."

In the nursery, Zimmerman checks the Book of Life, the ledger that lists all births, problems associated with them, discharge dates. He computes that in ten days he has examined forty-four babies in the nursery. Twenty-seven of them had some irregularity, from minor matters to serious ones. There were three withdrawal babies. Others had fevers or diarrhea or liver malfunctions, according to lab studies done. Although more than 50 percent is an atypical ratio—"The nursery is a constant source of pathology"—Zimmerman feels that many of the problems that arise in the nursery could be caught if the mothers had gone to the clinic regularly during pregnancy. That doesn't always happen with the mothers who deliver at Bellevue. Zimmerman voices his feelings about it to one of the nurses.

"A good percentage of them don't have any prenatal care. They don't get nutritional supplements, like vitamins and iron. The mothers are anemic. They don't come to the clinic, so we're not surprised when we get positive VD tests two weeks before delivery, which means that syphilis is passed on. The same with TB, with diabetes, with drug addiction. It's partly a socioeconomic matter. The mothers don't have a well-balanced diet. Babies born here are smaller. It's true. It's not that I want the mothers to eat in any traditional, middle-class way. I don't. They should eat what they can afford to eat, but alter the diet just enough to make sure that the baby is getting what it needs.

But how can we get that accomplished when the mothers don't really understand the value of coming to the clinic?

"If they came, we might be able to educate them, to monitor the pregnancy, to give them medication or know what medication they are taking, to watch for signs of infection, threats to the life of the mother or the child. Mothers should be in the best possible health, and in our population it just isn't true that they come to a clinic during pregnancy.

"Maybe that's why I believe we must make contact with the mothers while they're in the hospital. So when we make rounds, we don't just look at babies. We should talk to the mothers, answer their questions, try to get them to bring all their children in to the clinic. It's a problem for them, I know, but we don't arrange seven different appointments if the mother has seven kids, because the mother would go crazy. We try to get all of them seen in one day as a family group. It can be done, but we've got to make sure that the mothers know how important it is."

Zimmerman goes to lunch in the doctors' cafeteria, sitting at a table with several residents he doesn't know. They talk; he listens.

"Surgeons are turds," one of the residents mutters. "They make mistakes, then they always blame someone else. A patient they've operated on comes out gorked and dies, and they say, 'The nurse did it.' They're arrogant and aggressive and unpleasant."

Zimmerman keeps eating.

Another resident joins in. "They pull rank all the time. If a second-year resident in Surgery calls a first-year resident in Medicine, he let's the guy know who's who. They don't make entries on charts of patients on other services. They do you a favor to come and look and then they leave without making a note."

The first resident has not exhausted the subject. "One of the great ones, the gods of surgery, did one of those open-heart jobs and blew it," he says. "Know what? The word comes down, after the patient dies, that the nursing care put the guy away.

"When I was a medical student, I was in the OR one day for twelve straight hours. Not one of the surgeons spoke to me. I held the fucking retractor for hours, and when it was all over, no one even thanked me for helping. And that was the day, too, when the surgeon, trying to transplant a vein, lost it in the middle of the procedure and screamed all over the OR about our inefficiency. He was standing on the damned thing, so he had to pick it up in front of all of us. He washed it off in saline and stuck it into the patient."

Zimmerman keeps listening, but does not make a contribution to the diatribe. He finishes his meal and heads back to work.

In the ICU, Zimmerman stares at the twins, with another resident, and says, "Who knows, maybe there'll be a miracle." He takes a look at the new admission, the frail little black boy from the Brooklyn hospital. On the wall near the baby's bed is a quotation from Emily Dickinson:

> If I can stop one heart from breaking,
> I shall not live in vain;
> If I can ease one life the aching,
> Or cool one pain,
> Or help one fainting robin
> Unto his nest again,
> I shall not live in vain.

The tiny baby stares up at Zimmerman from his miniature bed. He is spread-eagled, face up, his thin legs wide apart. Since arriving last night, he has had several arrests and been revived. A tube is down his mouth; a respirator is sending oxygen into his lungs through it. He has not been responsive. A series of blood-gas tests and another series of X-rays show his pulmonary insufficiency. His mouth is open wide around the tube, as if it is not enough to give him the air he needs.

Suddenly, as Zimmerman is watching him, his tiny body jerks convulsively, as if he had been punched in the chest by an invisible adversary. A nurse sees it and shouts "arrest." A senior resident rushes over to join Zimmerman.

The baby is seizing, his legs contracting and his fists clenched. The cardiac monitor beside his isolette wails. The baby is turning blue. Zimmerman begins manual heart massage. On a child this small, he need only use his thumb, pushing on the baby's chest. Bicarb and epinephrine are administered, through a line already into the baby's umbilicus. Massage continues; the child does not respond. Zimmerman's forehead is covered with perspiration. The senior resident, leaning over the baby, is grimacing.

"That baby wants a cab to G-9," one of the nurses says. G-9 is the open air above the ICU.

"We have to try. We have to," the senior resident shouts. "Because you never know."

Zimmerman takes a syringe filled with epinephrine and gives an intracardiac injection. The baby has gone ominously pale. The cardiac monitor shows that the heart has stopped. Zimmerman stops massaging, exhausted. In the baby's open mouth, a small pool of blood is visible. At 3:20, Zimmerman gives up, reluctantly. The baby's mouth is open, the tube is removed. The mouth is filled to the brim with blood. The eyes are closed. A nurse suctions the blood from the mouth; a large clot comes out with it. Zimmerman walks over to another resident.

At the originating hospital, the parents of the baby were told that the baby was "good," but needed special care at Bellevue. Late last night, when the Bellevue residents suspected trouble, caution was suggested to the staff at the other hospital. Now someone at the other hospital will have to tell the mother, waiting for word of her child.

"It's not like he came in in good condition and then boom," one of the residents says to Zimmerman. "Nobody turned a back on this baby from the moment he got here. And if he had survived, the brain damage from the lack of oxygen would have made him a vegetable."

"The respirator didn't help him," Zimmerman says. "His blood gases were incompatible with life. One arrest after another without any trend to improve. You just wait for the inevitable. Once they have a pulmonary bleed, there's nothing you can do."

The body is taken by a nurse to a back room in the ICU. Several nurses leave, as the new shift begins to arrive. The residents return to other cases, other wards. Zimmerman phones the Brooklyn hospital, to transmit the bad news. When he finishes his conversation, he turns to a nurse and says, "The mother will be told by her doctor. She won't know what we did here. It'll be a void for her as it is for us. We don't even know her."

The phone rings, for Zimmerman. It is the baby's mother. She has been told. "It's very important," she tells Zimmerman, "that I have a picture of my baby. I'm not married and I want to have *something.*"

Yes, Zimmerman tells her, it can be done. The baby will be dressed and photographed.

He leaves the ICU, walks through the delivery area in OB, fills out discharge forms in the nursery, goes to the Premature Unit to discuss one of the babies with two cardiologists. After the discussion, he greets a mother who has come to take her daughter home.

The baby has had four exchange blood transfusions, had temporarily lost her suck reflex and had a slow heartbeat. She'll be seen in the Pediatrics clinic. Zimmerman phones for a final test result he wanted on the baby. He gets it. An EEG done earlier in the day shows signs of brain abnormality.

The mother dresses the baby in pink: booties, coat, bonnet. She seems serious, less joyful than other mothers might be.

Zimmerman has walked down the hall of the Premature Unit, away from the mother. He tells an intern, "She knows. Mothers know. The baby doesn't smile as soon as the other kids do. The baby doesn't do this or that when she thinks it should. *Something.* She knows. And we know, too, but we don't say anything, just as she won't say anything, at least now. The trouble is you don't know what form the abnormality might take."

The mother is ready to leave, and Zimmerman walks up to her, plucks the baby from her arms, hugs it, talks to it, kisses it and gives it back to her. The mother leaves, and Zimmerman heads for the ICU, to survey the population. A new admission, a premature girl, is grunting. Zimmerman can hear her from across the room. The sign of RDS, again. The names of the babies change, but the litany of their troubles does not.

Over breakfast at 7:45 A.M., Mary Williamson sits with another surgical resident, a friend, and talks about the episode in the recovery room yesterday, in which the surgeon had requested that his patient, in cardiac arrest, not be revived.

"There are several theories," Williamson says. "There's the eat-drink-and-be-merry theory. If you can't eat, drink and be merry, if you vegetate, maybe you shouldn't have your life prolonged. Then there's the theory that this is the only life you have, so you should hang onto it, even if that means living on a respirator. Then there is a third point of view: that this is *not* the only life you have."

The implication is that she adheres to the latter view. She

would not write a chart note stating that a patient shouldn't be revived, she says, because she feels our society isn't prepared to accept such judgments, but she knows that such judgments are made and she is prepared to make them.

The metaphysics of medicine must make way for the physical, however, and Williamson abandons the conversation to get to Operating Room 8 on the ninth floor, to begin the first of four operations she's scheduled for today.

They are: the revision of an amputation, the stripping and ligation of several varicose veins, a resection of a great toe and the removal of a perianal abscess.

The first patient is an old Puerto Rican woman whose leg became gangrenous as the result of an arteriosclerotic disease; it was amputated below the knee.

By 8:25, an anesthetist and an anesthesiologist have prepared the patient. Williamson removes the dressing wrapped around the stump of the right leg; the soft tissue has retracted and the bone is protruding, preventing the wound from closing properly. If part of the bone is removed, the skin and tissue can join, and heal.

Williamson washes the stump, and a first-year resident drapes the patient and wraps the leg in a sterile stocking, with the stump exposed. Under Williamson's direction, he trims off the edges of the wound with a scalpel and forceps, then separates the bone from the tissue around it. Williamson's instructions are economical: "A little more. A little more."

The scrub nurse hands her a Gigli saw, a long flexible wirelike saw with handles at both ends. It gets under bone easier than does a straight saw, Williamson points out to the resident. While she holds back the skin around the bone ("You don't want to saw the skin," she tells him), the resident glides the saw back and forth. A large piece of bone flies out, onto the floor.

"Wow, this thing really cuts," the resident says.

A gangly medical student arrives and announces his presence. "The gung-ho surgeon has arrived. You started without me?"

"You just missed the sawing," Williamson tells him.

"Oh, well. I walked into a door I thought was open," the student tells her, "and my knee doesn't bend the way it should. Just call me Hawkeye, though, and I'll do my best."

Using a kind of surgical pliers, the resident bites away at the protruding bone, then files it down. He cuts away more of the surrounding tissue. Now the skin can almost cover the bone. The resident resumes chipping away, bit by bit. The opening is irrigated with saline solution. Williamson packs it with gauze, puts in wire stitches, but doesn't tie them. Once the wound begins to heal, after a few days, and it remains clean, the stitches can be tied.

Williamson turns to the anesthetist. "She's okay?"

"Everything okay."

It is 9:45.

The medical student walks out of the OR with Williamson. He is boyish, awkward, ingratiating, known for asking blunt questions.

"What do you think about in there?" he wonders.

"Well, when it's a difficult or a new operation for me, I think about *it* and that's all," Williamson says. "When it's something I know well, I think about other patients or other operations I'll be doing. You know, like 'When can we operate on her?' or 'How is that lady doing?' or whatever. But most of the time, I'm working or helping and concentrating."

The medical student goes off to have his stiff knee checked. Williamson makes a few phone calls, checking with other residents on the status of other cases. She sits back in the room reserved for doctors, catching her breath. A resident she knows well strolls in, pulls up a chair, teases her about being a sublimated baseball fan from her childhood in Brooklyn.

For the first time all week, she seems able to talk about something other than medicine.

"When I was very small, I remember I hated baseball," she says. "My father, who was in the furniture business and still is, and my mother would sit around listening to the Dodgers on the radio, and if I made a sound, they'd tell me to be quiet. They wouldn't tolerate noise during a game. In fact, you could walk along our street in Flatbush and hear the Dodgers game coming out of every building.

"Finally, I just gave in and used to go to Ebbets Field with my friends, to get autographs. There would be a rumor that some of the players would sit in front of an open window at the park and we'd get up very early and be there by nine, just to wait under the window. In those days, the Yankees were for the upper class. For us, when the Dodgers and the Giants left town, it was never the same. No esprit. At Ebbets Field, you could meet down-to-earth people, good, ordinary people. You could talk to them. It was a real part of your life. The Dodgers were even a part of our fantasies."

A nurse interrupts, to tell Williamson that the next case is ready. It is 10:45. Williamson returns to the OR. The patient is a 34-year-old Puerto Rican woman with varicose veins to be removed. They cause pain, swelling, and can lead to ulceration. Williamson has removed some of them earlier and the scars are visible on one of the patient's legs. The woman has been given an epidural anesthetic; she is conscious but groggy.

Williamson paints both legs with Betadine. While one medical student holds up the woman's legs, four others hold sponges dipped in Betadine and help out.

"Is this a fondue party?" one of the students giggles.

"No, a marshmallow roast," Williamson says.

The patient is draped, exposing only her thighs and calves. Inked circles on her legs indicate the areas to be invaded. A small, narrow incision is made and a vein is seen. Two clamps are attached to it, and Williamson cuts between them. She loosens the vein from surrounding fat and twists it on a clamp.

"Twirl it like spaghetti and pull," she tells the students. "It's gross. Not a technically beautiful procedure."

She tells each student what she wants him to do, to assist. "Her problem is dilated superficial veins," she tells them. One medical student goes to work on the right leg, extracting small pieces of vein through shallow incisions he has made. Williamson, a resident and another student all work on the left leg. They use a long wire with a steel ball at the end of it. The wire is snaked into the vein, through an incision at one end, then pulled out through a lower incision. The ball forces the vein to coil on the wire and it comes out intact. A second vein is extracted the same way.

Williamson explains each step. It is a common complaint of medical students that they are allowed to be present on various services during their last two years of school, but they aren't always taught effectively. These students, on an eleven-week tour of Surgery, have not been neglected by Williamson.

Vessels are cauterized, the incisions sutured. The legs are wrapped.

It is 12:30 and the students dash off to lunch. Williamson notes that "at least today she didn't cry when we did it," and heads for a phone, instead of a meal, between operations.

Williamson's afternoon cases, the gangrenous toe and the perianal abscess, go smoothly, and a muscle biopsy she might have done has been rescheduled for next week, making it possible for Williamson to attend rounds this afternoon. She feels that rounds are as important as anything she does in the OR. She wants to know the patients and their histories before she sees them in the OR.

Today rounds are uneventful. The group of residents makes its way from the ICU to the wards, from bed to bed, discussing new developments, progress or lack of it, tentative OR scheduling for those patients cared for by Williamson and her corps of residents.

When she's done, it is after 6.

She's free to go home, but one of her friends, a senior resident, persuades her to have the week's last cup of coffee. Over it, she talks, without the distractions of the OR, about her life.

"I think I'm in a difficult position. I'm one person, remember, trying to unify my life and it isn't easy. I don't have a career the way most people do. I try to express my whole being and I try to give myself to others. I have to *function*. I know that. I try to function as both a human being and a doctor, without separating the two.

"I have to make quick decisions, and that pace doesn't always allow me to express the other things I believe and feel, those things outside of medicine. I'm not sure I've resolved that yet. I don't always have the time to be compassionate. Outside the hospital I live a life of prayer and contemplation. At home with the sisters I live with, there is a sharing of kindness and an understanding of the depth of human relationships. But I can't always participate as much as I'd like to. It has given me strength, though, when times have been bad, when I've felt wiped out.

"Many times I've prayed for my patients. I believe that there are miracles that aren't so pat, and some of them happen at Bellevue. By working together, we can bring a guy from being half dead to walking out of the hospital. That's a kind of miracle.

"I see God working every day. I pray for the wisdom to know the truth, what is right for the patient. I pray not to give up. You know, families have asked me to pray for patients. And I have.

I've prayed in the OR, too. One Jewish family once told me, in a wonderful way, that I was a believer. That's right. I am."

The evening shift at the AES begins innocuously. An old, wrinkled Oriental shuffles up to the triage nurse at the front desk.

"Have cold," he says. "Tired for week. Much sweeting."

"Sweating?" she asks.

"Sweating," he says, smiling.

The triage nurse tells him he can see a doctor in a few minutes.

An ambulance drives up, the rear doors open and a man hops out. Tom Spencer is there to greet him. The man is smiling and shoeless. The ambulance driver tells Spencer, "The guy doesn't speak English. I think he's Greek and I think he's thirty years old, because he held up three fingers and made an '0' with the other hand. He tried to tell me, in sign language, that he stuck his finger on a doorbell and got electrocuted." The smiling foreigner shakes Spencer's hand. Spencer recoils; there is alcohol on his breath. The man points to his own chest and grimaces.

"You've got pain there?" Spencer asks. The man smiles.

Spencer escorts him to the resuscitation room, helps him onto the table. A resident comes in. The man is feigning sleep at the sight of the doctor.

"Hey, wake up, man," the doctor shouts. "Talk to us. Sophocles. Aristotle." No reply. The doctor pokes him in the side. The man awakens, digs into his back pocket and produces several identification cards with Eastern European notations. He smiles and rattles on in a language no one understands. He shakes the doctor's hand, offers him his wristwatch.

"Maybe he speaks German?" Spencer asks.

A German-speaking nurse is summoned. She says a few words to him.

"Yes, he speaks a little German, he says, but he seems disoriented," she tells the others. "If I get it right, he rang a doorbell which had a short circuit, and he says he was frozen to it for fifteen minutes. He also says he knows he drank too much."

"Well, let's draw some blood," the resident says, "treat him like an American."

The man grabs his own arm and howls in pain.

"Either he's in pain or he's hallucinating," Spencer theorizes.

"There are times in this job when I feel like a veterinarian," the resident says. "Let's let him try to sleep it off and see how he does."

The man, now reasonably alert, is smiling, discoursing in some Eastern European tongue. Spencer finds him a bed in the corridor and lifts him onto it. The man sits up, watching what's going on in the AES like a spectator at a circus.

Down the hall two hospital policemen and a doctor are battling with an alcoholic, trying to tie him down to a bed. The doctor has his hands around the man's throat. "Don't move or I'll choke you to death," he says, suppressing a laugh. The man is tied down, given a multiple-vitamin formula, IV. On his chart, tucked into the bed, is the notation "Behavior at times bizarre."

Near the front desk, a black hospital policeman is talking to a young black patient with an Afro and in African garb.

The patient is bellowing, "Man, we ain't gonna get nothing without fighting."

"You mean like economic and political, man, then I say 'yes' to that," the policeman says.

"I mean like *killin'*, baby," the patient shouts.

"You mean like killin' cops, man, you can go shit." The patient retreats into the waiting room.

The police bring in an OD, a methadone addict, a woman who has taken chloral hydrate, a depressant used in Mickey Finns. She is holding her head, still awake. A Puerto Rican man in his forties, neatly dressed and projecting alcohol fumes, complains of an infected finger. A fat Puerto Rican woman tells the triage nurse that she's been suffering from prolonged constipation. She starts to laugh and the nurse laughs with her. Another alcoholic insists he has a hernia; the resident examining him agrees with him and admits him for surgery. A young, attractive woman makes her way to the rear desk in search of a particular resident; when she finds him, she smiles and tells him she thinks she ought to have a pregnancy test. He gets a urine sample and sends it off for analysis. She finds a chair and stares into space.

Tom Spencer, in and out of most of these cases, is on the verge of boredom for the first time all week. By 6 P.M., only twenty-five patients have been registered, nothing among them to test Spencer or the skills of the AES staff. It is like a first-aid station at a summer camp. Spencer goes to dinner.

When he gets back, he's greeted by a middle-aged alcoholic, a man who reaches Spencer by following invisible waves in the floor, very slowly.

"Doctor?" he asks.

"Nurse," Spencer says.

"Nurse? Nurse."

"Yes."

"I am here, nurse," he says, slurring the words, "because first of all I am in dire need of medication, pills you might say. In addition to that, I need a haircut. I hope I can get both here."

Spencer turns the man around, points to the front door.

"Ah, yes," the man says, "I understand perfectly." He walks out.

Spencer returns to the barefoot foreigner, who has now sobered up and is trying to tell his story. Two nurses and a resident are standing beside him. They seem to be playing charades, using sign language, bits of German, English, whatever seems to work.

"Yugoslav," the man says, solving one of the riddles.

"American one day," he grunts, holding up one finger.

The tests done on him are negative, but the resident is dubious about releasing him. "How can we send this guy back out there? He doesn't know where he is and this is New York. There can't be any place like this in Yugoslavia."

The man has grabbed a piece of paper and a pencil. He draws a crude map of Manhattan and traces a line down the East Side.

"A bus, a bus, that's what he's trying to tell us. He knows how to get home, but he can't remember the bus number," Spencer says. The man nods and starts to laugh, childishly.

At that precise moment, two people burst through the front door of the AES and spot him. The woman, short and stocky, pounds her way down the corridor to him; as he sees her coming, the smile on his face erupts into an expression of terror.

"This is what you came to America for, to get drunk," she shouts, punching him on the shoulder. She adds what is evidently a Yugoslav curse to reinforce her point. The man cringes.

"I am his sister-in-law and this is his brother," she says, turning to the nurses and doctor for a moment before resuming her attack.

"You lost your jacket and your shoes and your immigration papers," she screams. "From now on you will stay with us all the time."

Spencer gets him a pair of hospital slippers as the brother calls the police, to trace the lost immigration documents. The sister-in-law has tugged the man off his bed and is dragging him toward the front door.

"I guess we just released that guy," the resident says.

At the front door, the man, firmly in his sister-in-law's grip, wrenches free, turns around, waves and smiles.

An old woman edges around him and toward the front desk. She has been mugged and robbed and tells the triage nurse, tearfully, that her knee was injured and she wants some medication to calm her down. "My husband is home sick and I don't want him to know; I don't want to frighten him," she says.

A Puerto Rican woman, hysterical, runs in. Her son was shot while on the roof of their building on the Upper East Side. He is 11, and she doesn't know where he was taken. She wants to find him. Is he at Bellevue?

Spencer takes her to an examining room, so she can rest. A Puerto Rican nurse's aide tries to comfort her.

A few minutes later, the woman's sister arrives, her face bathed in tears. Spencer accompanies her to the examining room, where she tells her sister that her son is dead. The inimitable scream of loss can be heard throughout the quiet AES.

It is now 9:50. Two hospital police escort a man wearing blue hospital pajamas and a softball team T-shirt. He is carrying his shoes. They found him roaming around the hospital, but when they ask him where he came from, he says, "They're trying to shoot me," and quivers. He falls to the floor and assumes the fetal position. The triage nurse picks up the phone and calls Psychiatry. "Is one of your prize pupils missing?" she asks. They'll check and let her know.

"He must be from here, somewhere," one of the hospital policemen says, "but we don't know where."

A young Catholic chaplain walking through the AES on his nightly tour is approached by a 40-year-old man and several friends. The man's wife, he was told, had a heart attack at work and was taken to Bellevue. The man is flushed, troubled, shaking. The chaplain tells him he'll try to find out. He makes several phone calls without success, then one that produces a result. The chaplain turns to the man and says, "I'm sorry to have to tell you this. She died here and her body is at the Medical Examiner's. You'll have to go there to identify it."

"Oh my God, oh my God," the man chants. His friends support him. "She was such a good woman."

One of the friends takes the chaplain aside. "He is a very religious man, a good man, and if you can help us now, father, we would be grateful." The friends and the chaplain walk off together, surrounding the man, who continues to say, "She was such a good woman."

At 10:25, there is action. There has been a fire at Avenue C and Fifth Street. Five firemen, suffering from smoke inhalation, come stumbling through the front door. The aroma of smoke permeates the AES. A nervous woman, awaiting treatment, thinks that the AES is on fire. She screams, cries, vomits. Spencer runs over to her, to explain, to help.

The firemen stagger to the resuscitation room. Tests are done, to check the oxygen level in the blood, look for signs of respiratory distress, X-rays taken.

Five minutes later, four more firemen arrive by ambulance. Several more are due soon, they say. The place seems filled with firemen, their black uniforms and boots streaked with ashes.

At 10:40, the police bring in a beautiful young woman who drank too much Scotch and took too much Valium, simultaneously. A male friend is with her. She mumbles, "Don't be mad at me," over and over again. A nurse who has seen her come in turns to a nurse's aide beside her and says, "We never lose an OD here. The ones we lose are the nice people who *don't* abuse themselves."

A resident treats the woman with Ipecac; within a few minutes, she vomits. "She can go home as soon as she's fully awake," the resident tells her friend.

Staccato screams come from a patients' bathroom. Two nurse's aides are struggling with an unwilling woman, a Bowery alcoholic, so the doctor won't be overcome by her fumes or attacked by her lice when he examines her. The door to the bathroom bursts open and the woman emerges in the aides' arms, enraged but cleaner than she's ever been and wrapped in a new robe.

The pace, Spencer realizes, has been quickening; the sense of latent boredom he felt earlier has vanished.

At 11 P.M., two police cars speed up to the entrance. Each car carries a man, one white and one black. They were on a motorcycle on the FDR Drive when the bike either went out of control or was struck by a hit-and-run driver. The bike was

demolished; the two men were thrown and knocked unconscious. Spencer and several doctors get the two men directly
into the Emergency Ward.

The white man, in his twenties, bearded, has a fractured leg,
obvious, and a head trauma; his face is covered with blood. A
nurse starts to move his head. "Don't," a doctor screams at her.
"Put a neck brace on him." The black man is in worse condition,
with facial trauma, possible multiple fractures and lacerations
all over his body. Two teams of doctors and nurses work on both
men simultaneously. One of the policemen standing beside
them turns to a nurse and says, "I thought they'd be DOA for
sure." They are not. The doctors and nurses are working feverishly on both men. The tools of the EW are evident: suction, IV,
blood pressure, EKG, urinalysis, blood samples, antibiotics. A
doctor inserts a tube in the white man's bleeding mouth; the
blood snakes its way through the tube to a container on the
floor. "We need a Neuro consult," one of the doctors shouts. A
nurse runs to a phone.

"At most other hospitals," one of the policemen whispers to
Spencer, "they'd still be on stretchers." Within a few minutes,
the two men are on their way to the operating room. Spencer
returns to the AES, which is now noisy and busy.

A Puerto Rican teen-ager, accompanied by three friends, is
the eighty-first patient of Spencer's shift. He has a lacerated
hand, but seems calm about it, although his friends are restless.
They look nervously at several policemen who have lingered
after bringing in the victims of the bike crash. "He got beaten
up," one of the friends tells the triage nurse. She sends them on
to a doctor.

The doctor examines the hand, then asks, "How did it happen?"

"I take the Fifth Amendment," the teen-ager bellows, angrily.

The doctor screams, "Get him out of here. Get him out. I've
had enough of that kind of shit," and stalks off. A Puerto Rican
nurse's aide replaces him, bathes the boy's hand while the
friends pace outside the examining room. Their patience exhausted, they retrieve him from the room before she's finished
and the foursome run out of the AES. As they pass the front
desk, the triage nurse turns to a clerk and says, "I guess we
discharge the guy with the bloody hand."

It is midnight and the night staff has arrived. As Spencer walks out, one of the incoming nurses stops him and says, "You *better* get out of here. This is no place for a respectable person. This place is zoo-ey."

In the corridor from the AES to the main hospital, a resident, large, bearded and intense, is talking to another doctor.

"How can you *be* about this place? Angry. Sad. Hostile. Weary. The bathrooms are filthy. In a hospital, the bathrooms are filthy. For me, I suppose it doesn't matter. What the hell do I care? I'm going into academic medicine and most of what I see here I won't see again. That's the way it is. You leave here and go try to recover some of the money you've lost, so you practice middle-class medicine and you never see a Bowery drunk again. But I know I'll remember some of it and maybe it won't be the medicine, exactly.

"Last night I had a guy come in. Forty-three. Dirty. Scabby. A drunk. I wanted to know how it happened. That's the kind of schmuck I am. I have to know. So I asked him. He told me that when he was twenty-eight he was married and had three kids and one day his wife killed the kids and then killed herself. He wound up in a mental institution for a couple of years, then discovered that he could kill the pain with booze. So here he is and here I am, looking at him, trying to make him better, somehow.

"And when I did that one, I had to take care of a seventy-year-old man who had been mugged. Mugged. A seventy-year-old man. Why the hell did they do it to him? Why? I don't know and I'm not supposed to ask—right?—but I know the man is dying. His wife arrives and while she's talking to him, he dies, but she doesn't know it or doesn't want to know it, so she keeps talking to him. God Almighty, after that I went home and broke down.

"At another hospital, the patients might pay plenty and tell you what to do. So if I sound crazy about Bellevue, maybe I am crazy. I'm glad to be here, you can believe that."

"Why?"

"Why? Plenty of reasons why. The place has a history and a great one. That's number one. It's got size, which means it's got plenty of patients. They come here from everywhere, and most of them don't have a clue about what's bothering them. They're too poor to get help anywhere else, so that makes us important and it makes us responsible. That's fine with me. The place has a mystique, a reputation, a spirit, a sense of pride. Don't believe me. Go out and find some guy who did his residency here years ago and then find another who left three years ago and they'll probably say the same thing. They miss the Goddamned place.

"I'm glad to be here, sure. There were plenty of other hospitals in plenty of better neighborhoods. I wanted to be here. At Bellevue, the house staff has medical responsibility. That's important. You don't stand around, like you do at a fancy private hospital, being a flunky. Here, you *do* things. Bellevue is in a mixed socioeconomic area. That means a wide range of cases and problems, often untouched by medical hands before you get yours on them. And, finally, there's that fucking name. Bellevue. It *means* all I've said. And more."

It is midnight. Bernard Weinstein is alone in his office, alone in the entire Administration suite. He has walked around the hospital, then worked in silence for hours. Enough for one day, enough for a week.

He tosses papers into his attaché case and makes his way to his car. The maroon and white Chevy eases through Manhattan's late-night traffic toward the West Side, toward New Jersey.

Weinstein's head is full of details. The Waterside bridge debate. The child health station battle. The problems of the new Bellevue, its future, the bureaucratic combat ahead to get what he wants for it, what he thinks it needs. The HHC and what he must do to coexist with it. The medical records being moved this weekend. The zonked psychiatric patients he saw this afternoon. He remembers that someone in Psychiatry referred to "an ambulatory camisole." A strait jacket, he remembers, and smiles at the euphemism.

His concerns are like entries in a perpetual agenda, not typed neatly by his secretary, but remembered almost involuntarily.

Then he realizes he passed over the George Washington Bridge minutes ago and is almost home.

EPILOGUE

Administration: Bernard Weinstein continued to crusade for the completion of the new Bellevue; it had been dedicated and looked, from the outside, as if it had been completed, but was not finished inside. The new Director of Anesthesia took office, recruited some attendings. The residency program in Anesthesia regained A.M.A. approval. The prison ward remained on the eighteenth floor of the new hospital as planned and thrashed out. Weinstein stopped trying to fight the idea. Work on the interim location proceeded. The HHC and the Department of Health ruled that Bellevue should run the neighborhood child health station; Weinstein met with the neighborhood health organization to invite it to participate. The Waterside bridge debate continued. Multiple meetings with city officials were held. Letters were sent to politicians. A demonstration was held. But the matter remained unresolved. Both sides moved like sumo wrestlers, waiting for an advantage. The Physicians' Associates program was dead at Bellevue. Patient clothing was changed; new slippers and gowns, more colorful and attractive, replaced the old styles. Weinstein's article was published in the *Journal* of the American Hospital Association.

Psychiatry (Ward NO–6): Dirk Berger completed his residency at Bellevue and decided to remain there. As an attending, he could work at the Aberdeen Hotel and on the Bellevue wards, as well as with neighborhood agencies.

Howard Walker, the professor who attempted suicide, did well on NO–6. He stayed on the ward for several weeks, while he planned his future, then was discharged. He was followed in the clinic and went to a private psychiatrist.

Mrs. Sarah Morgan, the woman from the rural South, was transferred from NO–6 for exploratory surgery. It revealed metastatic cancer, inoperable. She didn't want to know why she was going to surgery. Following it, she returned to NO–6. Residents in Psychiatry applied for a room for her in a terminal-care home in the Bronx. She told them she preferred to die on NO–6. She did die there. A day later, her application for the nursing home was approved.

Jack McCurdy, the meek patient who had made a symbolic attempt on his wife's life, improved dramatically. He did well in work and volunteer programs. He was discharged after two months on the ward, was getting along well with his wife and seeing a resident in the clinic regularly.

Mrs. Elaine Green, the old speed freak, was sent from NO–6 to the Aberdeen, got drunk there, became "a suicidal risk" and was returned to NO–6 for six days. She was discharged to another hotel and has remained out of Bellevue.

Ken Kirshbaum was named one of two chief residents for his final year. Among his patients, Bobby Warren, the troubled boy, refused to live with his father, became unmanageable and was admitted to Bellevue. Kirshbaum tried to get him released, but the boy resisted his efforts. Sent on to Manhattan State, Warren told them, after two days, that he wasn't crazy. He was discharged and Kirshbaum remained in close touch with him.

Eleanor Golden divorced her husband, got a job, saw Kirshbaum weekly and is improving.

The 6-year-old boy was never brought in again by his mother, who told Kirshbaum that suicide was no longer a problem because she had bars installed on her windows.

The teen-age Puerto Rican boy who threatened his family with a knife was referred, with his entire family, for family therapy. They did not keep their appointment.

Peter Parker, the upper-middle-class young man Kirshbaum was concerned about, the one who resented standing in line for welfare checks, never returned to see Kirshbaum.

Maureen Barnes, the young woman who threatened to commit suicide on her thirtieth birthday, kept her promise. She took a mixture of ninety pills and slashed her wrists, but fortunately was found by police staggering around in front of her apartment building. She was taken to the Bellevue AES, and she became comatose, near death. Intensive care revived her and she was transferred to Psychiatry, where a new resident took on her case. She liked him, listened to him and was discharged after several weeks on the ward.

Chest Service: Lanie Eagleton completed his residency, and got a grant from the New York Lung Association to do research on asthmatics in a lab at Bellevue. He became an attending as well, working in the clinic and on the wards, with time to teach residents and interns.

The Guatemalan stonemason was picked up by his boss's wife, an intrigue that amused Eagleton, and the two returned to Guatemala. The man has not been heard from since.

The alcoholic man with TB and a collapsed lung was allowed to drain for four months. He improved remarkably and healed without surgery.

The old "Polish gentleman" died of silico-tuberculosis; he had been a miner and Eagleton assumed he had contracted the disease in the mines.

The middle-aged European man whom Eagleton saw in the clinic caught pneumonia and was admitted to one of the wards. When he was first seen there by Eagleton, he apologized for missing his clinic appointment.

The paranoid-schizophrenic with TB whom Eagleton saw in the clinic agreed to go to an alcoholic treatment center. He stayed there for three months, then fled to the streets again. He returned to the clinic to see Eagleton. He was coughing again, but refused to come into the hospital. Miraculously, his TB had become inactive (six months with negative cultures).

The black woman Eagleton treated in the clinic was taken off steroids and put on TB medication. She was doing well when she had a psychotic break and had to be admitted to Psychiatry.

DSCG, the new drug discussed by Dr. McClement at a conference, is being used in the clinic with good results. According to Eagleton, "McClement kept his word. We got our DSCG."

Obstetrics: The girl who was the subject of a debate between a resident and an attending, over the use of a vacuum abortion, was given Pitocin IV and aborted a fetus, dead and decaying.

Gynecology: The 83-year-old cancer patient left Bellevue two weeks after her surgery and was still alive six months later in a chronic-care hospital.

AES: The two motorcycle riders brought into the AES, then into the EW, the night when all the firemen were being treated, had distinctly separate fates. The bearded black man, unidentified, had a massive blood clot on the brain. An EEG was flat.

He lingered and died. His white companion, who appeared to be seriously injured on arrival, was not. He recovered and left Bellevue.

Neurology: Bruce Mack left Bellevue, completing his residency, to become a major in the U.S. Air Force for two years.

Mary Rollins, the young woman who had consumed methyl alcohol thinking it was vodka, lasted only a few days. At her death, the police initiated an inquiry into its circumstances. It was inconclusive.

Neurosurgery: Kal Post became Bellevue's chief resident. The 8-year-old boy whom Post saw in the Pediatrics ICU improved, was able to move, but did not speak. He was sent to Rehabilitation Medicine, then home.

The embolized man, subject of some controversy after that procedure was performed, recovered promptly. His seizures vanished and there was no need for surgery.

Post's own son, Alexander, prospered in the Premature Care Unit, was sent home, where he quickly got chubby.

Pathology: Eugene Fazzini lost fifty-five pounds and was still counting calories.

Emergency Ward: Lori Chiarelli's nursing textbook, written in collaboration with two others (a nursing instructor and the Assistant Nursing Director of Emergency Services), was completed.

The man with acute bacterial endocarditis developed a severe postoperative infection that required more than five weeks of intensive care. He recovered and was released.

The teen-age girl injured by a bus, who arrived at the EW with a badly mangled hand, underwent plastic surgery to put tendons, nerves and bones back into use. The hand, after surgery, was not as it once had been, but it was usable.

Medicine: Aaron Greenberg, the amputee whom George Feldman treated on a Home Care visit, was unable to care for himself at home while his wife was in Bellevue. He had a heart attack and was brought to the EW, where Feldman saw him again. A few days later, in Bellevue, he died. A social worker found a place in a nursing home for his wife.

The man with malignant lymphoma got worse on the ward; before radiation therapy could be initiated, he died.

The old Jewish woman in the Medical ICU, the one with severe lung trouble, never left the ICU. She died there.

Maria Diaz, the old woman Feldman saw on his Home Care afternoon, was hospitalized with pneumonia and bronchitis, was treated effectively and discharged.

The young Puerto Rican woman with the small kidney was discharged without surgery being done. According to Feldman, she faithfully took her medication, controlling her hypertension.

Pediatrics: Sol Zimmerman was slated to spend his third year as a senior resident, then enter the Air Force for two years.

The twins in the ICU had different fates. The girl, after more than six weeks on a respirator, swung her arm and dislodged her trach tube. Zimmerman, standing nearby, noticed that she was breathing room air successfully. He took her off the respirator. Within two weeks, she recovered sufficiently to go home. According to Zimmerman, of all the babies in his experience she was the one to spend the most time on a respirator and survive. Since her discharge, she's been admitted twice for pulmonary infections, dangerous for her, and her development has been slow, but no specific abnormalities have been seen.

Her brother, after nine weeks on a respirator, died when tracheal erosion took place (evident in a post-mortem), leading to respiratory and cardiac arrest. Attempts to revive him were unsuccessful.

The deformed boy-girl died in the ICU of progressive pulmonary disease, after returning to the ICU from the Premature Unit and being returned to a respirator as well.

The beautiful burned baby was sent to the New York Foundling Home, where her parents visited her, but didn't regain custody of her. Zimmerman filed a deposition with the Bureau of Child Welfare urging it to avoid returning the child to its parents. The baby never required skin grafts, recovering on her own to be an alert, healthy child, according to Zimmerman.

The baby with salmonella was treated successfully, discharged and seen in the clinic.

The baby in the Premature Unit who needed coronary surgery gained enough weight to permit it. It was successful and she's been doing "extraordinarily well" ever since.

Surgery: The young man suffering from severe burns lived for a month after the first pigskin graft was done, then died of sepsis (generalized infection).

The old woman who had the bilateral radical mastectomy

survived; no cancer was found elsewhere in her body; the lesion on her hip was benign. She was discharged.

Sister Mary Williamson left Bellevue for the missionary hospital in Ghana.

ACKNOWLEDGMENTS

People on all levels of life at Bellevue helped me. They did so knowing that I was writing a book about the hospital and they did so with a minimum of reticence. Patients, too, knew what I was doing and were extraordinarily cooperative. Doctors and nurses bore my questions patiently and helpfully and trusted me to write about them honestly. I hope I have justified that trust.

Bernard Weinstein, Bellevue's Executive Director, made it possible for me to roam through Bellevue freely, then allowed me to scrutinize his own role at the hospital. His staff was comparably helpful. Two of them, Jim Walsh and Kathleen Farrell, offered me guided tours, advice, consultations whenever I needed them. Dr. Joseph T. English, who headed the Health and Hospitals Corporation when I began researching this book, endorsed the project wholeheartedly, which got me on my way effectively. Layhmond Robinson, another HHC staff member, shared Dr. English's enthusiasm for the book and expressed it, to me and to others.

Buz Wyeth, my editor, was indispensable. Phil Liebowitz, a lawyer and friend, saw to it that I did not will my kidneys to Harper & Row when he helped me negotiate the book contract. Joan Whipple, R.N., answered many medical questions for me, happily. Wynn Kramarsky, medical consultant, offered supportive conversation when I needed it most, at the very beginning of my work on this book. And my daughter Tracy, as ever, provided invaluable support, as did my good friend Suzi Arensberg.